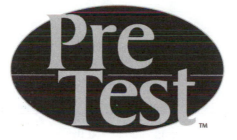

Clinical Vignettes for the USMLE Step 1

PreTest™ Self-Assessment and Review
Third Edition

Notice

Medicine is an ever-changing science. As new research and clinical experience broaden our knowledge, changes in treatment and drug therapy are required. The authors and the publisher of this work have checked with sources believed to be reliable in their efforts to provide information that is complete and generally in accord with the standards accepted at the time of publication. However, in view of the possibility of human error or changes in medical sciences, neither the authors nor the publisher nor any other party who has been involved in the preparation or publication of this work warrants that the information contained herein is in every respect accurate or complete, and they disclaim all responsibility for any errors or omissions or for the results obtained from use of the information contained in this work. Readers are encouraged to confirm the information contained herein with other sources. For example and in particular, readers are advised to check the product information sheet included in the package of each drug they plan to administer to be certain that the information contained in this work is accurate and that changes have not been made in the recommended dose or in the contraindications for administration. This recommendation is of particular importance in connection with new or infrequently used drugs.

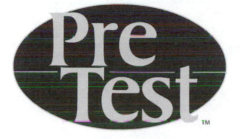

Clinical Vignettes for the USMLE Step 1

PreTest™ Self-Assessment and Review

Third Edition

McGraw-Hill
Medical Publishing Division

New York   Chicago   San Francisco   Lisbon   London   Madrid   Mexico City
Milan   New Delhi   San Juan   Seoul   Singapore   Sydney   Toronto

Clincal Vignettes for the USMLE Step 1

1 2 3 4 5 6 7 8 9 0   DOC/DOC   0 9 8 7 6 5 4

ISBN: 0-07-142291-9

This book was set in Berkeley by North Market Street Graphics.
The editor was Catherine A. Johnson.
The production supervisor was Phil Galea.
Project management was provided by North Market Street Graphics.
RR Donnelley was printer and binder.

This book is printed on acid-free paper.

Library of Congress Cataloging-in-Publication Data

Clinical Vignettes for the USMLE step 1 : preTest self-assessment and review.—3rd ed.
    p.; cm.
  Includes bibliographical references.
  ISBN 0-07-142291-9
  1. Medicine—Examinations, questions, etc. 2. Medical sciences—Examinations, questions, etc. 3. Physicians—Licenses—United States—Examinations—Study guides.
    [DNLM: 1. Medicine—Examination Questions. W 18.2 C6412 2004]
  R834.5.C563 2004
  610'.76—dc22
                                                                                2004058755

Contents

Preface

The current format of the United States Medical Licensing Examination (USMLE) Step 1 emphasizes clinical vignettes as the primary test questions. The examination is 400 questions, broken into eight blocks of 50 questions each. Examinees have one hour to complete each block.

Clinical Vignettes for the USMLE Step 1: Third Edition parallels this format. The book contains 400 clinical-vignette-style questions covering the basic sciences and was assembled based on the published content outline for the USMLE Step 1. The questions are divided into eight blocks of 50 questions. As on the Step 1 exam, each block tests the examinee in all basic science areas. Halfway through each block, a stopwatch set at 30 minutes is included to remind the examinee of the one-hour limit. Answers are in the second half of the book. Each answer is accompanied by a concise but comprehensive explanation and is referenced to a key textbook and/or journal article for further reading.

The questions in this book were culled from the nine PreTest™ Basic Science books. The publisher acknowledges and thanks the following authors for their contributions to this book:

Anatomy, Histology, & Cell Biology: Robert Klein, PhD, and George Enders, PhD

Behavioral Sciences: Michael H. Ebert, MD

Biochemistry & Genetics: Cheryl Ingram-Smith, PhD, and Kerry Smith, PhD

Microbiology: James Kettering, PhD

Neuroscience: Alan Siegel, PhD, and Heidi Siegel, MD

Pathology: Earl J. Brown, MD

Pathophysiology: Maurice A. Mufson, MD

Pharmacology: Marshal Shlafer, PhD

Physiology: James C. Ryan, PhD, and Michael Wang, PhD

McGraw-Hill
November 2004

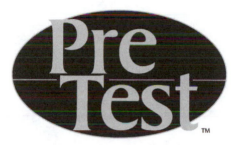

Clinical Vignettes for the USMLE Step 1

PreTest™ Self-Assessment and Review
Third Edition

Block 1

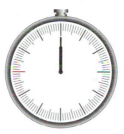

YOU HAVE **60** MINUTES TO COMPLETE **50** QUESTIONS.

Questions

1-1. An adult migrant farm worker in the San Joaquin Valley of California has been hospitalized for 2 weeks with progressive lassitude, fever of unknown origin, and skin nodules on the lower extremities. A biopsy of one of the deep dermal nodules shown in the photomicrograph below reveals the presence of what abnormality?

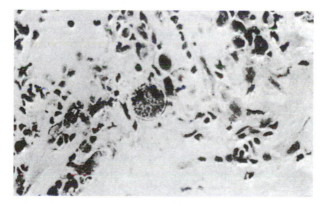

a. Russell bodies
b. Malignant lymphoma
c. Coccidioides spherule
d. Lymphomatoid granulomatosis
e. Erythema nodosum

1-2. A 35-year-old woman presents with slowly progressive weakness involving the left side of her face. She says she cannot completely close her left eye. Physical examination finds facial asymmetry characterized by flattening of the entire left side of her face, but no abnormalities are seen on the right side. A 1.5-cm mass is found involving the deep portion of the left parotid gland. At the time of surgery the mass is found to be infiltrating along the facial nerve. Which of the following histologic changes is most likely to be seen in a biopsy specimen taken from this mass?

a. A mixture of epithelial structures and mesenchyme-like stroma
b. A mixture of squamous epithelial cells and mucus-secreting cells
c. Atypical cells forming tubular and cribriform patterns
d. Infiltrating groups of vacuolated epithelial cells
e. Papillary folds composed of a double layer of oncocytic cells

1-3. A 26-year-old man contracted viral influenza with an unremitting fever of 39.5°C (103°F) for three days. Because spermatogenesis cannot occur above a scrotal temperature of 35.5°C (96°F), he was left with no viable sperm on his recovery. Approximately how much time is required for the return of viable sperm to the epididymis?

a. 3 days
b. 1 week
c. 5 weeks
d. 2 months
e. 4 months

1-4. A 70-year-old male was brought to the emergency room after experiencing headaches, nausea, and dizziness. An MRI revealed the presence of a brain tumor, which had produced a noncommunicating hydrocephalus. Which of the following is the most likely location of the tumor?

a. White matter of the cerebral cortex
b. Medial thalamus
c. Interventricular foramen
d. Pontine cistern
e. Cisterna magna

1-5. A 9-year-old child is brought to the emergency room with the chief complaint of enlarged, painful axillary lymph nodes. The resident physician also notes a small, inflamed, dime-sized lesion surrounding what appears to be a small scratch on the forearm. The lymph node is aspirated and some pus is sent to the laboratory for examination. A Warthin-Starry silver impregnation stain reveals many highly pleomorphic, rod-shaped bacteria. Which of the following is the most likely cause of this infection?

a. *Bartonella henselae*
b. *Brucella canis*
c. *Mycobacterium scrofulaceum*
d. *Y. enterocolitica*
e. *Y. pestis*

1-6. A 60-year-old man with aggressive rheumatoid arthritis will be started on an anti-inflammatory drug to suppress the joint inflammation. Published pharmacokinetic data for this drug include:

Bioavailability (*F*): 1.0 (100%)
Plasma half-life ($t_{1/2}$) = 0.5 h
Volume of distribution (V_d): 45 L

For this drug it is important to maintain an average steady state concentration 2.0 mcg/mL in order to ensure adequate and continued anti-inflammatory activity.

The drug will be given every 4 hours.

What dose will be needed to obtain an average steady-state drug concentration of 2.0 mcg/mL?

a. 5 mg
b. 100 mg
c. 325 mg
d. 500 mg
e. 625 mg

1-7. A 66-year-old woman complains of high fever, myalgias, and non-productive cough of 2 days' duration. She is fatigued also. She says that this is the second time in 2 years that she has become ill with the flu. On examination, her temperature is 102.2°F. Her lungs are clear to percussion and auscultation. Which immunoglobulin class predominates in the secondary antibody response?

a. IgA
b. IgG
c. IgM
d. IgE
e. IgD

1-8. A child presents with severe growth failure, accelerated aging that causes adult complications such as diabetes and coronary artery disease, and microcephaly (small head) due to increased nerve cell death. In vitro assay of labeled thymidine incorporation reveals decreased levels of DNA synthesis compared to controls, but normal-sized labeled DNA fragments. The addition of protein extract from normal cells, gently heated to inactivate DNA polymerase, restores DNA synthesis in the child's cell extracts to normal. Which of the following enzymes used in DNA replication is likely to be defective in this child?

a. DNA-directed DNA polymerase
b. Unwinding proteins
c. DNA polymerase I
d. DNA-directed RNA polymerase
e. DNA ligase

1-9. During a routine physical examination, a 32-year-old female is found to have second-degree heart block. Which of the following ECG recordings was obtained from the patient during her physical examination?

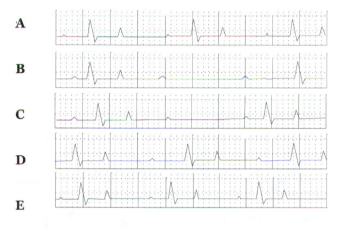

a. Recording A
b. Recording B
c. Recording C
d. Recording D
e. Recording E

1-10. A 65-year-old female found that she had weakness when attempting to flex her left knee and extend the hip. Neurophysiological analysis of the affected regions revealed a reduced number of motor units firing with fasciculations and slowed conduction velocity. There was no depression of tendon reflexes or muscle wasting. Likewise, plantar and abdominal reflexes were normal, and there was little sensory loss, nor were there any signs of sphincter disturbances. Which of the following is the best explanation for this disturbance?

a. Peripheral neuropathy of nerves on the left side of the body that exit the spinal cord at L4–S1
b. Damage of the neuromuscular junctions associated with nerves that exit the left side of the spinal cord between T8 and L3
c. Degeneration of nerve cells in the ventral horn of the left side of the spinal cord between T8 and T12
d. Degeneration of fibers contained in the lateral funiculus of the left side of the thoracic spinal cord
e. Damage to the dorsal horn of the spinal cord of the left side between L1 and L4

1-11. A 65-year-old man who just retired after having worked for many years as a shipyard worker presents with increasing shortness of breath. Pertinent medical history is that he has been a long time smoker. A CT scan of his chest reveals thick, pleural plaques on the surface of his lungs. The associated picture is from a bronchial washing specimen from this patient. The dumbbell-shaped structures in this picture were found to stain blue with a Prussian blue stain. What are these structures?

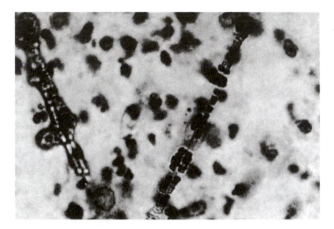

a. *Candida* species
b. Cholesterol crystals
c. Ferruginous bodies
d. Schaumann bodies
e. Silica particles

1-12. A patient presents with a complaint of muscle weakness following exercise. Neurological examination reveals that the muscles supplied by cranial nerves are most affected. You suspect myasthenia gravis. Your diagnosis is confirmed when lab tests indicate antibodies against which of the following in the patient's blood?

a. Acetylcholinesterase
b. Muscle endplates
c. Cranial nerve synaptic membranes
d. Cranial nerve presynaptic membranes
e. Acetylcholine receptors

1-13. A parent brought her child to a pediatric neurologist because the boy exhibited a number of serious neurologic signs. These included lack of coordination, especially around the region of the trunk, vomiting, lack of ability to develop new motor skills, headaches, and an enlarged cranium. Which of the following is the most likely diagnosis?

a. Pyramidal tract syndrome
b. Spina bifida
c. Anencephaly
d. Dandy-Walker syndrome
e. Meningomyelocele

1-14. A male patient who has been "surfing the Web" in search of an aphrodisiac or some other agent to enhance "sexual prowess and performance" discovers yohimbine. He consumes the drug in excess and develops symptoms of toxicity that require your intervention. You consult your preferred drug reference and learn that yohimbine is a selective α_2-adrenergic antagonist. Which would you expect as a response to this drug?

a. Bradycardia
b. Bronchoconstriction
c. Excessive secretions by exocrine glands (salivary, lacrimal, etc.)
d. Hypertension
e. Reduced cardiac output from reduced left ventricular contractility

1-15. A 55-year-old woman presents with pain in her right hip and thigh. The pain started approximately six months ago and is a deep ache that worsens when she stands or walks. Your examination reveals increased warmth over the right thigh. The only laboratory abnormalities are alkaline phosphatase 656 IU/L (normal 23 to 110 IU/L), elevated 24-hour urine hydroxyproline, and osteocalcin 13 ng/mL (normal 6 ng/mL). X-ray of hips and pelvis shows osteolytic lesions and regions with excessive osteoblastic activity. Bone scan shows significant uptake in the right proximal femur. Which of the following would you include in your differential diagnosis?

a. Paget's disease
b. Multiple myeloma
c. Osteomalacia
d. Osteoporosis
e. Hypoparathyroidism

1-16. A 36-year-old man presented at his physician's office complaining of fever and headache. On examination, he had leukopenia and increased liver enzymes, and inclusion bodies were seen in his monocytes. History revealed that he was an outdoorsman and remembered removing a tick from his leg. Which of the following diseases most likely caused the symptoms described?

a. Ehrlichiosis
b. Lyme disease
c. Q fever
d. Rocky Mountain spotted fever
e. Tularemia

1-17. A child presents with low blood glucose (hypoglycemia), enlarged liver (hepatomegaly), and excess fat deposition in the cheeks (cherubic facies). A liver biopsy reveals excess glycogen in hepatocytes. Deficiency of which of the following enzymes might explain this phenotype?

a. α-1,1-glucosidase
b. α-1,1-galactosidase
c. α-1,4-glucosidase
d. α-1,4-galactosidase
e. α-1,6-galactosidase

1-18. A person who was physically dependent on and an abuser of heroin is now maintained on methadone. He succumbs to temptation and buys an opioid on the street. He takes it and rapidly goes into withdrawal. Which of the following drugs did he take?

a. Meperidine
b. Heroin
c. Pentazocine
d. Codeine
e. Propoxyphene

1-19. The accompanying x-ray shows the shoulder of an 11-year-old female who fell off the monkey bars, extending her arm in an attempt to break her fall. The small arrows indicate a fracture in the area of the surgical neck of the humerus. The large arrows indicate which of the following?

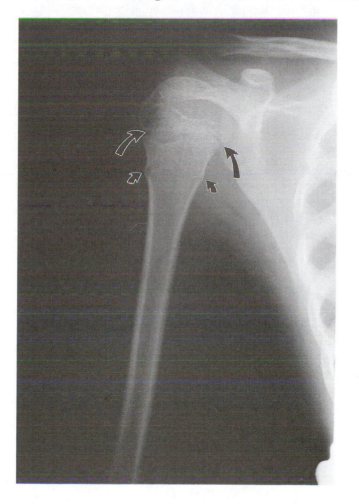

a. A fracture at the anatomic neck of the humerus
b. The glenohumeral joint
c. The joint space between the proximal humerus and the acromion of the scapula
d. The proximal humeral epiphyseal plate
e. What is commonly called a shoulder separation

1-20. A 75-year-old woman with congestive heart failure (CHF) is unable to climb a flight of stairs without experiencing shortness of breath. Digoxin is administered to improve cardiac muscle contractility. Within 2 weeks, she has a marked improvement in her symptoms. The direct cellular action of digoxin that accounts for its ability to improve cardiac output is inhibition of which of the following?

a. β_1-adrenergic receptor activation
b. Cyclic adenosine 5'-monophosphate (cAMP) synthesis
c. GTP binding to specific G proteins
d. Mitochondrial calcium (Ca^{2+}) release
e. Na^+-K^+-ATPase

1-21. A 28-year-old man complains of a painless mass in the left scrotum. His physician orders a CT scan of the pelvis and notes that the retroperitoneal lymph nodes are not involved. The patient has an orchiectomy done and the tumor is categorized as a nonseminoma. Which one of the following is secreted by nonseminoma germ cell tumors (GCT)?

a. α-fetoprotein (αFP)
b. Monoclonal immunoglobulin
c. CD30
d. Lactate dehydrogenase (LDH)
e. Carcinoembryonic antigen (CEA)

1-22. A patient taking a diuretic for several months presents with significantly elevated serum glucose levels and impaired carbohydrate tolerance (i.e., abnormally slow decline of blood glucose levels following a carbohydrate load). You suspect it is diuretic-induced. Which of the following is the most likely cause?

a. Acetazolamide
b. Amiloride
c. Chlorothiazide
d. Spironolactone
e. Triamterene

I-23. A 65-year-old man is diagnosed with a form of a peripheral neuropathy. What effect will this disorder have upon the patient?

a. A loss in motor function, but sensory functions will remain largely intact
b. A reduction in conduction velocity of the affected nerve
c. An increase in the number of Ranvier's nodes
d. Degeneration of myelin but the axon will typically remain intact
e. Signs of a UMN paralysis

I-24. A 16-year-old boy on the track team asks his pediatrician if he can take creatine on a regular basis in order to increase his muscle strength prior to a track meet. He wants to take creatine because

a. Creatine increases plasma glucose concentration
b. Creatine prevents dehydration
c. Creatine increases muscle glycogen concentrations
d. Creatine is converted to phosphocreatine
e. Creatine delays the metabolism of fatty acids

I-25. A five year-old boy sustains a tear in his gastrocnemius muscle when he is involved in a bicycle accident. Regeneration of the muscle will occur through which of the following?

a. Differentiation of satellite cells
b. Dedifferentiation of myocytes into myoblasts
c. Fusion of damaged myofibers to form new myotubes
d. Hyperplasia of existing myofibers
e. Differentiation of fibroblasts to form myocytes

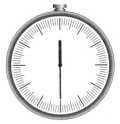

YOU SHOULD HAVE COMPLETED APPROXIMATELY 25 QUESTIONS AND HAVE 30 MINUTES REMAINING.

1-26. A 35-year-old man presents with weight loss, fever, and fatigue. Physical examination finds signs and symptoms of mitral valve disease. Further work-up finds a pedunculated mass in the left atrium. The tumor is resected and histologic sections reveal stellate cells in a loose myxoid background. Which of the following is the most likely diagnosis?

a. Chordoma
b. Fibroelastoma
c. Leiomyoma
d. Myxoma
e. Rhabdomyoma

1-27. An 18-year-old high school student in rural north Mississippi develops fever, cough, and chest pain. The cough, associated with weight loss, persisted. Because of poor performance at football practice, he was advised to see a physician. Lymph node biopsies stained with H and E studies revealed granulomatous inflammation and macrophages engorged with oval structures measuring 2 to 4 μ. Cultures incubated at room temperature grew powdery white colonies, which on microscopic study had tuberculate spores. The high school student acquired the infection from which of the following?

a. Another human via respiratory secretions
b. Bird excrement
c. Cat feces
d. Contaminated drinking water
e. Desert sand

1-28. A 27-year-old woman presents with headaches, muscle pain (myalgia), anorexia, nausea, and vomiting. She denies any history of drug or alcohol use, but upon further questioning she states that recently she has lost her taste for coffee and cigarettes. Physical examination reveals a slight yellow discoloration of her scleras, while laboratory results indicate a serum bilirubin level of 1.8 mg/dL, and aminotransferases (AST and ALT) levels are increased. Which of the following is the most likely diagnosis?

a. Gilbert's syndrome
b. Chronic hepatitis
c. Amebic liver abscess
d. Acute viral hepatitis
e. Acute hepatic failure

1-29. An older man with severe emphysema is found to have decreased amounts and abnormal mobility of α_1 antitrypsin (AAT) protein in his serum when analyzed by serum protein electrophoresis. Liver biopsy discloses mild scarring (cirrhosis) and demonstrates microscopic inclusions due to an engorged endoplasmic reticulum (ER). Which of the following is the most likely explanation for these findings?

a. Defective transport from hepatic ER to the serum
b. A mutation affecting the N-terminal methionine and blocking initiation of protein synthesis
c. A mutation affecting the signal sequence
d. Defective structure of the signal recognition particles
e. Defective energy metabolism causing deficiency of GTP

1-30. A 72-year-old male is evaluated by a physiatrist after a stroke. The patient is observed to suffer from dysmetria and ataxia. These neurological signs are most likely related to a lesion within which of the following regions of the brain?

a. Cerebellum
b. Medulla
c. Cortical motor strip
d. Basal ganglia
e. Eighth cranial nerve

1-31. A 30-year-old secretary who is a single mother with two preschool children has frequent symptoms of anxiety, tension, headaches, and insomnia. Which of the following behavioral interventions could be the most effective in relieving her symptoms?

a. Progressive muscle relaxation
b. Psychoanalytic psychotherapy
c. Hypnosis
d. Selective biofeedback
e. Interpersonal psychotherapy

1-32. A 27-year-old man sustains an injury to the lateral aspect of his left ankle in an accident about 6 weeks ago. The skin, which was lacerated, became erythematous and swollen, and over the few weeks since then he developed persistent pain in his ankle. His physician recommended local treatment to relieve the swelling, had x-rays of the ankle done, and started him on antibiotics. His physician concluded that he had an acute bacterial infection of the bone; these infections characteristically show which one of the following?

a. Necrotic bone
b. Prolonged clinical course
c. Predominantly mononuclear cells
d. Congested and thrombosed blood vessels
e. Granulation tissue

1-33. A 58-year-old woman presents with increased "fullness" in her neck. Physical examination finds nontender diffuse enlargement of her thyroid gland. Clinically she is found to be euthyroid and her serum TSH level is within normal limits. Sections from her enlarged thyroid gland reveal numerous, mainly enlarged follicles, most of which are filled with abundant colloid material. There are areas of fibrosis, hemorrhage, and cystic degeneration. No papillary structures are identified and neither colloid scalloping nor Hurthle cells are present. Which of the following is the most likely diagnosis?

a. Colloid carcinoma
b. Diffuse toxic goiter
c. Graves' disease
d. Hashimoto's thyroiditis
e. Multinodular goiter

1-34. A 45-year-old man complains of frequent "heartburn" and a mild chronic cough. On examination, he has gastroesophageal reflux disease (GERD). In addition to prescribing medications, which one of the following dietary recommendations would you make?

a. Avoid high-protein meals because they would increase lower esophageal sphincter (LES) pressure
b. Avoid fats, chocolates, and alcohol because they would decrease LES pressure
c. Eat high-carbohydrate foods to increase overall GI motility
d. Eat high-protein meals to decrease LES pressure
e. Avoid concentrated carbohydrates to decrease dopamine secretion

1-35. A premature male infant born at 29 weeks' gestation to a 22-year-old woman with gestational diabetes develops problems breathing about 14 h after delivery. Physical examination finds cyanosis, tachypnea, and nasal flaring. A chest x-ray reveals a bilateral diffuse reticular ("ground glass") appearance. His respiratory problems worsen and he is put on a ventilator. Which one of the following therapies should also be given at this time?

a. Dietary vitamin C
b. Intramuscular insulin
c. Intranasal vasopressin
d. Intratracheal surfactant
e. Intravascular epinephrine

1-36. A 16-year-old boy with breathing difficulty is seen in the emergency department. He is diagnosed with asthma and given urgent care. The next day he visits his primary physician, who starts him on therapy with albuterol, to be inhaled "as needed" (for acute symptom control—rescue therapy). After several weeks the patient says he needs to use the inhaler several times a day, nearly every day, because "breathing just gets real hard; I can't get much air in." The physician's assessment is that symptom severity and frequency are getting progressively and quickly worse.

Which *initial* therapeutic modification for outpatient management would be most reasonable, with the greatest likelihood of controlling the asthma?

a. Add an inhaled corticosteroid
b. Add cromolyn
c. Add oral prednisone
d. Add theophylline
e. Double the albuterol dose to be taken with each episode
f. Replace the albuterol with salmeterol

1-37. A divorced working mother takes her 4-year-old child to a day-care center. She has noticed that the child's frequent stools are nonbloody with mucus and are foul smelling. The child has no fever, but does complain of "tummy hurting." The increase of fat in the stool directs the pediatrician's concern toward a diagnosis of malabsorption syndrome associated with which of the following?

a. Amebiasis
b. Ascariasis
c. Balantidiasis
d. Enterobiasis
e. Giardiasis

1-38. A 29-year-old woman presents with frequent, debilitating migraine headaches. Sumatriptan is prescribed for abortive therapy. Not long after using the drug she is rushed to the hospital. Her vital signs are unstable, and she has muscle rigidity, myoclonus, generalized CNS irritability and altered consciousness, and shivering. You learn that for several months she had been taking another drug with which the triptan interacted. Which of the following was the most likely drug?

a. Acetaminophen
b. Codeine
c. Diazepam
d. Fluoxetine
e. Phenytoin

1-39. A 35-year-old woman during her first pregnancy develops oligohydramnios. At 34 weeks of gestation she delivers a stillborn infant with abnormal facial features consisting of wide-set eyes, low-set floppy ears, and a broad-flat nose. Which of the following abnormalities is most likely to be present in this still-born infant?

a. Absence of the thymus
b. Bilateral renal agenesis
c. Congenital biliary atresia
d. Cystic renal dysplasia
e. Urinary bladder exstrophy

1-40. A 24-year-old woman develops adult respiratory distress syndrome (ARDS) after near-drowning due to attempted suicide. Conventional mechanical ventilation together with prone positioning and inhaled nitric oxide do not provide sufficient oxygenation. Porcine surfactant is instilled via fiberoptic bronchoscope, and the partial arterial carbon dioxide pressure ($Paco_2$) and fraction of inspired oxygen (F_Io_2) ratio as well as shunt fraction (Qs/Qt) improve impressively. The improvements in respiratory function occurred because surfactant decreased which of the following?

a. Bronchiolar smooth-muscle tone
b. Arterial bicarbonate concentration
c. Lung compliance
d. The work of breathing
e. Functional residual capacity (FRC)

1-41. A patient was diagnosed with a form of epilepsy. One approach in treating this disorder is to give the patient a drug that would have a selective blocking action upon neurotransmitter receptors. Which of the following receptors would such a drug block in order to serve as an effective treatment procedure?

a. GABA receptors
b. Glutamate receptors
c. Nicotinic receptors
d. Serotonin receptors
e. Glycine receptors

1-42. A 36-year-old woman presents because of increasing pain in her hands and knees, which, she says, is worse in the morning. Physical examination finds her fingers to be swollen and stiff, and there is ulnar deviation of her metacarpophalangeal joints. A biopsy from her knee would likely show areas where histiocytes were palisading around irregular areas of necrosis, as seen in the picture below. The biopsy would also likely show proliferation and hyperplasia of the synovium with destruction of the articular cartilage. Which one of the following terms best describes these pathologic changes?

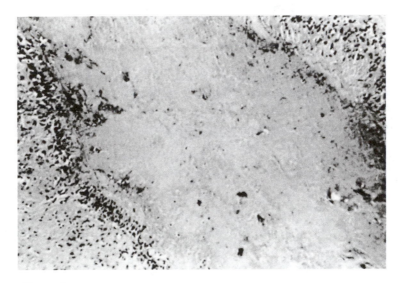

a. Eburnation
b. Gumma
c. Pannus
d. Spondylosis
e. Tophus

1-43. An 18-year-old male patient with acute lymphocytic leukemia fails all standard chemotherapies. Cells from an HLA-nonidentical donor are used to perform a bone marrow transplant. Prior to transplantation, the patient is given broad-spectrum antibiotics and an immunosuppressive regimen. Within two to four weeks, lymphocyte and granulocyte numbers begin to rise, confirming bone marrow cell engraftment. However, one month later, the patient develops diarrhea, jaundice, and a severe maculopapular rash. Physical exam reveals hepotomegaly and splenomegaly. Which of the following is most likely occurring?

a.   Acute rejection
b.   Chronic rejection
c.   Cyclosporine A toxicity
d.   Graft-versus-host disease (GVHD)
e.   Hyperacute rejection

1-44. A 43-year-old woman who has suffered from diabetes for 30 years comes into the clinic. Her hematocrit is 21 and she has a reduced RBC count. Her serum creatinine is 3.0 (normal 2.0 or below). She has a negative pregnancy test and is a nonsmoker. Which of the following would best explain her condition?

a.   Decreased hepatic production of erythropoietin leading to decreased numbers of circulating reticulocytes in the bloodstream
b.   Increased erythropoietin production by the liver resulting in increased numbers of reticulocytes
c.   Decreased renal erythropoietin production leading to reduced red blood cell production
d.   Decreased estrogen levels stimulating hepatic production of erythropoietin
e.   Decreased estrogen levels directly inhibiting red blood cell production by the bone marrow

1-45. A 5-year-old boy is being evaluated for recurrent epistaxis and other abnormal bleeding episodes, including excessive bleeding from the umbilical cord at birth. Laboratory studies reveal the following: decreased hemoglobin (with microcytic hypochromic red cell indices), normal platelet count, markedly prolonged prothrombin time (PT) and partial thromboplastin time (PTT), and unmeasurable thrombin time (TT). Platelet aggregation studies reveal a normal platelet response to ristocetin, but with other substances (including collagen, ADP, and epinephrine), this patient's platelets exhibit a primary wave defect. Based on these findings, which of the following is the most likely diagnosis?

a. Afibrinogenemia
b. Bernard-Soulier syndrome
c. Glanzmann's thrombasthenia
d. Gray platelet syndrome
e. Wiskott-Aldrich syndrome

1-46. A patient has multiple gastric ulcers but has done nothing about them. Shortly after consuming a large meal and large amounts of alcohol, he experiences significant GI distress. He takes an over-the-counter heartburn remedy. Within a minute or two he develops what he will later describe as a "bad bloated feeling." Several of the ulcers have begun to bleed and he experiences searing pain.

The patient becomes profoundly hypotensive from upper GI blood loss and is transported to the hospital. Endoscopy confirms multiple bleeds; the endoscopist remarks that it appears as if the lesions had been literally stretched apart, causing additional tissue damage that led to the hemorrhage. The drug or product the patient most likely took was:

a. An aluminum salt
b. An aluminum-magnesium combination antacid product
c. Magnesium hydroxide
d. Ranitidine
e. Sodium bicarbonate

1-47. Parents bring in their 2-week-old child fearful that he has ingested a poison. They had delayed disposing one of the child's diapers, and noted a black discoloration where the urine had collected. Later, they realized that all of the child's diapers would turn black if stored as waste for a day or so. Knowing that phenol groups can complex to form colors, which amino acid pathways are implicated in this phenomenon?

a.   The phenylalanine, tyrosine, and homogentisate pathway
b.   The histidine pathway
c.   The leucine, isoleucine, and valine pathway
d.   The methionine and homocystine pathway
e.   The arginine and citrulline pathway (urea cycle)

1-48. A 75-year-old male comes to your office for a complete history and physical examination accompanied by his daughter. He takes no medications. Your nurse immediately notifies you that his blood pressure is 190/100. He states, "Oh, don't worry about that; I check it at the grocery store and it has been high for 10 years. That's normal for me." Which of the following EKG findings would you expect?

a.   A tall R wave in V_1 with right axis deviation
b.   A wide QRS complex consistent with left or right bundle branch block
c.   ST segment elevation in most leads
d.   Tall left precordial R waves and deep right precordial S waves consistent with left ventricular hypertrophy
e.   Q-T interval prolongation

1-49. A 48-year-old male executive has had confirmed ischemic heart disease for several years. His symptoms are exacerbated significantly by stress. He agreed to join a controlled experimental program of 500 patients with heart disease to test the prevention of stress-related illness and death in patients with heart disease (the Ischemic Heart Disease Life Stress Monitoring Program). The experimental program was successful in lowering the stress on a case-by-case basis. This patient was much improved after the first year and the cardiac mortality rate in the experimental group had decreased by

a.   10%
b.   20%
c.   30%
d.   40%
e.   50%

1-50. During a routine breast self-examination, a 35-year-old woman is concerned because her breasts feel "lumpy." She consults you as her primary care physician. After performing an examination, you reassure her that no masses are present and that the "lumpiness" is due to fibrocystic changes. Which of the following pathologic findings is a type of nonproliferative fibrocystic change?

a. A blue-domed cyst
b. A radial scar
c. Atypical ductal hyperplasia
d. Papillomatosis
e. Sclerosing adenosis

BLOCK 2

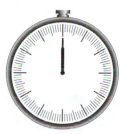

YOU HAVE 60 MINUTES TO COMPLETE 50 QUESTIONS.

Questions

2-1. A 39-year-old man presents to the emergency room complaining of tingling in his hands and muscle twitching. On admission, the patient is alert and stable, with an initial examination remarkable only for carpopedal spasm. Which of the following blood gas values will most likely be observed in this patient?

	Pa_{CO_2} (mM)	HCO_3^-
a.	50	40
b.	60	20
c.	40	30
d.	30	15
e.	20	20

2-2. A 22-year-old male who belongs to a weekend football league was running with the ball when a defender tackled him mid-lower limb from the side. After the tackle, he felt that the knee was hurt and went to the emergency room. From an MRI of the knee, the lateral meniscus is uniformly black; however, the medial meniscus has a tear (lucent area within the meniscus). Which of the following is the reason why the medial meniscus is more susceptible to damage than the lateral meniscus?

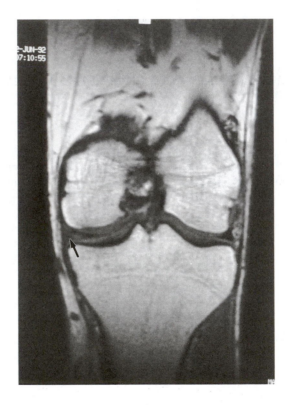

a. The medial meniscus is attached to the popliteus muscle tendon, which can move into a position making it more susceptible
b. The medial meniscus is attached to the medial (tibial) collateral ligament, which holds it relatively immobile, making it more susceptible
c. The medial meniscus is attached to the anterior cruciate ligament, which holds it relatively immobile, making it more susceptible
d. The only reason the medial meniscus is more susceptible to damage is that the knee usually gets hit laterally, causing more torsion on the medial meniscus

2-3. A 44-year-old traveling salesman was recently diagnosed with type 2 diabetes mellitus. The physician prescribed an exercise and diet plan, but this gentleman wouldn't be compliant. He habitually has a morning cup of coffee, gets in his car in the morning, and drives until he gets to his next appointment late afternoon. He says he rarely stops and eats in between.

The next approach is to use a single oral antidiabetic drug, but you are concerned about the drug causing or worsening hypoglycemia in this "meal-skipper." Which of the following drugs poses the greatest relative risk of causing or exacerbating hypoglycemia?

a. Acarbose
b. Glyburide
c. Metformin
d. Pioglitazone
e. Repaglinide

2-4. A 59-year-old woman is diagnosed with tuberculosis (TB). Before prescribing a drug regimen, you take a careful medication history because one of the drugs commonly used to treat TB induces microsomal cytochrome P450 enzymes in the liver. Which drug is it?

a. Ethambutol
b. Isoniazid
c. Pyrazinamide
d. Rifampin
e. Vitamin B_6

2-5. A couple comes to your urology office because of inability to conceive a wanted child after one year of unprotected sex. The wife had undergone a gynecological work up, including testing for 3 months showing a normal ovulation profile as confirmed by an ovulatory kit. The primary care physician describes the husband's physical exam as normal and had ordered a semen analysis and had forwarded the results to you. The semen volume was 0.5 mL, pH 6.8, and azospermic without any fructose. The husband has a brother, who has two children, one of whom has confirmed cystic fibrosis. You order a pelvic MRI to determine whether which of the following exist(s)?

a. Bilateral abdominal testicles
b. Hypospadias
c. Congenital absence of ejaculatory ducts and vas deferens
d. Congenital hydrocele
e. Congenital absence of the prostate gland

2-6. A 34-year-old male patient visits a physician with complaints of fatigue, weight loss, night sweats, and "swollen glands." The physician also observes that he has an oral yeast infection. Which of the following tests would most likely reveal the cause of his problems?

a. A human T-lymphotropic virus type I (HTLV-I) test
b. A test for *C. albicans*
c. A test for CD8 lymphocytes
d. A test for infectious mononucleosis
e. An HIV ELISA test

2-7. A 29-year-old woman is being evaluated to find the cause of her urine turning a dark brown color after a recent upper respiratory tract infection. She has been otherwise asymptomatic, and her blood pressure has been within normal limits. Urinalysis finds moderate blood present with red cells and red cell casts. Immunofluorescence examination of a renal biopsy reveals deposits of IgA within the mesangium. These clinical findings suggest that her disorder is associated with activation of the alternate complement system. Which of the following serum laboratory findings is most suggestive of activation of the alternate complement system rather than the classic complement system?

	Serum C2	Serum C3	Serum C4
a.	Decreased	Normal	Normal
b.	Normal	Decreased	Normal
c.	Normal	Normal	Decreased
d.	Decreased	Normal	Decreased
e.	Decreased	Decreased	Decreased

2-8. Previously, you treated a 44-year-old man, a former intravenous drug abuser, for acute hepatitis C infection. Several months later, it is clear that the patient has chronic hepatitis and may need therapy with interferon. Which long-term complications of hepatitis C infection must you discuss so that the patient can make an informed decision about treatment?

a. Hepatoma and cirrhosis
b. Hepatic adenoma
c. Sclerosing cholangitis
d. Hemochromatosis
e. Lymphoma or leukemia

2-9. A 41-year-old woman is admitted to the outpatient area of the hematology-oncology center for her first course of adjuvant chemotherapy for metastatic breast cancer following a left modified radical mastectomy and axillary lymph node dissection for infiltrating ductal carcinoma of the breast. Two biopsies were positive for cancer.

Following premedication with dexamethasone and ondansetron, she will receive combination chemotherapy with doxorubicin, cyclophospha-mide, and fluorouracil. Premedications include intravenous ondansetron and dexamethasone.

Twenty-four hours after the first course of chemotherapy she will start a 10-day regimen with filgrastim. Which of the following is the purpose of giving that drug?

a. Control of nausea and emesis
b. Potentiate the anticancer effects of the chemotherapeutic agents
c. Prevent doxorubicin-induced cardiotoxicity
d. Reduce the risk/severity of chemo-induced neutropenia, and related infections
e. Stimulate the gastric mucosa to repair damage caused by the chemotherapy drugs

2-10. A patient with elevated heart rate and blood pressure is examined by a battery of physicians and they conclude that his condition is due to a defi-ciency or loss of the carotid sinus reflex. What is a component of this reflex?

a. Baroreceptor afferent fibers from cranial nerve XI
b. Glossopharyngeal efferent fibers
c. Interneurons within the nucleus ambiguus of the medulla
d. Efferent fibers contained in the intermediate component of the facial nerve
e. Vagal efferent fibers

2-11. A 15-year-old boy attempts suicide with a liquid that he found in his parents' greenhouse. His dad used it to get rid of "varmints" around the yard. The toxin causes intense abdominal pain, skeletal muscle cramps, projectile vomiting, and severe diarrhea that leads to fluid and electrolyte imbalances, hypotension, and difficulty swallowing. On examination he is found to be volume depleted and is showing signs of a reduced level of consciousness. His breath smells "metallic." Which of the following proba-bly accounts for these symptoms?

a. Arsenic (As)
b. Cadmium (Cd)
c. Iron (Fe)
d. Lead (Pb)
e. Zinc (Zn)

2-12. A child with a large head, multiple fractures, and blue scleras (whites of the eyes) is evaluated for osteogenesis imperfecta (166200). One study involves labeling of collagen chains in tissue culture to assess their mobility by gel electrophoresis. Amino acids labeled with radioactive carbon 14 are added to the culture dishes in order to label the collagen. Which of the following amino acids would not result in labeled collagen?

a. Serine
b. Glycine
c. Aspartate
d. Glutamate
e. Hydroxyproline

2-13. A 21-year-old man was bitten by a tick in Oregon. Two years later, during the course of routine screening for an unknown ailment, a screening Lyme disease test was performed, which was negative. A western blot strip (IgG) showed the following pattern:

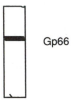

Gp66

Which of the following is the correct interpretation of the test?

a. The patient has acute Lyme disease
b. The patient has chronic Lyme disease
c. The patient should be tested for HIV on the basis of the western blot
d. The pattern may represent nonspecific reactivity
e. The screening test should be repeated

2-14. A 47-year-old man presents with headaches, muscle weakness, and leg cramps. He is not currently taking any medications. Physical examination finds a thin adult man with mild hypertension. Laboratory examination reveals slightly increased sodium, decreased serum potassium level, and decreased hydrogen ion concentration. Serum glucose levels are within normal limits. A CT scan reveals a large tumor involving the cortex of his left adrenal gland. Which of the following combinations of serum laboratory findings is most likely to be present in this individual?

a. Decreased aldosterone with increased renin
b. Decreased cortisol with decreased ACTH
c. Increased aldosterone with decreased renin
d. Increased cortisol with increased ACTH
e. Increased deoxycorticosterone with increased cortisol

2-15. A 37-year-old immunosuppressed patient presents with increasingly severe diarrhea, characterized by numerous watery and nonbloody stools every day. Additional clinical symptoms include abdominal cramping, nausea, flatulence, and occasional vomiting. Which one of the following laboratory tests would be the best method to diagnose infection with *Cryptosporidium parvum* in this individual?

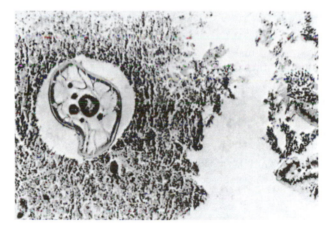

a. Examine the stool with an acid-fast stain
b. Measure vitamin B_{12} levels in the serum
c. Perform an anal "Scotch-tape" test
d. Quantitate the amount of fecal in a 24-h stool specimen
e. Test the absorption of D-xylose in the colon

2-16. A sibling donor is found for a patient with Tay-Sachs disease, and the physician writes to the patient's insurance company explaining the diagnosis of Tay-Sachs disease and the reasons for the bone marrow transplant. Not only does the insurance company refuse payment for transplantation, it also discontinues coverage for the family based on anticipated medical expenses. From the ethical perspective, these events fall under which of the following categories?

a. Patient confidentiality
b. Nondisclosure
c. Informed consent
d. Failure to provide ongoing care
e. Discrimination

2-17. A 35-year-old man has a prolactinoma and a history of severe peptic ulcer disease. There is a family history of pituitary tumors. The findings of what other diagnostic test at this time may be abnormal and potentially useful in diagnosis?

a. Fasting blood sugar
b. Serum calcium
c. Serum calcitonin
d. Urinary metanephrine
e. Serum ferritin

2-18. A 22-year-old male has just entered medical school and has decided to "assert himself" by beginning to smoke cigarettes. In an attempt to persuade him that smoking will damage his entire body, you inform him that the most immediate effect of cigarette smoking is

a. Lower lymphocyte function
b. Lower immune function
c. Mucociliary damage
d. Addiction to the nicotine
e. Destruction of the macrophages in his lungs

2-19. An elderly man, persuaded to have his eyes examined after a series of minor automobile accidents, was found to have a pituitary adenoma that was producing visual field defects. A pituitary adenoma that expands superiorly and compresses the central portion of the optic chiasm will result in which of the following?

a. Total blindness
b. Losses of left and right inferior fields of vision
c. Losses of left and right nasal fields of vision
d. Losses of left and right temporal fields of vision

2-20. A 59-year-old male with an ejection fraction of 15%, who is being treated with medications for his heart failure, is asked whether he would like to participate in a trial for an experimental drug. The drug being tested is designed to decrease the expression of phospholamban on ventricular muscle cells. Which one of the following would be increased by decreasing phospholamban?

a. The activity of the sodium-potassium pump
b. The diastolic stiffness of the ventricular muscle cells
c. The activity of the L-type calcium channels
d. The duration of the ventricular muscle action potential
e. The concentration of calcium within the SR

2-21. A patient with chronic open-angle glaucoma is treated with a topical ophthalmic β blocker. Which of the following is the most likely mechanism by which this drug lowers intraocular pressure?

a. Decreasing aqueous humor synthesis/secretion
b. Contracting the iris dilator muscles
c. Dilating the uveoscleral veins
d. Directly opening the trabecular meshwork
e. Contracting the circular pupillary constrictor muscle

2-22. An HIV-positive patient asks you if you can tell him the chances of his progressing to symptomatic AIDS. Which one of the following tests would be most useful?

a. CD4 lymphocyte count
b. HIV antibody test
c. HIV p24 antigen
d. HIV RT PCR
e. Neopterin

2-23. A 9-year-old boy is being evaluated for deafness. Physical examination reveals a child with short stature, coarse facial features (low, flat nose; thick lips; widely spaced teeth; facial fullness), a large tongue, and clear corneas. Laboratory examination reveals increased urinary levels of heparan sulfate and dermatan sulfate. Metachromatic granules (Reilly bodies) are found in leukocytes from a bone marrow biopsy. These leukocytes are also found to be deficient in iduronosulfate sulfatase. Which of the following is the most likely diagnosis?

a. Hunter's disease
b. Hurler's disease
c. I cell disease
d. Metachromatic leukodystrophy
e. Wolman's disease

2-24. A 4-year-old boy presents with a history of numerous fractures that are not related to excessive trauma. Physical examination reveals evidence of previous fractures along with abnormally loose joints, decreased hearing, and blue scleras. X-rays of the boy's arms reveal the bones to be markedly thinned. Which of the following is the most likely diagnosis?

a. Osteopetrosis
b. Osteoporosis
c. Osteomalacia
d. Osteogenesis imperfecta
e. Osteitis deformans

2-25. A 55-year-old man, who had been suffering from hypertension for the past eight years, experienced attacks of pain in the regions of the pharynx and ear, which were usually preceded by swallowing and coughing spells. These attacks, each of which lasted for an average of one minute, occurred a number of times; ultimately, this condition showed remission. Although the neurological examination was basically normal, a subsequent MRI was taken and revealed an abnormality at the base of the skull.

Which cranial nerve was most likely involved in this disorder?

a. Nerve V
b. Nerve VII
c. Nerve IX
d. Nerve XI
e. Nerve XII

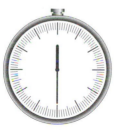

**YOU SHOULD HAVE COMPLETED APPROXIMATELY
25 QUESTIONS AND HAVE 30 MINUTES REMAINING.**

2-26. A 55-year-old man presents with increasing fatigue, weakness, anorexia and jaundice over the past several months. Physical examination finds mild ascites and gynecomastia. A liver biopsy reveals regenerative nodules of hepatocytes surrounded by fibrosis, as seen in the picture below. Which of the following is the source of the excess collagen deposited in these fibrotic bands?

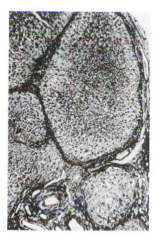

a. Hepatocytes

b. Kupffer cells

c. Ito cells

d. Endothelial cells

e. Bile duct epithelial cells

2-27. A patient with severe, acute trauma pain requires analgesia. The physician orders morphine. Which of the following coexisting conditions would pose the greatest risk from morphine's use in this case?

a. Acute pulmonary edema
b. Closed head injury
c. Compound fractures of both femurs
d. Hypertension
e. Opioid abuse, recent history of
f. Recent myocardial infarction

2-28. An individual is diagnosed with retinitis pigmentosa, which produces a defective opsin. Which of the following will most likely result from this deficit?

a. Degeneration of area 17 of the cerebral cortex
b. Degeneration of cone cells
c. Loss of central vision
d. Total loss of vision
e. Reduced response to light

2-29. A 36-year-old man, homosexual, had experienced an acute infection several months previously, characterized by fever, headache, malaise, and arthraligias. Examination at that time showed only axillary and cervical adenopathy. The chest roentgenogram was clear. Now, his tests for HIV are positive, but he feels well and he does not have AIDS. His physician will start anti-HIV therapy when

a. The CD4 T lymphocyte count is about 450 cells/μL and the viral load is 10,000 copies/μL
b. The patient feels that the medications will benefit him
c. The patient experiences another acute infection as he had before
d. The patient experiences any opportunistic infection
e. The patient starts a new monogamous relationship

2-30. A 22-year-old male receives a severe, traumatic compression injury to his radial nerve after a motorcycle crash. He shows an advancing Tinel's sign. Which of the following is true about regeneration of axons after his nerve injury?

a. It occurs in the absence of motor unit potentials
b. It occurs at a rate of 100 mm/day
c. It occurs by a mechanism that is dependent on the proliferation of Schwann cells
d. It occurs in conjunction with degeneration and phagocytosis of endoneurial tubes
e. It occurs in the segment distal to the damage

2-31. A 27-year-old man presents with a testicular mass, which is resected and diagnosed as being a yolk sac tumor. Which of the following substances is most likely to be increased in this patient's serum as a result of being secreted from the cells of this tumor?

a. Acid phosphatase
b. α-fetoprotein (AFP)
c. Alkaline phosphatase
d. β-human chorionic gonadotropin (β-hCG)
e. Prostate-specific antigen (PSA)

2-32. A 30-year-old male presents to the emergency room with shortness of breath and right-sided pleuritic chest pain. His chest x-ray in the emergency room is normal. An arterial blood gas is obtained while the patient is breathing room air. The results show a pH of 7.48, Pa_{co2} of 35, Pa_{o2} of 68, and an oxygen saturation of 92%. What is his A-a gradient?

a. 20
b. 30
c. 40
d. 50
e. 60

2-33. You have taken on a part-time responsibility as the company physician for a small factory that has a mixture of hourly workers, engineers, and executives. The company is under stress because of falling profits and competition with foreign manufacturers. You are aware of a number of stresses in the workplace from uncertainty about the future of the company to interpersonal conflict. Which of the following psychological stresses is likely to have the most adverse impact on physical health?

a. Regressiveness
b. Interpersonal conflict
c. Confusion
d. Uncontrollability
e. Fearfulness

2-34. A 25-year-old woman who has never been pregnant presents with amenorrhea for 3 months and a milky discharge from her nipple. She states that her menstrual cycles have been irregular for the past year. Laboratory tests show that her serum LH and estradiol levels are below normal, and a pregnancy test is negative. Which of the following is the most likely cause of these signs and symptoms?

a. Craniopharyngioma of the hypothalamus
b. Germinoma of the pineal gland
c. Islet cell adenoma of the pancreas
d. Medullary carcinoma of the thyroid gland
e. Prolactinoma of the pituitary gland

2-35. A 74-year-old female was brought to the hospital after she suffered a stroke. Several days later, a neurological examination revealed that she was unable to perform certain types of learned, complex movements (referred to as *apraxia*). Which region of the cerebral cortex was affected by the stroke?

a. Precentral gyrus
b. Postcentral gyrus
c. Premotor cortex
d. Prefrontal cortex
e. Cingulate gyrus

2-36. A healthy, 24-year-old man is prescribed sustained-release bupropion (Zyban) for smoking cessation. Twenty-one days after therapy he presents to his family physician with intermittent fever and a generalized rash, at which point the bupropion therapy is discontinued. A month later he develops a dry, intermittent cough and dyspnea. Blood gas analysis indicates a Pao_2 of 52 mmHg and a $Paco_2$ of 32 mmHg. Which of the following pulmonary function test results is consistent with a diagnosis of allergic bronchospasm?

a. An increased forced vital capacity
b. A decreased FEV_1/FVC
c. An increased diffusing capacity
d. A decreased residual volume
e. An increased breathing frequency

2-37. A patient who worked in an industrial setting presented to his ophthalmologist with acute conjunctivitis, enlarged and tender preauricular nodes, and early stages of keratitis. The differential diagnosis should include infection with which of the following viruses?

a. Adenovirus
b. Epstein-Barr virus
c. Parvovirus
d. Respiratory syncytial virus
e. Varicella-zoster virus

2-38. A 34-year-old man with anxiety has heard about buspirone and asks whether it might be suitable for him. According to the latest diagnostic criteria, the drug would be appropriate. However, before prescribing it you should know that buspirone does which of the following?

a. Causes a withdrawal syndrome that, if unsupervised, is frequently lethal
b. Requires almost daily dosage titrations in order to optimize the response
c. Seldom causes drowsiness
d. Has a significant potential for abuse
e. Is likely to potentiate the CNS depressant effects of alcohol, benzodiazepines, and sedative antihistamines (e.g., diphenhydramine), so such interactants must be avoided at all cost

2-39. A 32-year-old female complains of intermittent chest discomfort that occurs most frequently when she drinks lots of coffee to stay up to meet deadlines at work. She is referred to cardiology for an exercise stress test to rule out cardiac ischemia as the cause for her angina. The test will be considered positive if

a. Mean arterial blood pressure increases
b. ST segment depression occurs
c. Tachycardia develops
d. A diastolic murmur is heard
e. The QRS complex widens

2-40. A 65-year-old obese male presents with severe indigestion and chest pain after a spicy meal. A lactate dehydrogenase (LDH) level obtained to evaluate possible myocardial infarction is normal, but the laboratory recommends that LDH isozymes be performed. The managing physician knows that lactate dehydrogenase is composed of two different polypeptide chains arranged in the form of a tetramer. Assuming that all possible combinations of the different polypeptide chains occur, how many isozyme forms of lactate dehydrogenase must be measured?

a. Two
b. Three
c. Four
d. Five
e. Six

2-41. A 23-year-old woman complains of severe weakness. Her laboratory findings are markedly elevated indirect bilirubin, normal direct bilirubin, normal alkaline phosphatase and cholesterol, and an increase of urobilinogen in the urine. What disease is she likely to have with this pattern of laboratory findings?

a. Hemolytic anemia
b. Gilbert's syndrome
c. Hepatitis
d. Partial extrahepatic obstruction
e. Intravascular and extravascular hemolysis

2-42. A 35-year-old woman presents with the recent onset of shortness of breath. The only pertinent medical history is that she had rheumatic fever as a child. Physical examination finds the presence of a new cardiac murmur. Which of the following changes is a frequent consequence of chronic rheumatic fever?

a. Anitschkow cells in the endocardium
b. Aschoff bodies in the myocardium
c. Fibrin deposits in the pericardium
d. Rupture of the papillary muscle
e. Stenosis of the mitral valve

2-43. A 25-year-old medical student presented with a burst appendix. A peritoneal infection developed, despite prompt removal of the organ and extensive flushing of the peritoneal cavity. An isolate from a pus culture was a gram-negative rod identified as *Bacteroides fragilis*. Anaerobic infection with *B. fragilis* is characterized by which one of the following?

a. A black exudate in the wound
b. A foul-smelling discharge
c. A heme-pigmented colony formation
d. An exquisite susceptibility to penicillin
e. Severe neurologic symptoms

2-44. A 55-year-old man has heart failure. He is being treated with digoxin, furosemide, and triamterene. He presents with atrial fibrillation. Serum electrolyte levels are normal; serum digoxin concentrations are at the high end of the normal range. The arrhythmia is electrically converted. In addition to beginning anticoagulant therapy for prophylaxis of thromboembolism, the physician starts oral quinidine, at a usually effective dose.

Which of the following is the most likely outcome of adding the quinidine?

a. Development of signs and symptoms of quinidine toxicity (cinchonism)
b. Hyponatremia due to quinidine's ability to enhance diuretic-induced sodium loss
c. Onset of signs and symptoms of digoxin toxicity
d. Precipitous development of hypokalemia
e. Prompt suppression of cardiac contractility, onset of acute heart failure

2-45. A young man received a head injury in a football game, which later resulted in the development of seizure activity and the loss of his short-term memory. Which is the likely structure affected by this injury?

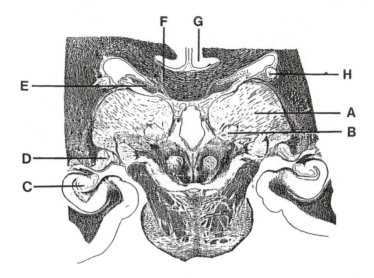

a. Structure A
b. Structure B
c. Structure C
d. Structure D
e. Structure E
f. Structure F
g. Structure G
h. Structure H

2-46. A first-year female medical student presents with patches of raised red skin covered by a flaky white buildup on her knees and elbows. The patches enlarge and become itchy and burning immediately before and during major exams during the first year of medical school. A biopsy from her skin is shown to the right. Which of the following is the underlying cause of this disorder?

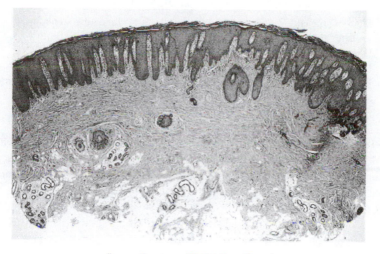

(Image Courtesy of Dr. Wolfram Sterry.)

a. Hyperplasia of dermal cells
b. A longer keratinocyte cell cycle
c. Production of cytokines by infiltrating inflammatory cells
d. Microabcesses of the dermis
e. Abnormal microcirculation in the epidermis

2-47. An asthma patient has symptom flare-ups during hay fever season. He visits the local superstore and purchases an over-the-counter antihistamine/allergy remedy containing diphenhydramine. After a few days of using it, his breathing becomes worse. You evaluate him and conclude that what the patient viewed as the allergy cure was actually the cause of the problems. Which of the following is the most likely mechanism by which the diphenhydramine worsened this patient's condition?

a. Blocking the endogenous bronchodilator effects of circulating epinephrine
b. Causing greater bronchoconstriction by releasing more ACh in the airways
c. Directly causing bronchoconstriction
d. Drying the airways, increasing mucus viscosity
e. Enhancing metabolic clearance of other asthma medications (lowering their serum levels)
f. Releasing histamine

2-48. An 18-year-old male patient appeared at the emergency room with a three-day history of fever, dry cough, difficulty breathing, and muscle aches and pains. His chest x-ray showed a diffuse left upper lobe infiltrate. The following question focuses on the etiology of "atypical" or community-acquired pneumonia.

M. pneumoniae pneumonia (walking pneumonia) may be rapidly identified by which of the following procedures?

a. Cold agglutinin test
b. Culture of respiratory secretions in HeLa cells after centrifugation of the inoculated tubes
c. Culture of respiratory secretions on monkey kidney cells
d. Detection of specific antigen in urine
e. Electron microscopy of sputum

2-49. A 19-year-old man presents with a rash that involves a large, irregular portion of his trunk. Examination reveals several annular lesions that have a raised papulovesicular border with central hypopigmentation. Examination of this area under a Wood's lamp reveals a yellow fluorescence. A scraping of this area viewed under the microscope after KOH is added reveals characteristic "spaghetti and meatball" forms. Which of the following is the cause of this skin lesion?

a. *Malassezia furfur*
b. *Molluscum contagiosum*
c. *Sarcoptes scabiei*
d. *Staphylococcus aureus*
e. *Trichophyton rubrum*

2-50. A 29-year-old man is brought to the emergency room after a traffic accident causing a traumatic brain injury. Within several hours he begins eating objects such as paper, is unable to maintain attention, and displays increased sexual activity. He is diagnosed with Klüver-Bucy syndrome, which is produced by bilateral lesions of which of the following regions of the brain?

a. Temporal lobe
b. Hypothalamus
c. Olfactory lobe
d. Hippocampus
e. Cingulate gyrus

BLOCK 3

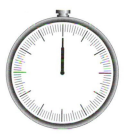

YOU HAVE 60 MINUTES TO COMPLETE 50 QUESTIONS.

Questions

3-1. A newborn with ambiguous genitalia and a 46,XY karyotype develops vomiting, low serum sodium concentration, and high serum potassium. Which of the following proteins is most likely to be abnormal?

a. 21-hydroxylase
b. An ovarian enzyme
c. 5α-reductase
d. An androgen receptor
e. A testicular enzyme

3-2. A 48-year-old man living in an underdeveloped country presents with pain in the left side of his face. Physical examination reveals a large, indurated area involving the left side of his jaw with multiple sinuses draining pus. This draining material contains a few scattered small yellow granules. This lesion was most likely caused by an infection with which one of the following organisms?

a. *Streptococcus pyogenes*
b. *Borrelia vincentii*
c. *Corynebacterium diphtheriae*
d. *Klebsiella rhinoscleromatis*
e. *Actinomyces israelii*

3-3. A 64-year-old man with arteriosclerotic heart disease (AHD) and CHF who has been treated with digoxin complains of nausea, vomiting, and diarrhea. His EKG reveals a bigeminal rhythm. The symptoms and EKG findings occurred shortly after another therapeutic agent was added to his regimen. A drug-drug interaction is suspected. Which of the following add-on agents most likely provoked the problem?

a. Lovastatin
b. Hydrochlorothiazide
c. Phenobarbital
d. Nitroglycerin
e. Captopril

3-4. A 44-year-old man has progressive weight loss, tiredness, diarrhea, and night sweats. On examination, he appears gaunt and his temperature is normal, his respiratory rate is 20, and his heart rate is 110 beats/min. A few bilateral crackles are present at the lung bases. His heart is not enlarged and the heart sounds are normal. He has mild dependent edema. His CD4 count is 40 cells/µL and his viral load is 87,000 copies/µL. Blood cultures are positive. Which is the most likely pathogen

a. *Chlamydia psittaci*
b. *Pneumocystis carinii*
c. *Mycobacterium tuberculosis*
d. *Mycobacterium avium* complex
e. *Toxoplasma gondii*

3-5. A 68-year-old woman is brought to the emergency room by paramedics after she was rescued from her burning house. Physical examination reveals a large area of burn affecting the majority of her right arm and portions of the upper right side of her chest. These burn areas are painful and appear to be red, weeping, blisters. No brown or black eschars are seen. Histologic sections of the burn areas reveal injury to the entire epidermis and the superficial portions of the dermis. Which of the following is the best classification for this type of burn?

a. Superficial epidermal first-degree burn
b. Superficial partial thickness second-degree burn
c. Deep partial thickness third-degree burn
d. Deep partial thickness fourth-degree burn
e. Full thickness fifth-degree burn

3-6. A 32-year-old male was admitted to the hospital with an initial diagnosis of heart failure. Cardiac catheterization was performed to measure cardiac output using the Fick principle. Use the following data to calculate the cardiac output. Pulmonary artery O_2 content = 20 ml/100 ml; Pulmonary vein O_2 content = 12 ml/100 ml; oxygen consumption = 280 ml/min.

a. 2.5 L/min
b. 3.5 L/min
c. 4.5 L/min
d. 6.0 L/min
e. 8.0 L/min

3-7. During the physical examination of a newborn child, it is observed that the genitalia are female, but masculinized. The genotype is determined to be 46,XX. Which of the following is the most likely cause of this condition?

a. Androgen insensitivity
b. Decreased blood ACTH levels
c. Atrophy of the zona reticularis
d. A defect in the cortisol pathway
e. Hypersecretion of vasopressin

3-8. After obtaining spinal fluid from a patient presenting with meningitis, a Gram stain is performed. Which of the following is the correct order of procedural steps when performing the Gram stain?

a. Fixation, crystal violet, alcohol/acetone decolorization, safranin
b. Fixation, crystal violet, iodine treatment, alcohol/acetone decolorization, safranin
c. Fixation, crystal violet, iodine treatment, safranin
d. Fixation, crystal violet, safranin
e. Fixation, safranin, iodine treatment, alcohol/acetone decolorization, crystal violet

3-9. A comatose laboratory technician is rushed into the emergency room. She dies while you are examining her. Her most dramatic symptom is that her body is literally hot to your touch, indicating an extremely high fever. You learn that her lab has been working on metabolic inhibitors and that there is a high likelihood that she accidentally ingested one. Which one of the following is the most likely culprit?

a. Barbiturates
b. Piericidin A
c. Dimercaprol
d. Dinitrophenol
e. Cyanide

3-10. A 40-year-old man develops depressed mood, anhedonia, initial and terminal insomnia, loss of appetite, a 10-lb weight loss, and difficulty with sexual arousal. The clinical features of the patient's psychiatric illness suggest dysfunction of the

a. Frontal lobes
b. Pituitary
c. Hippocampus
d. Hypothalamus
e. Corpus callosum

3-11. A 68-year-old man went to a sleep clinic after he had repeated episodes of loud snoring during sleep, coupled with sudden periods of restlessness and cessation of breathing. After extensive analysis, the physicians concluded that the patient's problem was not a result of obstructive sleep. Instead, it was judged that this condition reflected central sleep apnea due to loss of chemoreceptor sensitivity of the neuronal control mechanisms governing respiration. Which of the following sites within the CNS is most closely associated with these effects?

a. Dorsal horn of the thoracic spinal cord
b. Reticular formation of the medulla
c. Midbrain periaqueductal gray
d. Hippocampal formation
e. Border of occipital and parietal lobes

3-12. A patient with an allergic disorder experiences significant bronchoconstriction and urticaria. Histamine, released from mast cells, is incriminated as an important contributor to these responses. Which of the following drugs may pose extra risks for this patient—not because it has any bronchoconstrictor effects in its own right, but because it quite effectively releases histamine from mast cells?

a. Atropine
b. Isoproterenol
c. Neostigmine
d. Pancuronium
e. Propranolol
f. *d*-tubocurarine

3-13. A 23-year-old woman presents with progressive bilateral loss of central vision. You obtain a detailed family history from this patient and produce the associated pedigree (dark circles or squares indicate affected individuals). Which of the following transmission patterns is most consistent with this patient's family history?

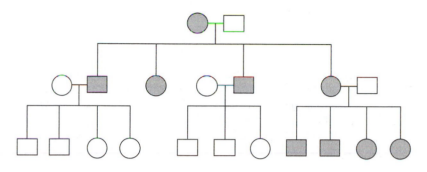

a. Autosomal recessive
b. Autosomal dominant
c. X-linked recessive
d. X-linked dominant
e. Mitochondrial

3-14. A 23-year-old male presents to the emergency department complaining of severe chest pain that is enhanced by inspiration. The pain is somewhat relieved by leaning forward. He reports he had a "cold" about 3 weeks ago, but feels otherwise healthy. You examine the patient and hear a very loud friction rub. Which of the following is true?

a. The friction rub is best heard if the patient is supine
b. The EKG findings include diffuse ST elevation and P-R depression
c. The presence of a pericardial effusion is inconsistent with the diagnosis
d. The friction rub never changes in intensity or quality
e. The diagnosis is often confused with myocardial infarction due to the large serum creatine phosphokinase level released in this disorder

3-15. A 49-year-old man is brought to the emergency room with severe gastric pain after ingesting a large quantity of unknown fluid. Laboratory results show the following:

plasma pH   = 7.03
bicarbonate   = 12 meq/L
potassium   = 6.3 mM
anion gap   = 32 meq/L
ionized calcium = 1 mM

His blood pressure is 80/40 mmHg and his pulse rate is 102 beats/min. The ECG shows sinus tachycardia and peaked T waves. The high anion gap is most likely caused by a higher-than-normal plasma concentration of which of the following?

a. Lactate
b. Potassium
c. Chloride
d. Bicarbonate
e. Citrate

3-16. Following an automobile accident in which a 23-year-old male received severe injuries to his head and parts of his body, he was admitted to the emergency room and then transferred to a rehabilitation center. Approximately a week after the accident, the patient became quite irritable

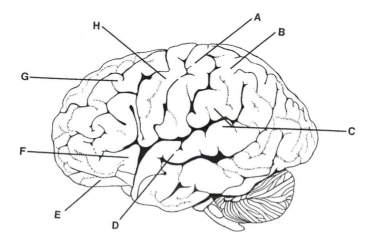

and scored poorly on card sorting, delayed alternation, and measures of intellectual skills. Which region of the brain in the illustration was most clearly affected by the accident and whose injury could most readily account for these deficits?

a. Region A
b. Region B
c. Region C
d. Region D
e. Region E
f. Region F
g. Region G
h. Region H

3-17. A 22-year-old woman marathon runner comes into the office complaining of amenorrhea for 8 months. There has been no weight change, and the serum pregnancy test is negative. She has never been pregnant. Menarche was at 13 years of age, and she had monthly menses until 8 months ago. Physical exam shows a women who is 66 inches tall, 90 pounds, and is otherwise fully normal. Why does she have amenorrhea?

a. Hypothyroidism
b. Prolactinoma
c. Early menopause
d. Resistance to LH and FSH
e. Excessive exercise

3-18. A 28-year-old man with a history of malaise and hemoptysis presents with the acute onset of renal failure. Laboratory examination reveals increased serum creatinine and BUN, but no antineutrophil cytoplasmic antibodies (ANCA) nor antinuclear (ANA) antibodies are present. Urinalysis reveals the microscopic presence of red blood cells and red blood cell casts, while a renal biopsy reveals crescents within Bowman's space of many glomeruli. Immunofluorescence reveals linear deposits of IgG and C3 along the glomerular basement membrane. Which of the following is the most likely diagnosis?

a. Alport syndrome
b. Diabetic glomerulopathy
c. Goodpasture's syndrome
d. Henoch-Schönlein purpura
e. Wegener's granulomatosis

3-19. A patient biopsy is reviewed by a pathologist. She diagnoses the tumor as originating from the cells delineated with the star (✩). The tumor would most likely produce which of the following? Refer to the photomicrograph below.

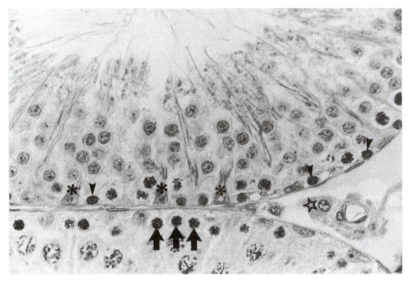

(Courtesy of Dr. George C. Enders.)

a. Calcitonin
b. Progesterone
c. Androgens
d. FSH
e. Parathyroid hormone

3-20. A patient with multiple medical problems is taking several drugs, including theophylline, warfarin, quinidine, and phenytoin. Despite the likelihood of interactions, dosages of each are adjusted carefully so their serum concentrations and effects are acceptable. However, the patient suffers some GI distress and purchases and begins consuming an over-the-counter "heartburn" remedy. He presents with excessive or toxic effects from all his other medications. He almost certainly took which OTC drug?

a. Cimetidine
b. Famotidine
c. Nizatidine
d. Omeprazole
e. Ranitidine

3-21. A 23-year-old woman presents with the recent onset of vaginal discharge. Physical examination reveals multiple clear vesicles on her vulva and vagina. A smear of material obtained from one of these vesicles reveals several multinucleated giant cells with intranuclear inclusions and ground-glass nuclei. These vesicles are most likely the result of infection with which one of the following organisms?

a. Cytomegalovirus (CMV)
b. Herpes simplex virus (HSV)
c. Human papillomavirus (HPV)
d. *Candida albicans*
e. *Trichomonas vaginalis*

3-22. When examining an AP chest film of one of your 57-year-old male patients with a systolic ejection-type cardiac murmur, you notice that the arch of the aorta forms a typical aortic knob on the left of the mediastinal border, but also appears as a bulge on the right upper mediastinal border, suggesting an enlarged ascending aorta. In addition, the left ventricular heart border appears prominent. There is no evidence of pulmonary hypertension in your patient. Your order an echocardiogram because you suspect your patient has which of the following?

a. Tetralogy of Fallot
b. Pulmonary valve stenosis
c. Atherosclerosis
d. Aortic valve stenosis
e. Defective tricuspid valve

3-23. A 54-year-old man with other well-treated medical disorders has erectile dysfunction. He takes a dose of sildenafil and shortly thereafter develops acute and severe hypotension. Upon arrival at the emergency department his blood pressure is very low, he is tachycardic, and an EKG shows changes indicative of acute myocardial ischemia. Which other medication was this man most likely taking?

a. Digoxin
b. Glipizide
c. Nitroglycerin
d. Propranolol
e. Testosterone

3-24. A patient presents to the physician's office to ask questions about color blindness. The patient is color-blind, as is one of his brothers. His maternal grandfather was color-blind, but his mother, father, daughter, and another brother are not. His daughter is now pregnant. What is the risk that her child will be color-blind?

a. 100%
b. 50%
c. 25%
d. 12.5%
e. Virtually 0

3-25. A full-term male infant displays projectile vomiting 1 h after suckling. There is failure to gain weight during the first 2 weeks. The vomitus is not bile-stained and no respiratory difficulty is evident. Examination reveals an abdomen neither tense nor bloated. Which of the following is the most probable explanation?

a. Congenital hypertrophic pyloric stenosis
b. Duodenal atresia
c. Patent ileal diverticulum
d. Imperforate anus
e. Tracheoesophageal fistula

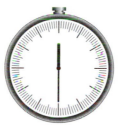

YOU SHOULD HAVE COMPLETED APPROXIMATELY 25 QUESTIONS AND HAVE 30 MINUTES REMAINING.

3-26. Several young adults camped in a wilderness area and received multiple mosquito bites. Ten days later, one had a sudden onset of headache, chills, and fever, and became stuporous 48 hours later. He was diagnosed with Saint Louis encephalitis (SLE) and, fortunately, recovered completely. Which of the following best describes SLE?

a. It is transmitted to humans by the bite of an infected tick
b. It is caused by a togavirus
c. It is the major arboviral cause of central nervous system infection in the United States
d. It may present initially with symptoms similar to influenza
e. Laboratory diagnosis is routinely made by cultural methods

3-27. The 19-year-old female is brought to the emergency room after being in a single-car accident just 20 min earlier in which she lost control of her car on black ice and hit a retaining column of an overpass at about 45 miles per hour. She was the only occupant and was wearing a seat belt but looks pale, has tachycardia and positional hypotension, is extremely nauseated, and is lying in the fetal position due to severe abdominal pain. She does not appear to have any broken bones and a cranial nerve test appears normal. You order an abdominal CT because you suspect which of the following?

a. That she is pregnant
b. That she has peritonitis from a ruptured spleen
c. That she has peritonitis from a ruptured gallbladder
d. That she has diverticulitis
e. That she has hemorrhoids

3-28. A young woman in her early twenties experiences loss of sensation in her legs and weakness in her limbs. A neurological examination further indicated some spasticity of the limbs as well. The neurologist provided a preliminary diagnosis of onset of multiple sclerosis. Assuming that this diagnosis is correct, which of the following can best account for the diminution of sensory and motor functions?

a. Loss of Schwann cells in peripheral neurons
b. An overall loss of dopaminergic release throughout the brain and spinal cord
c. Loss of peripheral cholinergic neurons
d. Demyelination of CNS neurons
e. Proliferation of oligodendrocytes

3-29. A male child presents with delayed development and scarring of his lips and hands. His parents have restrained him because he obsessively chews on his lips and fingers. Which of the following is likely to occur in this child?

a. Increased levels of 5-phosphoribosyl-1-pyrophosphate (PRPP)
b. Decreased purine synthesis
c. Decreased levels of uric acid
d. Increased levels of hypoxanthine-guanosine phosphoribosyl transferase (HGPRT)
e. Glycogen storage

3-30. A patient presents with a large wound to his right forearm that is the result of a chain saw accident. You treat his wound appropriately and follow him in your surgery clinic at routine intervals. Initially his wound is filled with granulation tissue, which is composed of proliferating fibroblasts and proliferating new blood vessels (angiogenesis). Which of the following substances is a growth factor that is capable of inducing all the steps necessary for angiogenesis?

a. Epidermal growth factor (EGF)
b. Transforming growth factor α (TGF-α)
c. Platelet-derived growth factor (PDGF)
d. Basic fibroblast growth factor (FGF)
e. Transforming growth factor β (TGF-β)

3-31. A couple is being evaluated for possible hematologic problems after the mother delivered a stillborn infant at 25 weeks of gestation. A Coombs' test was also performed on cord blood and the mother's blood and was negative on both specimens. The parents, both of whom are Vietnamese and 21 years of age, are found to have mild microcytic anemias with normal serum iron levels. Further work-up finds that each parent has α thalassemia trait, due to the deletion of two α-globin genes on one chromosome 16 (the other chromosome 16 being normal with two α-globin genes). Inheritance of the abnormal chromosome 16 from each parent in a subsequent pregnancy would most likely produce which one of the following disorders?

a.   Cooley's anemia
b.   Fanconi's anemia
c.   Hemoglobin H disease
d.   Hemolytic disease of the newborn
e.   Hydrops fetalis

3-32. A child has mononucleosis-like symptoms, yet the test for mononucleosis and the EBV titers are negative. Which of the following is one of the causes of heterophile-negative mononucleosis?

a.   Adenovirus
b.   Coxsackievirus
c.   Cytomegalovirus
d.   Herpes simplex virus
e.   Varicella-zoster virus

3-33. A 3-month-old baby is brought to her pediatrician for a check up. Stroking the plantar surface of the foot produces a reflex extension of the large toe rather than the expected flexion. The Babinski sign elicited by the physician indicates damage to which of the following?

a.   Spinal cord
b.   Brainstem
c.   Cerebellum
d.   Basal ganglia
e.   Pyramids

3-34. A 31-year-old man whom you treated for alcoholic intoxication at the emergency room 2 days ago comes to your office because he wants another opinion about his infertility. He has seen other physicians for this condition. Considering his excessive alcohol intake for the past decade, the likely site of his infertility is

a. Pretesticular
b. Testicular
c. Posttesticular
d. Idiopathic

3-35. Your new patient is a 45-year-old, recently divorced woman. She has just told you that her 25-year-old son returned home three days ago with AIDS, and that she has experienced severe chest pains when she thinks about it. She starts to tell you about some other disturbing symptoms, begins to cry, and looks away. Of the following, which would be the most appropriate immediate response to facilitate the interview?

a. Silence
b. "I know how you feel"
c. "Don't worry, it'll be OK"
d. "Why are you so upset? You know you can tell me anything"
e. "Are you thinking that you may have AIDS?"

3-36. A baby was born with an inherited autosomal recessive trait in which there was a delay in development, resulting in the occurrence of seizures and mental retardation. The child was diagnosed as having phenylketonuria (PKU). What is the likely neurochemical locus of this genetic defect?

a. Tyrosine
b. Tryptophan
c. Tryptophan hydroxylase
d. Dopamine
e. Phenylalanine (Phe) hydroxylase

3-37. A 60-year-old woman presents with a slowly enlarging 2.5-cm firm, irregular mass in the upper outer quadrant of her left breast. A biopsy from this mass is interpreted by the pathologist as being an infiltrating lobular carcinoma of the breast. Which of the following histologic features is most characteristic of this tumor?

a. Expansion of lobules by monotonous proliferation of epithelial cells
b. Large cells with clear cytoplasm within the epidermis
c. Large syncytium-like sheets of pleomorphic cells surrounded by aggregates of lymphocytes
d. Small individual malignant cells dispersed within extracellular pools of mucin
e. Small tumor cells with little cytoplasm infiltrating in a single-file pattern

3-38. A 47-year-old male is brought into the emergency room and is diagnosed with a small brainstem stroke. The patient presents with an inability to display reflex movements of the head in response to vestibular stimulation. Which structure is most likely affected by this lesion?

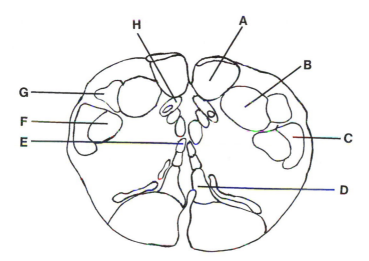

a. Structure A
b. Structure B
c. Structure C
d. Structure D
e. Structure E
f. Structure F
g. Structure G
h. Structure H

3-39. A 29-year-old male is admitted to the intensive care unit with pneumonia and requires supplemental oxygen. Lung function tests reveal: total lung capacity = 3.34 L (56% of predicted), residual volume = 0.88 L (54% of predicted), and force vital capacity = 1.38 L (30% of predicted). Which of the following characteristics will be approximately normal?

a. Lung compliance
b. Tidal volume
c. V/Q ratio
d. Diffusing capacity
e. FEV$_1$/FVC ratio

3-40. A single, 30-year-old woman presented to her physician with vaginitis. She complained of a slightly increased, malodorous discharge that was gray-white in color, thin, and homogenous. Clue cells were discovered when the discharge was examined microscopically. Which organism listed below was the most likely cause of her infection?

a. *Candida albicans*
b. *Trichomonas vaginalis*
c. *Escherichia coli*
d. *Gardnerella vaginalis*
e. *Staphylococcus aureus*

3-41. A small vascular lesion that affected the region of the ventromedial white matter of the cervical cord was discovered in a middle-aged man during a neurological examination. The neurologist came to the conclusion that the lesion affected the descending fibers of the medial longitudinal fasciculus (MLF). What deficit did the neurologist observe that led him to this conclusion?

a. The patient presented with a UMN paralysis
b. The patient displayed difficulties in regulating his head position in response to postural changes
c. The patient displayed an LMN paralysis
d. The patient displayed ataxia of movement
e. The patient experienced significant difficulties in regulating blood pressure and bladder functions

3-42. A 60-year-old man on long-term therapy with a drug develops hypertension, hyperglycemia, and decreased bone density. Blood tests indicate anemia. Stool samples initially were positive for occult blood and then developed a "coffee-grounds" appearance. Which of the following drugs is most likely responsible for the patient's symptoms?

a. Beclomethasone
b. Hydrochlorothiazide
c. Metformin
d. Pamidronate
e. Prednisone

3-43. A 19-year-old woman presents with urticaria that developed after she took aspirin for a headache. She has a history of chronic rhinitis, and physical examination reveals the presence of nasal polyps. This patient is at an increased risk of developing which one of the following pulmonary diseases following the ingestion of aspirin?

a. Asthma
b. Chronic bronchitis
c. Emphysema
d. Interstitial fibrosis
e. Pulmonary hypertension

3-44. A man who has a penile chancre appears in a hospital's emergency service. The VDRL test is negative. What is the most appropriate course of action for the physician in charge?

a. Perform dark-field microscopy for treponemes
b. Perform a Gram stain on the chancre fluid
c. Repeat the VDRL test in 10 days
d. Send the patient home untreated
e. Swab the chancre and culture on Thayer-Martin agar

3-45. A 15-year-old male patient presents with hematuria, hearing loss, lens dislocation, and cataracts. Genetic analysis shows a mutation of the COL4A5 gene. A renal biopsy is performed. In which area labeled **A–E** on the accompanying electron micrograph would you expect to see the primary site of damage?

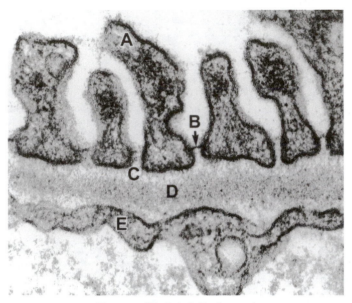

(Courtesy of Dr. Dale R. Abrahamson.)

a. Area A
b. Area B
c. Area C
d. Area D
e. Area E

3-46. A 45-year-old man with recurrent asthma is being treated with oral theophylline and prednisone, supplemented with an adrenergic bronchodilator (e.g., albuterol), inhaled "as needed." He has been exposed to *Haemophilus influenzae* by a family member, and is started on rifampin for prophylaxis against getting the infection himself. Which of the following is the most likely outcome of adding the rifampin?

a. Failure of rifampin prophylaxis due to induction of its metabolism by the theophylline
b. Increased risk of theophylline toxicity
c. Loss of asthma control, onset of asthma signs and symptoms
d. Rapid development of cholestatic jaundice and liver failure from acute rifampin toxicity
e. Sudden sodium and fluid retention, weight gain, from impaired prednisone metabolism

3-47. A 37-year-old man presents with a single, firm mass within the thyroid gland. This patient's father developed a tumor of the thyroid gland when he was 32 years of age. Histologic examination of the mass in this 37-year-old man reveals organoid nests of tumor cells separated by broad bands of stroma, as seen in the photomicrograph below. The stroma stains positively with Congo red stain and demonstrates yellow-green birefringence. Which of the following is the most likely diagnosis?

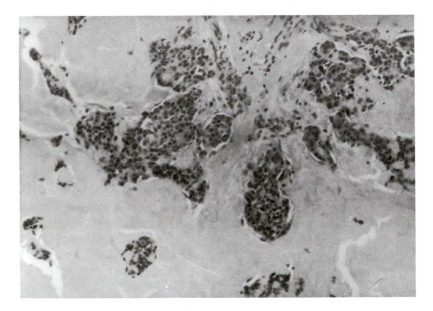

   a. Follicular carcinoma
   b. Papillary carcinoma
   c. Squamous cell carcinoma
   d. Medullary carcinoma
   e. Anaplastic carcinoma

3-48. A patient presents with food poisoning that is attributed to botulism (botulinus toxin poisoning). Which of the following is a correct characteristic, finding, or mechanism associated with this toxin?

a. Complete failure of all cholinergic neurotransmission
b. Favorable response to administration of pralidoxime
c. Impairment of parasympathetic, but not sympathetic, nervous system activation
d. Massive overstimulation of all structures having muscarinic cholinergic receptors
e. Selective paralysis of skeletal muscle

3-49. While in the ICU, you are called to evaluate seizure activity in a ventilator patient with nosocomial pneumonia. You review the situation including the medication record. The patient is currently receiving dopamine, one-half normal saline, imipenem/cilastatin, tobramycin, lisinopril, clonidine patch, and pantoprazole. The laboratory test results from this morning show normal electrolytes, a mildly elevated creatinine of 2.4 that is chronic, and the CBC shows an improving white blood count of 13,000. After stopping the acute seizure event, you determine the next step in preventing further seizures is

a. Stop dopamine
b. Stop clonidine
c. Intravenous phenytoin
d. Change antibiotic coverage
e. CT of the head

3-50. A 50-year-old man presents to the emergency room with severe "crushing" substernal chest pain that began approximately 5 h prior. He states that sometimes the pain extends into his left arm, and during the past hour he has become quite nauseated. Physical examination finds this man to be sweating profusely and in moderate distress. An ECG finds abnormal Q waves in several of the anterior leads. Which of the following substances is most likely to be elevated in this individual?

a. Alkaline phosphatase
b. Aspartate aminotransferase
c. Lactate dehydrogenase
d. Myoglobin
e. Troponin

BLOCK 4

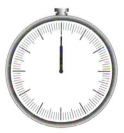

YOU HAVE **60** MINUTES TO COMPLETE **50** QUESTIONS.

Questions

4-1. An 82-year-old woman presents with headaches, visual disturbances, and muscle pain. A biopsy of the temporal artery is shown in the associated photomicrograph. Which of the following is the best next step in the management of this patient?

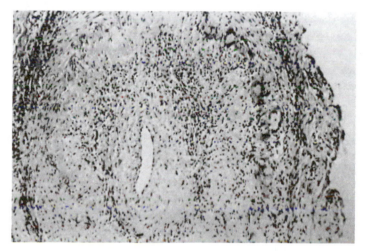

a. Administer corticosteroids
b. Verify with a repeat biopsy
c. Administer anticoagulants
d. Perform angiography
e. Order an erythrocyte sedimentation rate

4-2. A 32-year-old woman undergoing surgery for appendicitis develops malignant hyperthermia. Malignant hyperthermia is a life-threatening increase in metabolic rate that occasionally occurs when volatile anesthetics are used during surgery. It is caused by a mutation of the ryanodine receptor. Which one of the following best explains why a mutation of the ryanodine receptor can produce malignant hyperthermia?

a. A sustained release of calcium from the sarcoplasmic reticulum of skeletal muscle
b. Presynaptic terminals of alpha motoneurons undergo rapid repetitive firing
c. Skeletal muscle cells are unable to repolarize
d. A sudden cooling of the body causes uncontrollable shivering
e. Serum thyroxine levels increases to abnormally high levels

4-3. A 37-year-old man suffers extensive burns of both lower extremities. He received allografts of skin, but these were rejected starting about 11 days after the graft procedure. The main cause of rejection is

a. B cell–mediated IgG antibody response
b. B cell antibody switching response of IgM to IgG antibodies
c. IgE-mediated release of mast cells
d. T cell–mediated reaction, mainly CD8-positive cytotoxic T cells
e. Nitric oxide release by macrophages

4-4. A 25-year-old man with difficulty sleeping and poor appetite associated with weight loss is placed on amitriptyline. This drug is classified as which of the following?

a. MAO inhibitor
b. Tricyclic nonselective amine reuptake inhibitor
c. Heterocyclic nonselective amine reuptake inhibitor
d. Selective serotonin reuptake inhibitor
e. α_2-adrenergic receptor antagonist

4-5. A 6-month-old boy is brought into the pediatric clinic. He weighs 12 lb, 2 oz and is 22 in. tall. Neither his height nor his weight is on the growth chart for his age; mean weight and height for a 6-month-old are 17 lb, 4 oz and 26.5 in., respectively. Through functional tests, you determine that he is suffering from an inherited condition known as I-cell disease and is missing UDP N-acetylglucosamine: lysosomal enzyme N-acetylglucosamine-1-phosphotransferase, which is more conveniently referred to as phosphotransferase. You recall from your cell biology that the phosphotransferase enzymes phosphorylate mannose to form mannose-6-phosphate. Electron microscopy is performed on a biopsy, and blood tests are completed. Which of the following explains the altered cell biological processes in this patient?

a. Lysosomal enzymes missorted back to the Golgi apparatus
b. Peroxisomal proteins missorted to other organelles
c. Abnormal KDEL sequence on vesicles
d. Absence of SNARE proteins on vesicles
e. Secretion of lysosomal enzymes into the blood

4-6. A 64-year-old woman has had several episodes of transient ischemic attacks (TIAs). Aspirin would be a preferred treatment, but she has a history of severe "aspirin sensitivity" manifest as intense bronchoconstriction. What would be a suitable alternative to the aspirin?

a. Acetaminophen
b. Aminocaproic acid
c. Clopidogrel
d. Dipyridamole
e. Streptokinase

4-7. A patient presented with loss of pain sensation from one side of the face. It was discovered that it was probably due to a small brainstem lesion. Where was the likely locus of this lesion?

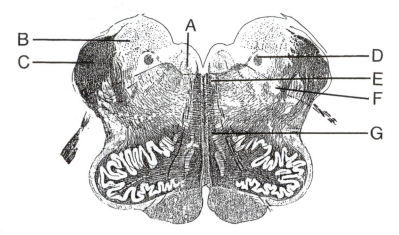

a. Area A
b. Area B
c. Area C
d. Area D
e. Area E
f. Area F
g. Area G

4-8. Mr. Baker, a 40-year-old stockbroker, is stressed and worried because he feels he has many of the personality and physical characteristics that place him at risk for coronary heart disease. His physical examination, laboratory results, symptoms, and electrocardiogram tapes confirm that he is indeed at moderate risk. To assess which of his personality and behavioral patterns could put him at an even higher risk, it would be best to test him with the

a. Millon Behavioral Health Inventory
b. Cohen Perceived Stress Scale
c. Rosenman and Friedman Type A Structured Interview
d. Jenkins Activity Survey of Type A Behavior
e. Cook-Medley Hostility Inventory

4-9. Parents bring their newborn daughter to you for consultation about diagnosis and management. Their first two children, a boy and a girl, have a complete form of albinism (203100) with pink irides, blond hair, and pale skin. Which of the following represents your correct advice concerning the newborn child?

a. A 1/8 risk for albinism and skin cancer from DNA deletions
b. A 1/8 risk for albinism and skin cancer from DNA cross-linkage
c. A 1/4 risk for albinism and skin cancer from DNA point mutations
d. A 1/4 risk for albinism and skin cancer from DNA deletions
e. A 1/4 risk for albinism and skin cancer from DNA cross-linkage

4-10. A 52-year-old man presents with symptoms of gastric pain after eating. During work-up, a 3-cm mass is found in the wall of the stomach. This mass is resected and histologic examination reveals a tumor composed of cells having elongated, spindle-shaped nuclei. The tumor does not connect to the overlying epithelium and is found only in the wall of the stomach. Which of the following is the cell of origin of this tumor?

a. Adipocyte
b. Endothelial cell
c. Glandular epithelial cell
d. Smooth-muscle cell
e. Squamous epithelial cell

4-11. A 28-year-old menstruating woman appeared in the emergency room with the following signs and symptoms: fever, 104°F (40°C); WBC, 16,000/μL; blood pressure, 90/65 mmHg; a scarlatiniform rash on her trunk, palms, and soles; extreme fatigue; vomiting; and diarrhea.

Culture of the menstrual fluid in the case cited would most likely reveal a predominance of which of the following?

a. *C. difficile*
b. *C. perfringens*
c. *G. vaginalis*
d. *S. aureus*
e. *S. epidermidis*

4-12. A 52-year-old male patient, who has smoked two packs of cigarettes per day for the past 38 years, presents with diminished breath sounds detected by auscultation accompanied by faint high-pitched rhonchi at the end of each expiration and a hyperresonant percussion note. He is afebrile. In addition, he shows discomfort during breathing and is using extra effort to involve accessory muscles to lift the sternum. The diminished lung sounds in this patient are primarily due to which cellular events?

a. Monocytic infiltration leading to collagenase destruction of bronchiolar connective tissue support
b. Neutrophilic infiltration leading to destruction of bronchiolar and septal elastic fibers
c. Monocytic infiltration leading to breakdown of the bronchiolar smooth muscle
d. Neutrophilic infiltration leading to excess production of antiprotease activity in the lung parenchyma
e. Monocytic infiltration leading to excess production of antiprotease activity in the lung parenchyma

4-13. A 20-year-old man with absence seizures is treated with ethosuximide. Which of the following is the principal mechanism of action of ethosuximide?

a. Sodium channel blockade
b. Increase in the frequency of the chloride channel opening
c. Increase in GABA
d. Calcium channel blockade
e. Increased potassium channel permeability
f. NMDA receptor blockade

4-14. A patient had been seeing a physician for almost a year because she complained of pain in her shoulder. After extensive analysis, the physician determined that the pain in her shoulder reflected referred pain that arose from another source. In this case, which of the following best explains the basis for the referred pain?

a. Inhibitory fibers that block transmission of pain impulses along a given pathway and then transfer the impulses to a different pathway associated with a different part of the body
b. A massive discharge along a given pathway that results in the activation of a separate pathway because of the principle of divergence
c. A convergence of primary afferent fibers from a given region onto second-order neurons that normally receive primary afferents from a different body part
d. The disruption of lateral spinothalamic fibers
e. The blockade of substance P from primary afferent terminals

4-15. A 19-year-old offensive tackle for a major university football team fractures his right femur during the first game of the season. He is admitted to the hospital and over the next several days develops progressive respiratory problems. Despite extensive medical intervention, he dies three days later. At the time of autopsy oil red O–positive material is seen in the small blood vessels of the lungs and brain. Which of the following is the most likely diagnosis?

a. Air emboli
b. Amniotic fluid emboli
c. Fat emboli
d. Paradoxical emboli
e. Saddle emboli

4-16. A 67-year-old female is brought to the emergency room because she fainted at the gym during her daily aerobic workout. A prominent systolic murmur is heard and a presumptive diagnosis of aortic stenosis is made. Which of the following is consistent with that diagnosis?

a. A decreased pulse pressure
b. An increased arterial pressure
c. A decreased left ventricular diastolic pressure
d. An increased ejection fraction
e. A decreased cardiac oxygen consumption

4-17. A 50-year-old woman is recently diagnosed with type 2 diabetes mellitus. Exercise and diet do not provide adequate glycemic control, so drug therapy is needed. The physician contemplates prescribing metformin. Which of the following statements about this drug is correct?

a. Beneficial and unwanted actions are unaffected by liver function status
b. Lactic acidosis occurs frequently, but it is seldom serious
c. Metformin-induced hypoglycemia seldom occurs
d. Useful, as monotherapy, for both type 1 and type 2 diabetes
e. Weight gain is a common and unwanted side effect

4-18. A 30-year-old woman complains of recent onset of easy bruising without trauma. She has had menometrorrhagia for several years. On physical examination, she has a normal blood pressure and multiple bruises on her upper and lower extremities. On laboratory examination, her platelet count is <100,000 cells/cm², hemoglobin 13 g/dL, creatinine 0.9 mg/dL, and blood urea nitrogen (BUN) 15 mg/dL. She likely has

a. Idiopathic thrombocytopenic purpura (ITP)
b. Splenectomy
c. von Williebrand's disease
d. Hemolytic uremic syndrome
e. Thrombotic thrombocytopenic purpura (TTP)

4-19. A 5-year-old girl is brought in with severe vomiting that has developed suddenly 5 days after she has had a viral infection. Upon questioning, her parents indicate that she was given aspirin for several days to treat a fever that occurred with the viral illness. She is hospitalized and quickly develops signs of cerebral edema. Liver tissue reveals marked steatosis. Which of the following is the most likely diagnosis?

a. α_1 antitrypsin deficiency
b. Dubin-Johnson syndrome
c. Hepatitis D infection
d. Reye's syndrome
e. Wilson's disease

4-20. A 2-month-old male infant, who was born at term without any prenatal abnormalities, is being evaluated for possible visual problems. He is noted to have an abnormal white light reflex involving his right eye, and examination finds a large mass that has almost completely filled the posterior chamber of this eye. Which of the following cells are most likely to be seen proliferating in histologic sections from this mass?

a. Benign fibroblasts and endothelial cells
b. Foamy macrophages with cytoplasmic clear vacuoles
c. Plasmacytoid cells within a dense Congo red–positive stroma
d. Small cells forming occasional rosette structures
e. Spindle-shaped cells with cytoplasmic melanin

4-21. A 5-year-old Egyptian boy receives a sulfonamide antibiotic as prophylaxis for recurrent urinary tract infections. Although he was previously healthy and well nourished, he becomes progressively ill and presents to your office with pallor and irritability. A blood count shows that he is severely anemic with jaundice due to hemolysis of red blood cells. Which of the following would be the simplest test for diagnosis?

a. Northern blotting of red blood cell mRNA
b. Enzyme assay of red blood cell hemolysate
c. Western blotting of red blood cell hemolysates
d. Amplification of red blood cell DNA and hybridization with allele-specific oligonucleotides (PCR-ASOs)
e. Southern blot analysis for gene deletions

4-22. A teenage baseball player was hit in the base of the skull by a loose bat. The patient is hoarse and complains of difficulty swallowing. The cranial x-ray indicates a basal skull fracture that passes through the jugular foramen. The examining physician notes a large hematoma behind the ear on the injured side. If the nerves passing through the jugular foramen were severed as a result of the cranial fracture, which of the following muscles would remain functional?

a. Palatoglossus muscle
b. Sternomastoid muscle
c. Styloglossus muscle
d. Stylopharyngeus muscle
e. Trapezius muscle

4-23. A woman goes into premature labor, and the physician administers ritodrine. Which of the following is the main mechanism of action by which this drug slows or suppresses uterine contractions?

a. Blocks prostaglandin synthesis
b. Blocks uterine oxytocin receptors
c. Inhibits oxytocin release from the posterior pituitary
d. Inhibits oxytocin synthesis in the hypothalamus
e. Stimulates α-adrenergic receptors
f. Stimulates β_2-adrenergic receptors

4-24. A 39-year-old man presented with sudden, influenza-like symptoms. He stated that he worked in a slaughterhouse, and several of his coworkers had similar symptoms. Early stages of pneumonia were detected. A rickettsial etiology was suspected. Which of the following characterizes Q fever?

a. Has an incubation period of four to six weeks
b. Is an acute febrile illness caused by *Coxiella burnetii*
c. Is an illness confined to the upper respiratory tract
d. Is most commonly found in tropical regions
e. Is transmitted by the bite of an arthropod

4-25. A young woman is being unfairly singled out in the workplace by being repeatedly criticized regarding her work, even though other employees are not held to the same standard. Coping effort on her part, associated with the negative emotions of embarrassment and feeling harassed, is likely to result in the preferential synthesis and release of

a. Corticotropin
b. Norepinephrine
c. Epinephrine
d. Catecholamines
e. Cortisol

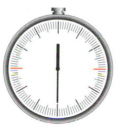

YOU SHOULD HAVE COMPLETED APPROXIMATELY 25 QUESTIONS AND HAVE 30 MINUTES REMAINING.

4-26. After displaying progressive memory loss over a period of several months, an elderly patient was referred to a neurologist, who concluded that the patient was suffering from Alzheimer's disease. Several years later, the patient died and an autopsy was performed, indicating a significant loss of cholinergic neurons in specific regions of the forebrain. Which structure most likely exhibited the greatest loss of cholinergic neurons?

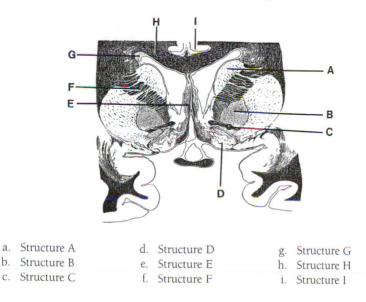

a. Structure A

b. Structure B

c. Structure C

d. Structure D

e. Structure E

f. Structure F

g. Structure G

h. Structure H

i. Structure I

4-27. You are taking an initial health history from a 22-year-old woman who just moved to your town. She is remarkably fit and healthy, but is wearing two hearing aids for binaural (bilateral) high-frequency hearing loss. You inquire about the possible reason(s) for this. She says she lost most of her hearing after receiving an antibiotic for a severe infection when she was 19, but cannot recall the specific drug. Which of the following drugs was most likely responsible for her hearing loss?

a. Aminoglycoside (e.g., gentamicin)
b. Cephalosporin, first-generation
c. Cephalosporin, third-generation
d. Fluoroquinolone (e.g., ciprofloxacin)
e. Penicillin

4-28. A 62-year-old white male was admitted to the hospital complaining of shortness of breath. His medical history indicated he had smoked one pack of cigarettes per day for the past 40 years. Recently, he has been on immunosuppressive therapy for severe arthritis. A biopsy specimen of the lung was obtained, and septate hyphae that formed V-shaped branches were observed. Culture on agar showed conidia with spores in radiating columns (see photo). Which of the following is most likely consistent with these diagnostic findings?

a. Aspergillosis
b. Emphysema
c. Lung cancer
d. *Pneumocystis carinii* pneumonia
e. Viral pneumonia
f. Zygomycosis

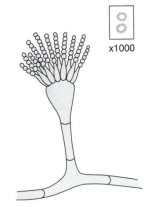

x1000

(Reproduced, with permission, from Brooks GF et al.
Jawetz's Medical Microbiology,
22e. New York: McGraw-Hill, 2001, 534.)

4-29. A patient with edema fails to respond adequately to maximum recommended dosages of chlorthalidone. Which of the following is the most appropriate and most fruitful next step?

a. Add hydrochlorothiazide
b. Add metolazone
c. Replace chlorthalidone with furosemide
d. Replace chlorthalidone with hydrochlorothiazide
e. Try increasing the chlorthalidone dose anyway

4-30. A 54-year-old man presents with left-sided costovertebral pain and gross hematuria. A large mass is found in the upper pole of one of his kidneys, as seen in the picture below. Which of the following histologic changes is most likely to be seen when examining microscopic sections from this mass?

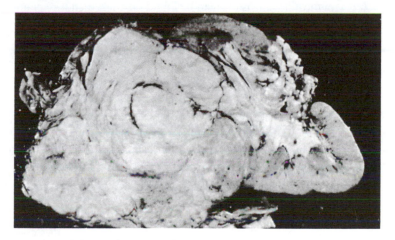

a. Groups and sheets of transitional epithelial cells
b. Immature tubules and abortive glomerular formation
c. Large cells with prominent eosinophilic cytoplasm containing numerous mitochondria
d. Malignant undifferentiated mesenchymal cells
e. Uniform cells with clear cytoplasm containing glycogen and lipid

4-31. A 17-year-old male who is being treated with the macrolide antibiotic erythromycin complains of nausea, intestinal cramping, and diarrhea. The side effects are the result of the antibiotic binding to receptors on GI tract enteric nerves and smooth-muscle cells that recognize which gastrointestinal hormone?

a. Gastrin
b. Motilin
c. Secretin
d. Cholecystokinin
e. Enterogastrone

4-32. A 57-year old man complains of long-standing respiratory distress. He worked for most of his adult life in a locomotive repair shop. On examination he does not have fever, palpable lymph nodes, or abnormal lung findings. Which one of the following is likely to be found on chest roentgenogram?

a. Pulmonary vascular prominence
b. Pleural blebs
c. Enlarged right ventricle
d. Acute bronchopneumonia
e. Diffuse interstitial pulmonary fibrosis with irregular or linear opacities

4-33. A patient received a single dose of succinylcholine for preoperative intubation. Skeletal muscle paralysis during a 3-h surgery is maintained by a long-acting nondepolarizing type (i.e., curare-like) neuromuscular blocker. Surgery is over and the plan is to reverse the skeletal muscle paralysis.

What adjunct is administered first to block unwanted effects of the reversing agent on smooth muscles and glands, and then what drug is used to actually reverse the skeletal muscle paralysis?

a. Atropine to control smooth muscle, cardiac, and gland responses, then neostigmine to reverse skeletal muscle paralysis
b. Belladonna alkaloids to block smooth muscle, cardiac, and gland responses, then pralidoxime to restore skeletal muscle function
c. β-blocker first to control cardiac responses, physostigmine for reversal
d. Epinephrine first to control smooth muscle and glands, acetylcholine to reactivate skeletal muscle
e. Physostigmine to control smooth muscles and glands, succinylcholine again for reversal

4-34. A 22-year-old varsity hockey player visits you because he has excessive bruising after a game 2 days before. His knee had been bothering him, so he took two aspirin tablets before the game. Other than getting checked 10 times during the game, he denies any excessive or unusual trauma. As you ponder the etiology you order several blood tests. Which test or finding do you expect to be abnormal?

a. Activated partial thromboplastin time (APTT)
b. Bleeding time
c. INR (International Normalized Ratio)
d. Platelet count
e. Prothrombin time

4-35. A 4-year-old boy is being evaluated for the acute development of multiple hemorrhagic areas on his skin and gums. Examination of his peripheral blood reveals a markedly increased white cell count to 50,000, the majority of which are lymphoid cells having prominent nucleoli. A bone marrow biopsy reveals the marrow to be diffusely infiltrated by these same cells and a diagnosis of acute lymphoblastic lymphoma is made. Special stains on these malignant cells demonstrate cytoplasmic staining for mu heavy chain. They lack surface immunoglobulin, but do express nuclear TdT staining and surface markers for CD19 and CD20. These malignant cells have the staining characteristics of what type of cell?

a. Lymphoid stem cell
b. Pre-pre B cell
c. Pre-B cell
d. Immature B cell
e. Virgin B cell

4-36. Louise is an 86-year-old woman who has had difficulty with high blood pressure, high cholesterol, diabetes, strokes, and blood clots in her legs for many years. One day, her grandson arrived at her apartment in a senior citizen center for his weekly visit and found her lying unconscious on the floor. He immediately called an ambulance to take her to the nearest emergency room. The paramedics in the ambulance gave Louise some medications, including glucose, but she did not awaken. She was taken to the nearest emergency room, where a physician was called to evaluate her. She was breathing on her own and had a pulse, but could not be aroused to any stimulus. Her arms and legs were stiff and would not move in response to a painful stimulus. Her eyes moved in response to moving her head. Finally, in response to a very loud shout and pinch on the arm, she briefly opened her eyes; however, she immediately shut them again. Further attempts to arouse Louise were unsuccessful. She was taken for a CT scan of her head, and then taken to an intensive care unit.

What was the cause of the stiffness in Louise's arms and legs?

a. Infarction of the corticospinal tracts bilaterally in the pons
b. Damage to the basal ganglia
c. Infarction of the precentral gyrus
d. Infarction of the internal capsules bilaterally
e. Thalamic infarction

4-37. A 44-year-old woman presents with anorexia and weight loss. Physical examination reveals a slightly decreased blood pressure along with increased skin pigmentation. Laboratory examination reveals a low cortisol with increased ACTH. After further work-up the diagnosis of adrenal cortical failure is made. One year later this woman is found to have hyperglycemia and after appropriate work-up the diagnosis of type 1 diabetes mellitus is made. Which of the following abnormalities is this individual most likely to develop?

a. Autoimmune destruction of the thyroid gland
b. Bacterial infection of the antrum of the stomach
c. Fungal infection of the oral cavity
d. Metabolic hyperfunction of the parathyroid glands
e. Neoplastic development in the anterior pituitary

4-38. A 27-year-old man presents to the emergency room with right heart failure and respiratory acidosis. Arterial blood gas analysis reveals a normal A - a gradient. Which of the following is the most likely cause of this patient's respiratory acidosis?

a. Left heart failure
b. Pulmonary edema
c. Airway obstruction
d. Hypoventilation
e. Anemia

4-39. A 52-year-old woman has an infarct involving a branch of the posterior communicating artery, causing damage to the ventral anterior (VA), ventrolateral (VL), dorsomedial, and anterior thalamic nuclei. Which of the following is the most likely clinical manifestation of this infarct?

a. Hemiparesis and neuropsychological impairment
b. Loss of sleep and apnea
c. Loss of appetite and thermoregulation
d. Total blindness of the contralateral eye
e. Marked endocrine dysfunction

4-40. An adolescent presents with shortness of breath during exercise and is found to be anemic. A hemoglobin electrophoresis is performed that is depicted in the figure below. The adolescent's sample is run with controls including normal, sickle trait, and sickle cell anemia hemoglobin samples and serum. The adolescent is determined to have an unknown hemoglobinopathy. Which one of the lanes contains the adolescent's sample?

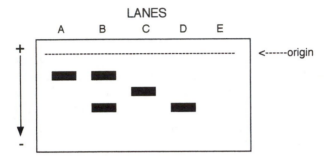

Electrophoretic Hemoglobin Patterns

a. Lane A
b. Lane B
c. Lane C
d. Lane D
e. Lane E

4-41. A 48-year-old male is brought to the emergency room by ambulance due to sudden shortness of breath and left-side chest and back pain. EKG and blood work suggest normal cardiac function and no evidence of a heart attack. He has diminished lung sounds on the left side and extreme tenderness in the mid-back on the left side about 6 cm off the midline. History reveals that he was kneed in the back during a game one week ago while playing goalie. He is 5 ft 10 in and 165 lbs. His urine is normal in color, smell, and volume. An AP chest film suggests fluid in the left pleural space at the costophrenic recess. You order a thorax and abdomen CT to look for which of the following?

a. Enlarged right ventricle consistent with pulmonary hypertension
b. A cracked rib
c. Cardiac tamponade
d. Appendicitis
e. Inflamed gallbladder

4-42. A butcher who is fond of eating raw hamburger develops chorioretinitis; a Sabin-Feldman dye test is positive. This patient is most likely infected with which of the following?

a. Giardiasis
b. Schistosomiasis
c. Toxoplasmosis
d. Trichinosis
e. Visceral larva migrans

4-43. A 53-year-old man presents with increasing gastric pain and is found to have a 3-cm mass located in the anterior wall of his stomach. This mass is resected and histologic examination reveals a tumor composed of cells having elongated, spindle-shaped nuclei. The tumor does not connect to the overlying gastric epithelium and is instead found only in the wall of the stomach. The tumor cells stain positively with CD117, but negatively with both desmin and S-100. Special studies find that these tumor cells have abnormalities of the KIT gene. Which of the following is the most likely diagnosis?

a. Ectopic islet cell adenoma (VIPoma)
b. Gastrointestinal stromal tumor (GIST)
c. Submucosal leiomyoma ("fibroid tumor")
d. Lymphoma of mucosa-associated lymphoid tissue (MALToma)
e. Nonchromaffin paraganglioma (chemodectoma)

4-44. A 37-year-old Asian male was admitted to the hospital complaining of shortness of breath. He denied use of cigarettes, although did admit a previous history of intravenous drug abuse. His chest films showed a diffuse ground glass pattern. A specimen was obtained by bronchoalveolar lavage, and distinctive thin-walled trophozoites and thick-walled spherical cysts containing four to eight nucleii were observed using methenamine-silver stain. The most likely diagnosis of his illness is which of the following?

a. AIDS-related lymphoma
b. Aspergillosis
c. Blastomycosis
d. Histoplasmosis
e. *P. carinii* pneumonia

4-45. A 23-year-old girl is admitted to the hospital with a 3-month history of malaise and generalized muscle cramps. Laboratory results reveal: serum sodium of 144 mmol/L, serum potassium of 2.0 mmol/L, serum bicarbonate of 40 mmol/L, and arterial pH of 7.5. Which of the following is the most likely cause of this patient's hypokalemic alkalemia?

a. Hyperaldosteronism
b. Hyperventilation
c. Persistent diarrhea
d. Renal failure
e. Diabetes

4-46. A child develops chronic diarrhea and liver inflammation in early infancy when the mother begins using formula that includes corn syrup. Evaluation of the child demonstrates sensitivity to fructose in the diet. Which of the following glycosides contains fructose and therefore should be avoided when feeding or treating this infant?

a. Sucrose
b. Oaubain
c. Lactose
d. Maltose
e. Streptomycin

4-47. A 40-year-old patient with a recent viral infection presents with a significantly tender gland, low radioiodine uptake, and signs and symptoms of thyrotoxicosis. This presentation is most likely

a. Graves' disease
b. Subacute thyroiditis
c. Toxic multinodular goiter
d. Hashimoto's thyroiditis
e. Toxic adenoma

4-48. A 63-year-old man is being examined 6 months after a stroke damaged part of his dominant parietal lobe. He is unable to balance his checkbook and has trouble writing his name. Further examination finds that he cannot name and identify each of his fingers, and he gets confused when trying to identify body parts on his right and left sides. Which of the following is the most likely diagnosis?

a. Déjérine-Roussy syndrome
b. Gerstmann's syndrome
c. Parinaud's syndrome
d. Wallenberg's syndrome
e. Weber's syndrome

4-49. An 8-year-old African girl develops a rapidly enlarging mass that involves a large portion of the right side of her maxilla. A smear made from an incisional biopsy of this mass reveals malignant cells with cytoplasmic vacuoles that stain positively with oil red O. Histologic sections from this biopsy reveal a diffuse, monotonous proliferation of small, noncleaved lymphocytes. In the background are numerous tingible-body macrophages that impart a "starry-sky" appearance to the slide. Which of the following viruses is most closely associated with this malignancy?

a. Cytomegalovirus (CMV)
b. Epstein-Barr virus (EBV)
c. Herpes simplex virus (HSV)
d. Human immunodeficiency virus (HIV)
e. Human papillomavirus (HPV)

4-50. A toddler is brought to you with swelling of the hands and face. The mother says he was well but fell from his bike 2 weeks ago. Examination shows an elevated blood pressure and an infected wound of his shin. Urinalysis shows numerous RBC. Which statement applies?

a. Hypertension due to sodium retention
b. The causative organism is *Staphylococcus*
c. Complement levels will remain depressed for up to 6 months
d. The child will likely develop chronic renal failure if untreated
e. The facial swelling is due to nephrotic syndrome

BLOCK 5

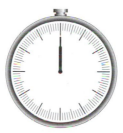

YOU HAVE 60 MINUTES TO COMPLETE 50 QUESTIONS.

Questions

5-1. A patient complained of severe abdominal pain on several occasions, but no cause could be identified. She was recently diagnosed with polyarteritis nodosa, so you ordered the abdominal arteriogram below to determine whether there were abdominal vascular changes that would explain her abdominal pain. On this arteriogram there is a tortuous vessel indicated by the arrow. What is this vessel?

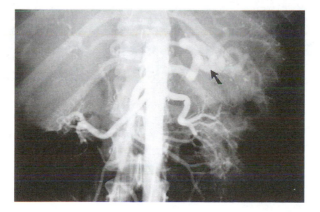

a. Left gastric artery
b. Superior mesenteric artery
c. Splenic artery

d. Right gastric artery
e. Right gastro-omental artery

5-2. A 23-year-old woman presents to her gynecologist for a routine physical examination that includes a Pap smear. Her sexual history includes many sexual partners beginning at an early age, but she has never been pregnant. Physical examination is unremarkable. The Pap smear returns as abnormal with the presence of atypical squamous epithelial cells of undetermined significance (ASCUS). She returns for a 6-month follow-up and a repeat pelvic exam is performed. Her cervix is painted with iodine and an area near the cervical os is present that does not stain with iodine. This area is flat and not papillary. Several biopsies are obtained from this pale area, and a representative histologic section is seen in the picture below. This histologic section shows koilocytosis, which is most characteristic of infection with which one of the following organisms?

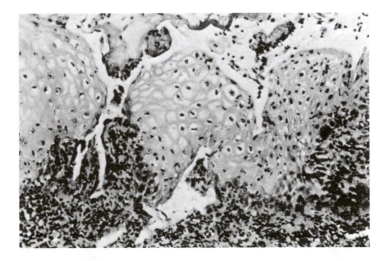

   a. Cytomegalovirus
   b. Epstein-Barr virus
   c. Herpes simplex virus
   d. Human papillomavirus
   e. Parvovirus B19

5-3. A 50-year-old man asks for help in establishing an effective weight loss program. He has been 40 lbs overweight for several years. In planning a weight loss intervention, the most effective self-management procedure is

a. Information control
b. Self-monitoring
c. Self-punishment
d. Self-reward
e. Enlisting social support

5-4. The vertebral angiogram in the figure reveals the effects of a severe motorcycle accident upon a 21-year-old woman. As a result of the accident, from which of the following does she most likely suffer?

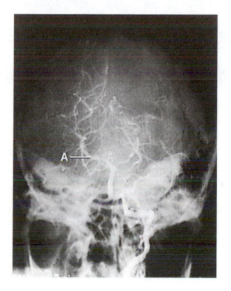

a. A UMN paralysis of the right side of the body
b. A right homonymous hemianopsia
c. A left upper quadrantanopia
d. Aphasia
e. Dyskinesia

5-5. A 39-year-old man with aortic insufficiency and a history of multiple antibiotic resistances is given a prophylactic intravenous dose of antibiotic before surgery to insert a prosthetic heart valve. As the antibiotic is being infused, the patient becomes flushed over most of his body. Which of the following antibiotics is most likely responsible?

a. Erythromycin
b. Gentamicin
c. Penicillin G
d. Tetracycline
e. Vancomycin

5-6. A newborn infant has severe respiratory problems. Over the next few days, it is observed that the baby has severe muscle problems, demonstrates little development, and has neurological problems. A liver biopsy reveals a very low level of acetyl-CoA carboxylase, but normal levels of the enzymes of glycolysis, gluconeogenesis, the citric acid cycle, and the pentose phosphate pathway. Which of the following is the most likely cause of the infant's respiratory problems?

a. Low levels of phosphatidyl choline
b. Biotin deficiency
c. Ketoacidosis
d. High levels of citrate
e. Glycogen depletion

5-7. A patient will be started on primaquine to treat active *Plasmodium vivax* malaria, specifically to target the hepatic forms of the parasite. Before you administer the drug you should screen the patient to assess their relative risk of developing which of the following "most common and severe" adverse responses to the primaquine?

a. Cardiac conduction disturbances
b. Hemolytic disease
c. Nephrotoxicity
d. Retinopathy
e. Seizures, convulsions

5-8. A man has prostate cancer that will be treated with leuprolide. Which of the following drugs must be used adjunctively when we start chemotherapy?

a. An aromatase inhibitor (e.g., anastrozole)
b. Flutamide
c. Prednisone or another potent glucocorticoid
d. Tamoxifen
e. Testosterone

5-9. A young girl has had repeated infections with *Candida albicans* and respiratory viruses since she was three months old. As part of the clinical evaluation of her immune status, her responses to routine immunization procedures should be tested. In this evaluation, the use of which of the following vaccines is contraindicated?

a. BCG
b. *Bordetella pertussis* vaccine
c. Diphtheria toxoid
d. Inactivated polio
e. Tetanus toxoid

5-10. A 45-year-old man was riding a snowmobile and hit a snow-covered rocky outcropping. While recovering from the accident, he slipped and fell on the outcropping and now is experiencing pain in the gluteal region. In this CT scan, the dark linear structure indicated by the arrow is which of the following?

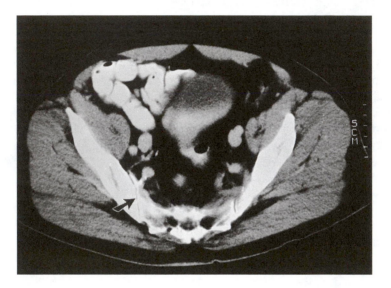

a. A fracture of the ilium
b. The sacroiliac joint
c. A spinal nerve
d. The superior gluteal artery
e. The inferior gluteal artery

5-11. A 43-year-old woman comes to your office complaining of pruritus, mainly of the soles and palms, and fatigue. She has minimal jaundice and steatorrhea. Laboratory tests show a slightly elevated bilirubin, an elevated alkaline phosphatase, and a positive IgG antimitochondrial antibody test. The likely diagnosis is

a. Extrahepatic biliary tract obstruction
b. Alcoholic hepatitis
c. Viral hepatitis
d. Primary biliary cirrhosis
e. Carcinoma of the liver

5-12. A 46-year-old woman who has been a type I diabetic for 35 years, visits your family medicine office. She has foot ulcers on both her right and her left feet. You prescribe Beclaperin gel, a prescription drug for the treatment of diabetic foot ulcers. It contains platelet-derived growth factor (PDGF). Which of the following is the most likely mechanism for the action of PDGF in the improvement of wound healing?

a. Acceleration of chemotaxis of monocytes-macrophages
b. Inhibition of vascular smooth-muscle cell proliferation
c. Inhibition of fibroblast proliferation
d. Inhibition of granulation tissue formation
e. Secretion of type II collagen

5-13. A 41-year-old woman is seen in the psychiatric clinic for a follow-up appointment. She has been taking an antidepressant for 3 weeks with some improvement in mood. However, she complains of drowsiness, palpitations, dry mouth, and feeling faint on standing. Which of the following antidepressants is she most likely taking?

a. Amitriptyline
b. Bupropion
c. Fluoxetine
d. Trazodone
e. Venlafaxine

5-14. A 63-year-old woman was brought into the emergency room by her son, who suspected she had suffered a stroke the previous night. Subsequent examination revealed spastic hemiplegia on the left side with hyperreflexia and a positive Babinski's sign. The left side of the patient's face was paralyzed below the eye, and the right eye was turned out and down. The right pupil made direct and consensual responses to light, but the left pupil was fixed and unresponsive. There were no apparent sensory deficits. Which is the most likely location of the lesion?

a. Left motor cortex
b. Right sensory cortex
c. Right midbrain
d. Left thalamus
e. Right thalamus

5-15. A 25-year-old mother, looking tired and harassed, brings her 5- and 7-year-old daughters to see you for rather severe colds and 100° F temperatures. She apologizes for not having brought them in for the past two years, but tells you that she just could not afford it. You notice that the daughters look pale, underweight, and somewhat undernourished. In talking with the mother, you learn that her husband abandoned her two years ago and her only means of support is a job as a clerk in a busy discount store. You wonder how many other families in your practice are in this difficult situation. Later that day, you call the headquarters of the American Academy of Family Physicians and learn that in America the percentage of youngsters living with just one parent is

a. 5%
b. 10%
c. 15%
d. 20%
e. 25%

5-16. As part of the management of a 28-year-old male with acute onset of Crohn's disease of the small bowel, you decide to treat him with a new cocktail of mouse-human chimeric antibodies to reduce his intestinal inflammation and cachexia. To what set of proteins may these antibodies be directed?

a. IL-1, IL-2, IL-3
b. IL-2, IL-12, TNF-α
c. IL-2, TGF-β, TNF-α
d. IL-1, IL-6, TNF-α
e. IL-2, IL-3, IL-12

5-17. A patient who has been treated for Parkinson's disease for about a year presents with purplish, mottled changes to her skin. Which of the following is the most likely cause?

a. Amantadine
b. Bromocriptine
c. Levodopa (alone)
d. Levodopa combined with carbidopa
e. Pramipexole

5-18. A patient is hospitalized and waiting for coronary angiography. His history includes angina pectoris that is brought on by "modest" exercise (there is no evidence of coronary spasm), accompanied by transient electrocardiographic changes consistent with myocardial ischemia. In the hospital he is receiving nitroglycerine and morphine (slow intravenous infusions), plus oxygen via nasal cannula.

He suddenly develops episodes of chest discomfort. Heart rate during these episodes rises to 170 to 190 beats/min; blood pressure reaches 180–200/110–120 mm Hg, and prominent findings on the EKG are runs of ventricular ectopic beats that terminate spontaneously, plus ST-segment elevation.

Although there are several things that need to be done for immediate care, administration of which one of the following is most likely to remedy (at least temporarily) the majority of these signs and symptoms and pose the lowest risk of doing further harm?

a. Aspirin
b. Captopril
c. Furosemide
d. Labetalol
e. Lidocaine
f. Nitroglycerin (increased dose as a bolus)
g. Prazosin

5-19. A 13-year-old boy presents with a slowly enlarging lesion that involves the distal portion of his right femur. He denies any history of trauma to this site. X-rays reveal a large destructive lesion that focally lifts the periosteum to form a triangular shadow between the cortex and the raised end of the periosteum (Codman's triangle). Laboratory examination reveals elevated serum levels of alkaline phosphatase. Which of the following histologic changes is most likely to be seen in a biopsy specimen taken from this bone lesion?

a. Multiple blood filled spaces that are not lined by endothelial cells
b. Haphazard arrangement of immature bony trabeculae forming "Chinese letters"
c. Lobules of hyaline cartilage with few cells
d. Malignant anaplastic cells secreting osteoid
e. Thick bone trabeculae with osteoclasts that lack a normal ruffled border

5-20. A 47-year-old man walks into the emergency room because of feeling very weak, tired, short of breath, and dizzy. He has numbness and tingling of his fingers. He appears pale and sallow. On examination, his heart rate is 132. His sclerae and nailbeds are pale. His heart is enlarged and he has dependent edema of his ankles. Laboratory findings include a negative Coombs' test and a hemoglobin of 4 g/dL. Which of the following is the most likely diagnosis?

a. Traumatic hemolytic anemia
b. Autoimmune anemia
c. Blood loss
d. Pernicious anemia
e. Iron-deficiency anemia

5-21. A 28-year-old woman is brought to the emergency room after developing hypokalemic paralysis. Arterial blood gas analysis shows a PaO_2 of 102 mmHg and a pH of 7.1. She is diagnosed with type I renal tubular acidosis caused by Sjögren's syndrome (an autoimmune tubulointerstitial nephropathy that damages the H^+-ATPase on the distal nephron). Which of the following laboratory measurements will most likely be normal in this patient?

a. Net acid excretion
b. Aldosterone secretion
c. Serum bicarbonate
d. Urine ammonium
e. Anion gap

5-22. Gary is a 35-year-old man who was previously healthy until one day he noticed that his right leg was weak. As the day progressed, he found that he was dragging the leg behind him when he walked, and he finally asked a friend to drive him home from work because he was unable to lift his right foot up enough to place it on the gas pedal. He also noticed that his left leg felt a little bit numb. Finally, his wife convinced him to go to the emergency room of his local hospital.

When Gary arrived at the emergency room, he was having a great deal of difficulty walking. The physician who examined him asked him when this had begun, and when Gary thought about it in more depth, he realized that perhaps this had started slowly several days before and he had ignored the symptoms. Gary's language function, cranial nerves, and motor and sensory examinations of his arms were within normal limits. When the physician examined Gary's right leg, it was markedly weak, with very brisk reflexes in the knee and ankle. Vibration and position sense in the right leg were absent. Pain and temperature testing were normal in the right leg, but these sensations were absent on the left leg and abdomen to the level of his umbilicus. Reflexes in the left leg were normal, but when the physician scratched the lateral portion of the plantar surface on the bottom side of Gary's right foot, the great toe moved up. The remainder of Gary's examination was normal.

What area of Gary's nervous system was damaged?

a. Brainstem
b. Cervical spinal cord
c. Thoracic spinal cord
d. Frontal lobe
e. Peripheral nerves

5-23. A 44-year-old woman presents with the new onset of seizures along with increasing frequency of severe headaches. Her medical history is otherwise unremarkable. Physical examination finds bilateral neurologic defects. Work-up reveals a large, ill-defined, necrotic mass that involves both the right and left cerebral cortex. Histologic sections from this lesion reveal a hypercellular tumor with pseudopalisading of tumor cells around large areas of serpentine necrosis. Marked vascular endoneural proliferation is present. Numerous atypical nuclei and mitoses are seen. This tumor is best classified as what type of high-grade neoplasm?

a. Astrocytoma
b. Lymphoma
c. Medulloblastoma
d. Oligodendroglioma
e. Schwannoma

5-24. A female patient falls on an icy sidewalk and complains of her thumb hurting. You take her x-ray and show her there are no fractures. However, she asks what the small light circles (arrow) on the x-ray are. You explain they are sesamoid bones in the tendon of which of the following?

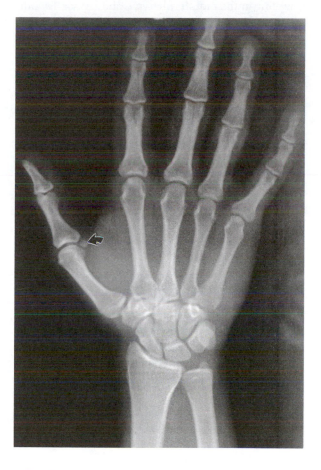

a. Flexor pollicis longus
b. Flexor pollicis brevis
c. Adductor pollicis
d. Abductor pollicis longus
e. Abductor pollicis brevis

5-25. A 30-year-old male presents to the emergency room with difficulty breathing and abdominal pain. Upon physical exam, you notice diffuse areas of nondependent, nonpitting swelling without pruritus, with predilection for the face, especially the perioral and periorbital areas. You also notice swelling in the mouth, pharynx, and larynx. Laboratory analysis of blood drawn from this patient indicates a complement problem. Which of the following is most likely?

a. High C1 and normal level of C1 esterase inhibitor
b. High C1 esterase inhibitor and low C4
c. Low C4 and high C2
d. High C4, C2, and C3
e. Low C1 esterase inhibitor and low C4

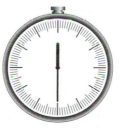

YOU SHOULD HAVE COMPLETED APPROXIMATELY 25 QUESTIONS AND HAVE 30 MINUTES REMAINING.

5-26. A 65-year-old woman presents to the hospital with increasing confusion. Pertinent clinical history is that she had been taking large amounts of laetrile as part of a metabolic therapy program consisting of a special diet and high-dose vitamin supplementation. Physical examination finds weakness of her arms and legs along with bilateral ptosis. Her skin has a cherry-red color, and the strong odor of bitter almonds is present. Which of the following is the most likely diagnosis?

a. Arsenic ingestion
b. Carbon monoxide toxicity
c. Carbon tetrachloride exposure
d. Cyanide poisoning
e. Ethylene glycol ingestion

5-27. A patient with a history of hypertension, heart failure, and peripheral vascular disease has been on oral therapy with drugs suitable for each for about 3 months. He runs out of the medication and plans to have the prescriptions refilled in a week.

Within a day or two after stopping his medications he experiences an episode of severe tachycardia accompanied by tachyarrhythmias, and an abrupt rise of blood pressure to 240/140 mmHg—well above pretreatment levels. He complains of chest pain, anxiety, and a pounding headache. Soon thereafter he suffers a hemorrhagic stroke.

Abruptly stopping which of the following drugs is most likely to account for these responses?

a. ACE inhibitors
b. Clonidine
c. Digoxin
d. Hydrochlorothiazide
e. Nifedipine (a long-acting formulation)
f. Warfarin

5-28. Morris is a 79-year-old man who was brought to the emergency room because his family was worried that he suddenly was not using his right arm and leg and seemed to have a simultaneous behavior change. He was unable to write a reminder note to himself, even with his left hand, and he put his shoes on the wrong feet. A neurologist was called to the ER to examine the patient. A loud bruit was heard with a stethoscope over the left carotid artery in his neck. When asked to show the neurologist his left hand, he pointed to his right hand, since it could not move. The neurologist asked him to add numbers, and he was unable to do this, despite having spent his life as a bookkeeper. Morris was unable to name the fingers on either hand, and he could not form any semblance of a letter using his left hand. Morris's eyes did not blink when the neurologist waved his hands close to them in the left temporal and right nasal visual fields. The right lower two-thirds of his face drooped. There was some asymmetry of his reflexes between the right and left sides, and there was a positive Babinski response of his right toe.

Where in the CNS is the damage?

a. Right frontal and parietal lobes
b. Left frontal and parietal lobes
c. Right frontal lobe
d. Left frontal lobe
e. Right temporal lobe

5-29. A 10-year-old boy is brought to the emergency room after fainting during soccer practice. He often complained that he was tired and had difficulty catching his breath. The presence of a systolic murmur and the ventricular and aortic pressure waves illustrated below suggest which diagnosis?

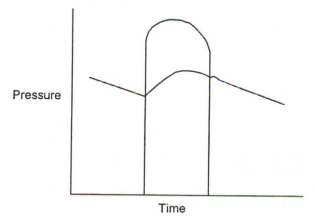

a. Aortic regurgitation
b. Aortic stenosis
c. Congestive heart failure
d. Mitral regurgitation
e. Atherosclerosis

5-30. A 25-year-old woman in her fifteenth week of pregnancy presents with uterine bleeding and passage of a small amount of watery fluid and tissue. She is found to have a uterus that is much larger than estimated by her gestational dates. Her uterus is found to be filled with cystic, avascular, grapelike structures that do not penetrate the uterine wall. No fetal parts are found. Which of the following is the most likely diagnosis?

a. Partial hydatidiform mole
b. Complete hydatidiform mole
c. Invasive mole
d. Placental site trophoblastic tumor
e. Choriocarcinoma

5-31. A 64-year-old male was admitted to the hospital with edema and congestive heart failure. He was found to have diastolic dysfunction characterized by inadequate filling of the heart during diastole. The decrease in ventricular filling is due to a decrease in ventricular muscle compliance. Which one of the following proteins determines the normal stiffness of ventricular muscle?

a. Calmodulin
b. Troponin
c. Tropomyosin
d. Titin
e. Myosin light chain kinase

5-32. An elderly individual was admitted to a hospital after a long period in which the family had complained that he showed increasing incidences of disorientation coupled with memory loss. The patient was diagnosed with Alzheimer's disease and a few years later, after further physical and mental deterioration, the patient died. An autopsy was taken of his brain and regional brain chemistry and neuropathology identified.

Which of the following would represent likely sites where the neuropathology could be identified?

a. Cerebellar cortex, hypothalamus, red nucleus
b. Substantia nigra, midbrain periaqueductal gray, ventrolateral thalamus
c. Nucleus gracilis, deep pontine nuclei, vestibular nuclei
d. Cerebral cortex, basal nucleus of Meynert, hippocampus
e. Fastigial nucleus, subthalamic nucleus, superior colliculus

5-33. A 59-year-old man with a history of coronary artery disease and severe mitral regurgitation has surgery to replace his mitral valve. Postoperatively there were no complications until 6 months after the surgery when he presented with increasing fatigue. Work-up finds a normocytic normochromic anemia that is due to fragmentation of red blood cells by his artificial heart valve. Which of the following red cell abnormalities is most indicative of intravascular hemolysis and is most likely to be seen when examining a peripheral blood smear from this patient?

a. Drepanocytes
b. Heinz bodies
c. Pappenheimer bodies
d. Schistocytes
e. Target cells

5-34. A woman with a cardiac arrhythmia is being treated long-term with amiodarone. This drug can cause biochemical changes and clinical signs and symptoms that resemble those associated with which of the following endocrine diseases/disorders?

a. Addisonian crisis
b. Cushing's syndrome
c. Diabetes insipidus
d. Diabetes mellitus
e. Hypothyroidism
f. Ovarian hyperstimulation syndrome

5-35. A 35-year-old woman with fever, weight loss, fatigue, and painful joints and muscles presents to her physician's office. The physician notes that she has marked photosensitivity and a rash on the cheeks and over the bridge of her nose. Laboratory tests reveal anemic conditions and the presence of anti-DNA antibodies. Which one of the following is the correct diagnosis for this patient?

a. Goodpasture's syndrome
b. Grave's disease
c. Hashimoto's disease
d. Juvenile onset diabetes mellitus
e. Myasthenia gravis
f. Pernicious anemia
g. Rheumatoid arthritis
h. Systemic lupus erythematosus (SLE)

5-36. A middle-aged man presents with congestive heart failure with elevated liver enzymes. His skin has a grayish pigmentation. The levels of liver enzymes are higher than those usually seen in congestive heart failure, suggesting an inflammatory process (hepatitis) with scarring (cirrhosis) of the liver. A liver biopsy discloses a marked increase in iron storage. In humans, molecular iron (Fe) is which of the following?

a. Stored primarily in the spleen
b. Stored in combination with ferritin
c. Excreted in the urine as Fe^{2+}
d. Absorbed in the intestine by albumin
e. Absorbed in the ferric (Fe^{3+}) form

5-37. A 4-year-old boy presents with mild fatigue and malaise. Several other children in the day-care center he attends 5 days a week have developed similar illnesses. Physical examination finds mild liver tenderness, but no lymphadenopathy is noted. Laboratory examination finds mildly elevated serum levels of liver enzymes and bilirubin. The boy recovers from his mild illness without incident. Which of the following organisms is the most likely cause of this child's illness?

a. Cytomegalovirus (CMV)
b. Epstein-Barr virus (EBV)
c. Group A β-hemolytic streptococcus
d. Hepatitis A virus
e. Hepatitis B virus

5-38. A 57-year-old obese white female was referred to your clinic due to a sore throat characterized by a white pseudomembranous lesion of epithelial cells and organisms. The patient's history revealed type 1 diabetes mellitus and recent penicillin use for a severe bacterial infection in her right foot. *C. albicans* was recognized in microscopic examination of infected tissues by the presence of which of the following?

a. Abundance of septate rhizoids
b. Asci containing two to eight ascospores
c. Metachromatic granules
d. Spherules containing endospores
e. Yeasts and pseudohyphae

5-39. A man who has been at the local tavern, drinking alcohol heavily, is assaulted. He is transported to the hospital. Among various findings is an infection for which prompt antibiotic therapy is indicated. Given his high blood alcohol level, which antibiotic(s) should be avoided because of a high potential of causing a serious disulfiram-like reaction that might provoke ventilatory or cardiovascular failure? Assume that were it not for the alcohol consumption, the antibiotic prescribed would be suitable for the infectious organisms that have been detected.

a. Amoxicillin
b. Cefoperazone or cefotetan
c. Erythromycin ethylsuccinate
d. Linezolid
e. Penicillin G

5-40. A 19-year-old woman comes to the office complaining of galactor-rhea. She has never been pregnant. Which hormone is the most likely to be responsible for this situation?

a. Prolactin
b. Estrogen
c. Progesterone
d. Thyroxine
e. Cortisol

5-41. Upon neurological testing, a 55-year-old male who had recovered from a stroke was unable to make smooth, purposeful movements involving mainly his left arm. The movements were jerky and lacked coordination. Which lettered option on the illustration below most closely corresponds to the affected region.

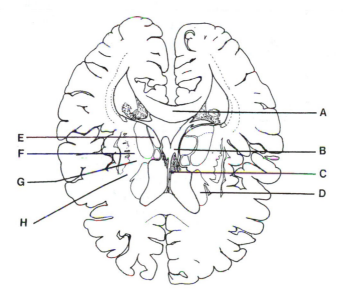

a. Region A
b. Region B
c. Region C
d. Region D

e. Region E
f. Region F
g. Region G
h. Region H

5-42. A 5-year-old girl presents with a several day history of localized swelling in the right side of her neck. There is no recent history of sore throat. Physical examination finds a low-grade fever, and one very tender, firm, slightly enlarged lymph node is palpated in the right cervical region. A CBC reveals a mild leukocytosis. A fine needle aspiration of the lymph node reveals scattered neutrophils. Which of the following is the most likely diagnosis?

a. Bacterial lymphadenitis
b. Granulomatous lymphadenitis
c. Necrotizing lymphadenitis
d. Toxoplasmic lymphadenitis
e. Tuberculous lymphadenitis

5-43. A 65-year-old man presents with bone pain and is found to have hypocalcemia and increased parathyroid hormone. Surgical exploration of his neck finds all four of his parathyroid glands to be enlarged. Which of the following disorders is the most likely cause of this patient's enlarged parathyroid glands?

a. Primary hyperplasia
b. Parathyroid adenoma
c. Chronic renal failure
d. Parathyroid carcinoma
e. Lung carcinoma

5-44. An adolescent presents with abdominal discomfort, abdominal full-ness, excess gas, and weight loss. Blood glucose, cholesterol, and alkaline phosphatase levels are normal. There is no jaundice or elevations. The stool tests positive for reducing substances. Which of the following is the most likely diagnosis?

a. Diabetes mellitus
b. Starvation
c. Nontropical sprue
d. Milk intolerance
e. Gallstones

5-45. A 77-year-old man is brought to your office by his daughter, who visited him at his home today and found him slightly confused and "clumsy." He complains of a moderate generalized headache and some shortness of breath, but denies the other symptoms described by his daughter. His only other complaint is a sore neck, present since he slipped on the steps last week while going to his basement to check his furnace, which he thinks hasn't been working correctly. On examination he is mildly tachycardic, and he has a subtle but discernible reddish appearance to his mucous membranes. The most likely diagnosis is

a. Acquired spinal stenosis (cervical)
b. Normal pressure hydrocephalus
c. Carbon monoxide poisoning
d. TIA
e. Muscle tension headache

5-46. A 3-month-old boy is found dead in his crib by his parents. He is lying in the prone position, which is the same position he was placed in by his parents for an afternoon nap. He had been healthy without any clinical problems. Pertinent medical history is that he was born at 38 weeks of gestation and had a slightly low birth weight. An autopsy fails to reveal any anatomic reason for his death. Which of the following is the most likely cause of death in this child?

a. Acute bacterial meningitis
b. Hemorrhagic encephalopathy syndrome
c. Severe combined immunodeficiency syndrome
d. Shaken baby syndrome
e. Sudden infant death syndrome

5-47. A 20-year-old man presents with low back pain and stiffness. Radiographic examination finds extensive calcification of the vertebral and paravertebral ligaments, producing a "bamboo spine." Rheumatoid factor is not identified in his peripheral blood. This patient's abnormalities are most likely the result of a disorder that is most closely associated with which one of the following HLA types?

a. HLA-A3
b. HLA-B27
c. HLA-BW47
d. HLA-DR3
e. HLA-DR4

5-48. A couple is referred to the physician because their first three pregnancies have ended in spontaneous abortion. Chromosomal analysis reveals that the wife has two cell lines in her blood, one with a missing X chromosome (45,X) and the other normal (46,XX). Her chromosomal constitution can be described as

a. Chimeric
b. Monoploid
c. Trisomic
d. Mosaic
e. Euploid

5-49. A 12-year-old boy is brought to your office by his mother because he developed a painless rash on his face and legs. The rash began as red papules and then became vesicular and pustular and finally it coalesced in honeycomb-like crusts. The boy does not have fever, but he does have several insect bites and he is unwashed and dressed in dirty clothes. This rash is likely to be

a. Herpes simplex
b. Shingles
c. Impetigo
d. Scarlet fever
e. Erysipelas

5-50. A 65-year-old slightly cyanotic male presents to his physician complaining of dizziness and fatigue. A blood test reveals a hematocrit of 62, leading to the diagnosis of polycythemia vera. Treatment consists of periodic phlebotomy to reduce the hematocrit. The reduction in hematocrit is beneficial because it

a. Reduces blood viscosity
b. Increases arterial oxygen saturation
c. Reduces blood pressure
d. Increases cardiac output
e. Decreases oxygen-carrying capacity

BLOCK 6

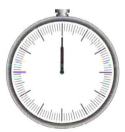

You Have 60 Minutes to Complete 50 Questions.

Questions

6-1. A 24-year-old woman presents with increasing pain and swelling in the posterior region of her neck. Physical examination finds a red, hot, swollen area measuring approximately 1 cm in greatest dimension. The skin is intact in this area, but surgical exploration finds a cavity that is filled with purulent material. Cultures from this material grow *Staphylococcus aureus*. Histologic sections reveal liquefactive necrosis filled with numerous neutrophils and necrotic tissue. These histologic findings best describe which one of the following pathological processes?

a.   Abscess formation
b.   Epithelial erosion
c.   Fibrinous inflammation
d.   Serous inflammation
e.   Ulcer formation

6-2. An 82-year-old woman is brought to the emergency room complaining of extreme thirst and generalized weakness. She has consumed a large amount of orange juice to quench her thirst. Laboratory analysis reveals a significant hyperkalemia. Which one of the following changes in nerve membranes will most likely be observed?

a. The membrane potential will become more negative
b. The sodium conductance will increase
c. The potassium conductance will increase
d. The membrane will become more excitable
e. The Na-K pump will become inactivated

6-3. You are volunteering in a hospital in a very poor part of the world. Their drug selection is limited. A patient presents with acute cardiac failure, for which your preferred drug is dobutamine, given intravenously. However, there is none available. Which other drug, or combination of drugs, would be a suitable alternative? (All these drugs are available in parenteral formulations.)

a. Dopamine (at a very high dose)
b. Ephedrine
c. Ephedrine plus propranolol
d. Norepinephrine plus phentolamine
e. Phenylephrine plus atropine

6-4. A couple presents for genetic counseling after their first child is born with achondroplasia (100800), a dwarfing syndrome. The physician obtains the following family history: the husband (George) is the first-born of four male children, and George's next-oldest brother has cystic fibrosis (219700). The wife is an only child, but she had DNA screening because a second cousin had cystic fibrosis and she knows that she is a carrier. There are no other medical problems in the couple or their families. The physician should now draw the pedigree with the female member of any couple on the left. The generations are numbered with Roman numerals and individuals with Arabic numerals; individuals affected with achondroplasia or cystic fibrosis are indicated. Which of the following risk figures applies to the next child born to George and his wife?

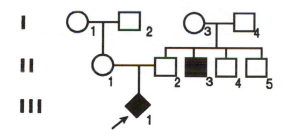

a. Achondroplasia ½, cystic fibrosis ¼
b. Achondroplasia ½, cystic fibrosis ⅛
c. Achondroplasia virtually 0, cystic fibrosis ¼
d. Achondroplasia virtually 0, cystic fibrosis ⅙
e. Achondroplasia virtually 0, cystic fibrosis ⅛

6-5. A 5-year-old child arrives at the emergency department minutes after being bitten by a black widow spider. You immediately inject gamma globulin in the form of an antivenom. This type of immunization is referred to as which of the following?

a. Artificial active immunization
b. Artificial passive immunization
c. Natural active immunization
d. Natural passive immunization
e. Adoptive immunization

6-6. A 25-year-old male reports to his physician that he has not been able to sleep for over two days and has been having "strange reactions." These reactions are most apt to be caused by

a. Increased levels of blood cortisol
b. Physiologic stress in response to sleep deprivation
c. The effects of the rebound phenomenon
d. Perceptual distortions
e. Feelings of excessive tiredness

6-7. An immigrant family from rural Mexico brings their 3-month-old child to the emergency room because of whistling inspiration (stridor) and high fever. The child's physician is perplexed because the throat examination shows a gray membrane almost occluding the larynx. A senior physician recognizes diphtheria, now rare in immunized populations. The child is intubated, antitoxin is administered, and antibiotic therapy is initiated. Diphtheria toxin is often lethal in unimmunized persons because it

a. Inhibits initiation of protein synthesis by preventing the binding of GTP to the 40S ribosomal subunit
b. Binds to the signal recognition particle receptor on the cytoplasmic face of the endoplasmic reticulum receptor
c. Shuts off signal peptidase
d. Blocks elongation of proteins by inactivating elongation factor 2 (EF-2, or translocase)
e. Causes deletions of amino acid by speeding up the movement of peptidyl-tRNA from the A site to the P site

6-8. A 51-year-old man who had an allogeneic bone marrow transplant about 2 months ago complains of anorexia and an erythematous maculo-papular rash. On physical examination, he is jaundiced and he has hepatosplenomegaly. The cause of his disease is

a. B cell–mediated IgG antibody response
b. Transplanted MHC I proteins that match the recipient's cells
c. IgE-mediated release of mast cells
d. Transplanted allogeneic T cells
e. Nitric oxide release by macrophages

6-9. A 45-year-old man asks his physician for a prescription for sildenafil to improve his sexual performance. Because of risks from a serious drug interaction, this drug should not be prescribed, and the patient should be urged not to try to obtain it from other sources, if he is also taking which of the following drugs?

a. An angiotensin-converting enzyme inhibitor
b. A β-adrenergic blocker
c. A nitrovasodilator (e.g., nitroglycerin)
d. A statin-type antihypercholesterolemic drug
e. A thiazide or loop diuretic

6-10. A 28-year-old woman comes into the emergency room exhibiting dyspnea and mild cyanosis, but no signs of trauma. Her chest x-ray is shown below. The most obvious abnormal finding in the inspiratory posteroanterior chest x-ray of this patient (viewed in the anatomic position) is a left pneumothorax (collapsed lung) as is evident by the dark appearance of the left lung and the shifting of the heart to the right. What structure is indicated by the arrow?

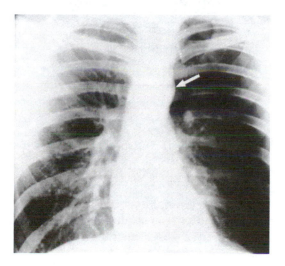

a. Bilateral expansion of the pleural cavities above the first rib
b. Grossly enlarged heart
c. Aortic arch
d. Pulmonary trunk
e. Left ventricle

6-11. An individual suffered a stroke involving part of his midbrain and, when tested by an audiologist, it was revealed that he had lost some ability in auditory discrimination, acuity, and ability to localize sound in space. The loss of which structure could possibly account for these deficits?

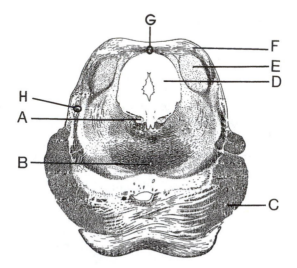

a. Structure A
b. Structure B
c. Structure C
d. Structure D
e. Structure E
f. Structure F
g. Structure G
h. Structure H

6-12. A 3-week-old child develops fever and lethargy, has a full fontanelle, and just about 1 h ago had a seizure. Cultures of the blood and of the CSF grew the same organism. The most likely pathogen is

a. *Neisseria meningitidis*
b. *Streptococcus pneumoniae* (pneumococcus)
c. Gram-negative bacilli
d. Staphylococci
e. *Hemophilus influenzae*

6-13. You have referred a patient in your practice for a nighttime sleep study because of his complaint of excessive daytime fatigue. When REM sleep is disrupted or interrupted, a tiredness can develop during waking hours. The proportion of REM sleep that you would expect in a normal sleep study is

a. 5%
b. 10%
c. 20%
d. 30%
e. 40%

6-14. An 18-year-old woman presents with amenorrhea and is found to have normal secondary sex characteristics and normal-appearing external genitalia. Her first menstrual period was at age 13, and her cycle has been unremarkable until now. She states that her last menstrual period was 8 weeks prior to this visit. A urine test for hCG is positive. Which of the following is the most likely diagnosis?

a. Ectopic pregnancy
b. Intrauterine pregnancy
c. Stein-Leventhal syndrome
d. Turner's syndrome
e. Weight loss syndrome

6-15. A patient with myocardial infarction is treated with nitroglycerin to dilate his coronary arteries. Which of the following best describes the action of nitroglycerin?

a. Methylation occurs to produce *S*-adenosylmethionine
b. GTP hydrolysis accomplishes oxidation of LDL proteins
c. Arginine is converted to a neurotransmitter that activates guanyl cyclase
d. Acetyl CoA and choline are condensed to form a neurotransmitter
e. Tyrosine is converted to serotonin

6-16. Emma was a 64-year-old woman who had heart disease for many years. While carrying chemicals down the stairs of the dry-cleaning shop where she worked, she suddenly lost control of her right leg and arm. She fell down the stairs and was able to stand up with some assistance from a coworker. When attempting to walk on her own, she had a very unsteady gait, with a tendency to fall to the right side. Her supervisor asked her if she was all right, and noticed that her speech was very slurred when she tried to answer. He called an ambulance to take her to the nearest hospital. The physician who was called to see Emma in the emergency room noted that her speech was slurred as if she were intoxicated, but the grammar and meaning were intact. Her face appeared symmetric, but when asked to protrude her tongue, it deviated toward the left. She was unable to tell if her right toe was moved up or down by the physician when she closed her eyes, and she couldn't feel the buzz of a tuning fork on her right arm and leg. In addition, her right arm and leg were markedly weak. The physician could find no other abnormalities in the remainder of Emma's general medical examination.

Where in the nervous system did the damage occur?

a. Right lateral medulla
b. Occipital lobe
c. Left lateral medulla
d. Right cervical spinal cord
e. Left medial medulla

6-17. A 45-year-old woman makes an appointment to see her physician because she is having breathing difficulties when she lies down at night. An S_3 gallop is heard upon auscultation. Her signs and symptoms are most likely due to

a. Hypertension
b. Mitral regurgitation
c. Cor pulmonale
d. Cardiac pericarditis
e. Left heart failure

6-18. A 38-year-old woman presents with intermittent pelvic pain. Physical examination reveals a 3-cm mass in the area of her right ovary. Histologic sections from this ovarian mass reveal a papillary tumor with multiple, scattered small, round, laminated calcifications. Which of the following is the basic defect producing these abnormal structures?

a. Bacterial infection
b. Dystrophic calcification
c. Enzymatic necrosis
d. Metastatic calcification
e. Viral infection

6-19. A medical technologist visited Scandinavia and consumed raw fish daily for two weeks. Six months after her return home, she had a routine physical and was found to be anemic. Her vitamin B_{12} levels were below normal. What is the most likely cause of her vitamin B_{12} deficiency anemia?

a. Cysticercosis
b. Excessive consumption of ice-cold vodka
c. Infection with the fish tapeworm *D. latum*
d. Infection with Parvovirus B19
e. Infection with *Yersinia*

6-20. A 45-year-old male is seen in your office after discharge from the hospital. He suffered an anterior wall myocardial infarction and is asking you about modifying his risk factors. Which of the following is true?

a. Smoking is not a risk factor for development of atherosclerotic coronary disease
b. Hypertension is not a risk factor for development of atherosclerotic coronary disease
c. A fasting lipid profile is not important in risk factor modification
d. The goal of LDL-lowering should be to a value less than 100 mg/dL
e. Diabetes mellitus does not need to be closely monitored

6-21. A 37-year-old woman who has a clinical picture of fever, splenomegaly, varying neurologic manifestations, and purplish ecchymoses of the skin is found to have a hemoglobin level of 10.0 g/dL, a mean corpuscular hemoglobin concentration (MCHC) of 48, peripheral blood polychromasia with stippled macrocytes, and spherocytes, with a blood urea nitrogen level of 68 mg/dL. The findings of coagulation studies and the patient's fibrin-degradation products are not overtly abnormal. Which of the following is the most likely diagnosis?

a. Idiopathic thrombocytopenic purpura
b. Thrombotic thrombocytopenic purpura
c. Disseminated intravascular coagulopathy
d. Submassive hepatic necrosis
e. Waterhouse-Friderichsen syndrome

6-22. A hyperuricemic patient who is asymptomatic (no gouty arthritis or other expected signs or symptoms; merely elevated serum uric acid concentrations) is started on probenecid. In a couple of days he develops acute gout. Which of the following is the most likely explanation for this patient's symptoms?

a. Accelerated synthesis of uric acid by the probenecid
b. Co-precipitation of probenecid and urate in the joints
c. Idiosyncratic response
d. Probenecid-induced systemic acidosis, favoring uric acid crystallization
e. Reduced renal excretion of uric acid

6-23. A 55-year-old female arrives to your emergency room the day after St. Patrick's Day coughing up bright red blood. She has frequented your emergency room before. History includes alcohol consumption. Using abdominal percussion you determine that her liver extends 5 cm below the right costal margin at the midclavicular line. You call in a gastroenterologist because you suspect that the bright red blood is most likely the result of which of the following?

a. Hemorrhoids
b. Colon cancer
c. Duodenal ulcer
d. Gastric ulcer
e. Esophageal varices

6-24. A 2-week-old neonate presents with regurgitation and persistent, severe projectile vomiting. An olive-like epigastric mass is felt during physical examination. A chest x-ray does not reveal the presence of bowel gas in the chest cavity. This infant's mother did not have polyhydramnios during this pregnancy. Which of the following is the most appropriate treatment for this infant's condition?

a. Oral medication with omeprazole and clarithromycin
b. Oral medication with vancomycin or metronidazole
c. Surgery to cut a hypertrophied stenotic band at the pylorus
d. Surgery to remove a mass of the adrenal gland
e. Surgery to resect an aganglionic section of the intestines

6-25. A 12-year-old boy has sudden onset of fever, headache, and stiff neck. Two days before, he swam in a lake that is believed to have been contaminated with dog excreta. Leptospirosis is suspected. What laboratory tests are most appropriate at this time to determine whether he has been infected with leptospira?

a. Agglutination test for leptospiral antigen
b. Counterimmunoelectrophoresis of urine sample
c. Gram stain of urine specimen
d. Spinal fluid for dark-field microscopy and culture in Fletcher's serum medium
e. Urine culture on EMB and Thayer-Martin agar

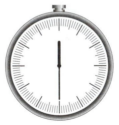

YOU SHOULD HAVE COMPLETED APPROXIMATELY 25 QUESTIONS AND HAVE 30 MINUTES REMAINING.

6-26. You have a patient who has been consuming extraordinarily large amounts of alcohol for several years. He goes into acute withdrawal and manifests nystagmus and bizarre ocular movements and confusion (Wernicke's encephalopathy). Although this patient's alcohol consumption pattern has been accompanied by poor nutrient intake overall, you specifically manage the encephalopathy by administering which of the following?

a. α-tocopherol (vitamin E)
b. Cyanocobalamin (vitamin B_{12})
c. Folic acid
d. Phytonadione (vitamin K)
e. Thiamine (vitamin B_1)

6-27. Your patient was examined by a neurologist after complaining that he kept having a sensation of smell that he could not clearly define. A subsequent MRI revealed the presence of a brain tumor and that the patient was experiencing uncinate hallucinations. The tumor was most likely situated in which of the following regions?

a. Uncal region
b. Medial dorsal thalamic nucleus
c. Parietal cortex
d. Hypothalamus
e. Midbrain periaqueductal gray

6-28. A 47-year-old woman with choriocarcinoma is treated with very high doses of methotrexate (MTX). You anticipate significant host cell toxicity in response to the high MTX dose, and so immediately after giving the anti-cancer drug you administer which of the following?

a. Deferoxamine
b. Leucovorin
c. *N*-acetylcysteine
d. Penicillamine
e. Vitamin K

6-29. A 5-year-old girl is brought to the doctor's office by her mother, who states that the girl has been drinking a lot of water lately and has been urinating much more often than normal. Physical examination reveals a young girl whose eyes protrude slightly. An x-ray of her head reveals the presence of multiple lytic bone lesions involving her calvarium and the base of her skull, a biopsy of which reveals aggregates of Langerhans cells with intracytoplasmic Birbeck's granules. Which of the following sets of laboratory values is most consistent with the expected findings for this girl's disorder?

	Serum Sodium	**Urine**
a.	Hypernatremia	Low osmolarity and low specific gravity
b.	Hypernatremia	High osmolarity and high specific gravity
c.	Hyponatremia	Low osmolarity and low specific gravity
d.	Hyponatremia	High osmolarity and high specific gravity
e.	Normal	Normal osmolarity and normal specific gravity

6-30. A 27-year-old man presents with fever, abdominal pain, muscle pain, and multiple tender cutaneous nodules. No pulmonary signs are found. A biopsy from one of the skin lesions is seen in the photomicrograph below. Involvement of small vessels by inflammation is not found. Laboratory tests are negative for P-ANCAs and C-ANCAs. Which of the following is most likely to be present in this patient's serum?

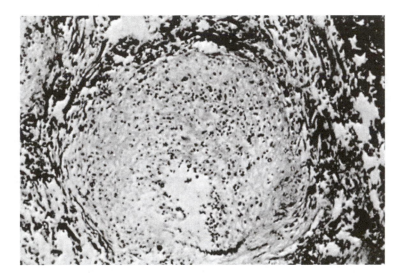

a. CMV antigen
b. *Cryptococcus* antigen
c. Hepatitis B antigen
d. *Histoplasma* antigen
e. *Pneumocystis* antigen

6-31. A 22-year-old male who belongs to a weekend football league pre-sents in the ER. He was running with the ball when a defender tackled him in the midthigh. The patient reports that when he got up, his thigh hurt, so he sat out the rest of the game. When walking to the car, his posterior thigh was extremely painful and swollen. After his shower, he noticed it was becoming discolored with increased swelling. You are concerned about the presence of a hematoma and a disruption of the arterial blood flow to the hamstring muscles. An arteriogram is performed and the vessels in ques-tion (arrows) show good filling by contrast. These blood vessels are which of the following?

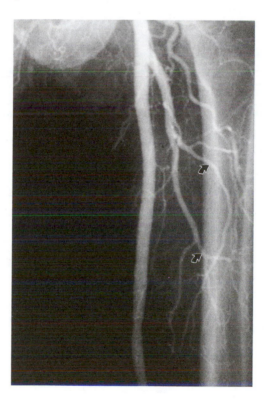

a. Descending branches of the inferior gluteal artery
b. Perforating branches of the deep femoral artery
c. Perforating branches from the obturator artery
d. Perforating branches of the femoral artery
e. Posterior femoral artery

6-32. A 49-year-old male showed changes in emotional behavior over the past few months. Several characteristics of his behavior included heightened sexuality, a very placid appearance, and making physical contact with almost anything that he could touch. The neurologist's diagnosis was that the patient was exhibiting a Klüver-Bucy syndrome. An MRI was given to the patient and a small vascular lesion was detected. Which of the following structures is most likely to contain the lesion?

a. Septal area
b. Amygdala
c. Cingulate gyrus
d. Medial hypothalamus
e. Lateral hypothalamus

6-33. A 43-year-old female presents with chief complaints of bulky and frequent diarrhea and weight loss. She experiences recurrent episodes of abdominal distension terminated by passage of stools. Laboratory data reveals a microcytic anemia, decreased serum calcium, and decreased serum albumin. After additional tests she is diagnosed with gluten-sensitive enteropathy. Her generalized decrease in intestinal absorption can be attributed to which of the following?

a. Decreased intestinal motility
b. Increased migrating motor complexes
c. Decreased intestinal surface area
d. Increased enterohepatic circulation of bile
e. Decreased gastric emptying

6-34. A patient exhibiting multiple facial tics, aggressive outbursts of behavior, and spontaneous repetitive foul language. This syndrome is managed appropriately with which of the following drugs?

a. Clozapine
b. Haloperidol
c. Levodopa
d. Thioridazine
e. Trazodone

6-35. A 2-year-old girl is being evaluated for strikingly yellow skin and is found to have elevated serum levels of indirect bilirubin. After appropriate work-up the diagnosis of type II Crigler-Najjar syndrome is made. She is then treated with phenobarbital, which causes hyperplasia of the smooth endoplasmic reticulum in hepatocytes and decreases the serum indirect bilirubin levels. Which of the following enzymes is most likely to be deficient in this child?

a. Aspartate aminotransferase
b. Bilirubin-UDP-glucuronyl transferase
c. Galactosylceramide beta-galactosidase
d. Gamma-glutamyl transpeptidase
e. L-iduronosulfate sulfatase

6-36. An elderly woman was brought to see an audiologist after complaining about some hearing difficulties. The audiologist noted that she was suffering from unilateral deafness and referred her to a neurologist for further examination. On the basis of his examination, damage to which of the following structures could account for her present condition?

a. The auditory cortex of one side
b. The lateral lemniscus of one side
c. Cranial nerve VIII on one side
d. The medial geniculate
e. The medial lemniscus

6-37. A 72-year-old woman comes to your office with chest pain that radiates to her jaw. The pain awakened her at 2 A.M.; the time is now 10 A.M. She has not been pain free since. Her EKG shows ST elevation in the antero-septal leads (V_1–V_4). Which of the following statements is true?

a. The creatine phosphokinase (CPK) level will probably be normal
b. The troponin level will be normal
c. The myoglobin level will be elevated
d. She will definitely develop Q waves on her surface electrocardiogram, regardless of therapy
e. The MB isoenzyme of creatine phosphokinase will probably be normal

6-38. A previously well 18-year-old girl is admitted to the ICU because of altered mental status. She does not respond to instructions and her arms are postured in a flexor position. Laboratory data reveal a serum sodium concentration of 125 mmol/L. Her friends indicate that the patient had taken ecstasy at a party the night before, and because she was extremely thirsty the next morning, she had consumed a lot of water in a short period of time. Assuming that the reduction in osmolarity is entirely due to water consumption and that her initial weight was 60 kg, approximately how much water would she have had to drink to produce the observed hyponatremia?

a. 5 L
b. 6 L
c. 7 L
d. 8 L
e. 9 L

6-39. A 2-year-old child was admitted to the hospital with acute meningitis. The Gram stain revealed gram-positive, short rods, and the mother indicated that the child had received "all" of the meningitis vaccinations. What is the most likely cause of the disease?

a. *H. influenzae*
b. *L. monocytogenes*
c. *N. meningitidis*, group A
d. *N. meningitidis*, group C
e. *S. pneumoniae*

6-40. A 4-year-old African boy develops a rapidly enlarging mass that involves the right side of his face. Biopsies of this lesion reveal a prominent "starry sky" pattern produced by proliferating small, noncleaved malignant lymphocytes. Based on this microscopic appearance, the diagnosis of Burkitt's lymphoma is made. This neoplasm is associated with chromosomal translocations that involve which one of the following oncogenes?

a. *bcl-2*
b. *c-abl*
c. *c-myc*
d. *erb*-B
e. N-*myc*

6-41. A recalcitrant patient with type 2 diabetes mellitus is noncompliant with medication and diet recommendations nearly all the time. However, he thinks he's smart enough to fool the physician into thinking otherwise: he takes his medication and eliminates nearly all carbohydrate intake for a few days before each clinic visit, knowing he will get a finger-stick for a spot check of serum glucose levels. The simplest, most cost-effective, and most informative way for the physician to assess for past noncompliance and long-term glycemic control would be to perform or measure which of the following?

a. Clinical lab assay of glucose in venous blood sample (rather than glucometer testing of blood from a finger stick)
b. Glucose tolerance test
c. HbA$_{1C}$
d. Serum levels of the antidiabetic drug
e. Urine ketone levels (in a sample donated at the time of clinic visit)
f. Urine glucose levels

6-42. An obese 18-year-old male patient presents with small firm testes, a small penis, little axillary and and facial hair, azoospermia, gynecomastia, and elevated levels of plasma gonadotropins. He has had difficulty in social adjustment throughout high school, but this has worsened and he has been referred for genetic and endocrine screening. The karyotype from peripheral blood leukocytes would most likely show how many Barr body/bodies?

a. Zero
b. One
c. Two
d. Three
e. Four

6-43. A 65-year-old man presents with bradykinesia, tremors at rest, and muscular rigidity. Physical examination reveals the patient to have a "mask-like" facies. In this patient, from which one of the following sites would biopsies most likely reveal intracytoplasmic eosinophilic inclusions within neurons?

a. Basal ganglia
b. Caudate nucleus
c. Hippocampus
d. Midbrain
e. Substantia nigra

6-44. A child with severe epilepsy, autistic behavior, and developmental delay has characteristics of a condition known as Angelman's syndrome. Because of the syndromic nature of the disorder and the developmental delay, a karyotype is performed that shows a missing band on one chromosome 15. Which of the following best describes this abnormality?

a. Interstitial deletion of 15
b. Terminal deletion of 15
c. Pericentric inversion of 15
d. Paracentric inversion of 15
e. 15q−

6-45. A jaundiced 1-day-old premature infant with an elevated free bilirubin is seen in the premature baby nursery. The mother had received an antibiotic combination for a urinary tract infection (UTI) 1 week before delivery. Which of the following is the most likely cause of the baby's kernicterus?

a. A fourth-generation cephalosporin
b. An aminopenicillin (e.g., amoxicillin)
c. Azithromycin
d. Erythromycin
e. A sulfonamide
f. A tetracycline

6-46. A 35-year-old female patient presents with weakness and spasticity in the left lower extremity, visual impairment and throbbing in her left eye, difficulties with balance, fatigue, and malaise. There is an increase in cerebrospinal fluid (CSF) protein, elevated gamma globulin, and moderate pleocytosis. MRI confirms areas of demyelination in the anterior corpus callosum. Which of the following cells are specifically targeted in her condition?

a. Microglia
b. Oligodendrocytes
c. Astrocytes
d. Schwann cells
e. Axons of multipolar neurons

6-47. A 71-year-old woman presents with increasing chest pain and occasional syncopal episodes, especially with physical exertion. She has trouble breathing at night and when she lies down. Physical examination reveals a crescendo-decrescendo midsystolic ejection murmur with a paradoxically split second heart sound (S₂). Pressure studies reveal that the left ventricular pressure during systole is markedly greater than the aortic pressure. Which of the following is the most likely diagnosis?

a. Aortic regurgitation
b. Aortic stenosis
c. Constrictive pericarditis
d. Mitral regurgitation
e. Mitral stenosis

6-48. An elderly male presents with urinary frequency. Laboratory examination shows an elevated serum creatinine. On physical examination you detect an enlarged prostate. Which other finding is most likely?

a. Pain on urination
b. Oliguria
c. Hypokalemia
d. Metabolic acidosis
e. Normal renal ultrasound

6-49. A 23-year-old man is brought to the emergency room after collapsing during basketball practice. On admission he is lethargic and appears confused. His coach reports that he was drinking a lot of water during practice. His symptoms are most likely caused by increased

a. Intracellular tonicity
b. Extracellular tonicity
c. Extracellular volume
d. Intracellular volume
e. Plasma volume

6-50. A 35-year-old male patient presents with numerous subcutaneous hemorrhages. History and physical exam reveal that he has been taking sedormid (a sedative) for the past week. Laboratory tests indicate normal hemoglobin and white blood cell levels with significant thrombocytopenia (very low platelet count). You suspect that he has developed a drug-induced type II hypersensitivity reaction. This reaction may occur if the drug does which of the following?

a. Activates T cytotoxic cells
b. Acts as a hapten
c. Induces mast cell degranulation releasing mediators such as histamine, leukotrienes, and prostaglandins
d. Induces oxygen radical production through the respiratory burst pathway
e. Persists in macrophages

BLOCK 7

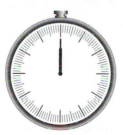

YOU HAVE 60 MINUTES TO COMPLETE 50 QUESTIONS.

Questions

7-1. A 70-year-old man presents to you because he has not been feeling well for several months. He mainly complains of malaise and achiness. He takes ibuprofen occasionally for these symptoms. His urine shows protein and erythrocyte casts. A 24-h urine shows 1 g of protein per day. His creatinine clearance is 24 mL/min. About 4 months ago, his serum creatinine was normal. The most likely diagnosis is

a. Amyloidosis
b. Light-chain deposition disease
c. Nonsteroidal induced interstitial nephritis
d. Vasculitis

7-2. A 41-year-old man is seen by his physician complaining of "always feeling tired" and having "vivid dreams when he is sleeping." He is referred to the hospital's sleep center for evaluation. He is diagnosed with narcolepsy based on his clinical history and the presence of rapid eye movements (REM) as soon as he falls asleep. Which one of the following signs will be observed when the patient is exhibiting REM sleep?

a. Hyperventilation
b. Loss of skeletal muscle tone
c. Slow but steady heart rate
d. High amplitude EEG wave
e. Decreased brain metabolism

7-3. A Nigerian medical student studying in the United States develops hemolytic anemia after taking the oxidizing antimalarial drug pamaquine. Which of the following is the most likely cause of this severe reaction?

a. Glucose-6-phosphate dehydrogenase deficiency
b. Concomitant scurvy
c. Vitamin C deficiency
d. Diabetes
e. Glycogen phosphorylase deficiency

7-4. A 55-year-old woman undergoes surgery. She receives several drugs for preanesthesia care, intubation, and intraoperative skeletal muscle paralysis; and a mixture of inhaled anesthetics to complete the balanced anesthesia. Toward the end of the procedure she develops hyperthermia, hypertension, hyperkalemia, tachycardia, muscle rigidity, and metabolic acidosis.

Which of the following drugs is most likely to have participated in this reaction?

a. Fentanyl
b. Halothane
c. Ketamine
d. Midazolam
e. Propofol

7-5. A second-year medical student was asked to see a nursing home patient as a requirement for a physical diagnosis course. The patient was a 79-year-old man who was apparently in a coma. The student wasn't certain of how to approach this case, so he asked the patient's wife, who was sitting at the bedside, why this patient was in a coma. The wife replied, "Oh, Paul isn't in a coma. But he did have a stroke." Slightly confused, the student leaned over and asked Paul to open his eyes. He opened his eyes immediately. However, when asked to lift his arm or speak, Paul did nothing. The student then asked Paul's wife whether she was certain that his eye opening was not simply a coincidence and whether he really was in a coma, since he was unable to follow any commands. Paul's wife explained that he was unable to move or speak as a result of his stroke. However, she knew that he was awake because he could communicate with her by blinking his eyes. The student appeared rather skeptical, so Paul's wife asked her husband to blink once for "yes" and twice for "no." She then asked him if he was at home, and he blinked twice. When asked if he was in a nursing home, he blinked once. The student then asked him to move his eyes, and he was able to look in his direction. However, when the student asked him if he could move his arms or legs, he blinked twice. He also blinked twice when asked if he could smile. He did the same when asked if he could feel someone moving his arm. The student thanked Paul and his wife for their time, made notes of his findings, and returned to class.

Where in the nervous system could a lesion occur that can cause paralysis of the extremities bilaterally, as well as in the face, but not of the eyes?

a. High cervical spinal cord bilaterally
b. Bilateral thalamus
c. Bilateral basal ganglia
d. Bilateral basilar pons
e. Bilateral frontal lobe

7-6. A 35-year-old obese woman of normal height is found to have hyperglycemia that lasts for several hours following a meal. Further work-up reveals normal fasting serum glucose levels. Physical examination is otherwise unremarkable. Which of the following is the most likely cause of this patient's postprandial hyperglycemia?

a. Antibodies to insulin
b. Decreased functioning of hepatocyte nuclear factor
c. Decreased production of glucagon
d. Excess production of cortisol
e. Impaired release of insulin

7-7. A 55-year-old man who is a longtime alcoholic comes to the emergency room after vomiting small amounts of bright red blood four times today. Which of the following is the most likely diagnosis?

a. Ulcerative colitis
b. Acute pancreatitis
c. Acute pharyngitis
d. Pulmonary embolus
e. Esophageal varices

7-8. A patient presents to the emergency room with vomiting, diarrhea, high fever, and delirium. Upon physical exam, you notice large, painful buboes and disseminated intravascular coagulation. Laboratory diagnosis of aspirate taken from the bubo reveals bipolar staining resembling a safety pin. As part of your treatment, you immediately give which of the following?

a. Ceftazidine
b. Ceftriaxone
c. Penicillin
d. Streptomycin
e. Vancomycin

7-9. A 65-year-old man presents with several enlarged lymph nodes in his left supraclavicular region. Physical examination reveals painless lymphadenopathy in this region. No other abnormalities are found. A biopsy from one of these enlarged lymph nodes, which is shown in the associated picture, reveals effacement of the normal lymph node architecture by numerous nodules of uniform size that are found crowded within the cortex and medulla of the lymph node. Tingible-body macrophages are not seen in these nodules. Which of the following is the most likely diagnosis?

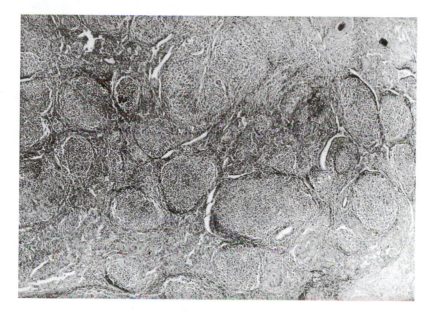

a. Follicular non-Hodgkin's lymphoma
b. Lymphocyte predominate Hodgkin's disease
c. Metastatic adenocarcinoma
d. Reactive follicular hyperplasia
e. Small lymphocytic lymphoma

7-10. An Asian child has severe anemia with prominence of the forehead (frontal bossing) and cheeks. The red cell hemoglobin concentration is dramatically decreased, and it contains only β-globin chains with virtual deficiency of α-globin chains. Which of the following mechanisms is a potential explanation?

a. A transcription factor regulating the α-globin gene is mutated
b. A regulatory sequence element has been mutated adjacent to an α-globin gene
c. A transcription factor regulating the β-globin gene is mutated
d. A transcription factor regulating the α- and β-globin genes is deficient
e. A deletion has occurred surrounding an α-globin gene

7-11. Helen is a 76-year-old woman who has had high blood pressure and diabetes for more than 10 years. One day, as she was reaching for a jar of flour to make an apple pie, her right side suddenly gave out, and she collapsed. While trying to get up from the floor, she noticed that she was unable to move her right arm or leg. Helen attempted to cry for help because she was unable to reach the telephone; however, her speech was slurred and rather unintelligible. She lay on the floor and waited for help to arrive. Helen's son began to worry about his usually prompt mother when she didn't arrive with her apple pie. After several attempts to telephone her apartment without getting an answer, he drove there and found her lying on the floor. She attempted to tell him what had happened, but her speech was too slurred to comprehend. Assuming that his mother had had a stroke, the son called an ambulance to take her to the nearest emergency room. A neurology resident was called to see Helen in the emergency room because the physicians there likewise thought that she had had a stroke. The resident noted that Helen followed commands very well, and, although her speech was very slurred, it was fluent and grammatically correct. The lower two-thirds of her face drooped on the right, but when she was asked to raise her eyebrows, her forehead appeared symmetric. Her tongue pointed to the right side when she was asked to protrude it. Her right arm and leg were severely, but equally, weak; her left side had normal strength. She felt a pin and a vibrating tuning fork equally on both sides.

Where in the CNS did Helen's stroke occur?

a. Left precentral gyrus
b. Right precentral gyrus
c. Left basilar pons or left internal capsule
d. Right putamen or globus pallidus
e. Left thalamus

7-12. A 38-year-old woman presents with increasing frequency of severe headaches. The previous day she had a seizure that lasted several minutes. Her past medical history is otherwise unremarkable, and she has no previous history of seizure activity. She is admitted to the hospital and a CT scan of her head finds a 2-cm mass attached to the dura in her right frontal area. Which of the following histologic changes is most likely to be seen in a biopsy specimen taken from this tumor?

a. Antoni A areas with Verocay bodies
b. A whorled pattern with psammoma bodies
c. Endothelial proliferation with serpentine areas of necrosis
d. "Fried-egg" appearance of tumor cells without necrosis
e. True rosettes and pseudorosettes

7-13. An irritable 18-month-old toddler with fever and blister-like ulcerations on mucous membranes of the oral cavity refuses to eat. The symptoms worsen and then slowly resolve over a period of two weeks. Assuming that the etiological agent was herpes simplex virus type 1, which of the following statements is applicable?

a. Antivirals do not provide any benefit
b. The virus remains latent in the trigeminal ganglia
c. Recurrence is likely to result in a generalized rash
d. Polyclonal B cell activation is a prominent feature
e. The child is at high risk for developing cancer later in life

7-14. A 65-year-old female has experienced a slow onset of rheumatoid arthritis in her hands and shoulder joints over the past 10 years. Treatment has slowed the progress of the disease. Her arthritis is not severe and she stays active, but she has scheduled an office visit for help with what she admits to be stress problems and anxiety. Even before her examination you suspect that the principle source of her psychosocial stress is

a. Loss of coping skills
b. Loss of self-esteem
c. Physical disability
d. Uncontrollable bouts of pain
e. Concern for her future

7-15. During a visit to her gynecologist, a patient reports she received vitamin A treatment for her acne unknowingly during the first two months of an undetected pregnancy. Which organ systems in the developing fetus are most likely to be affected?

a. The digestive system
b. The endocrine organs
c. The respiratory system
d. The urinary and reproductive systems
e. The skeletal and central nervous systems

7-16. A patient on the trauma-burn unit receives a drug to ease dressing changes. They experience good, prompt analgesia, but despite the absence of pain sensation their heart rate and blood pressure rise much as if the sympathetic nervous system were activated by painful responses. As the effects of the drug develop their skeletal muscle tone progressively increases. They appear awake at times because their eyes periodically open. As drug effects wear off they hallucinate and behave in a very agitated fashion. Which drug was given?

a. Fentanyl
b. Ketamine
c. Midazolam
d. Succinylcholine
e. Thiopental

7-17. A patient who has been taking an oral antihypertensive drug for about a year develops a positive Coombs' test. Which of the following is the most likely cause?

a. Captopril
b. Clonidine
c. Labetalol
d. Methyldopa
e. Prazosin

7-18. A 50-year-old multiparous woman comes to your office to rule out cancer. She reports a growing mass in the anterior wall of her vagina. Upon physical examination you detect a soft, bulging, very compressible, mass on the anterior surface of the vagina. When you push on the bulging mass she feels the need to urinate. You order a CT because you suspect which of the following?

a. Rectocele
b. Cystocele
c. Cervical cancer
d. Didelphic uterus
e. Indirect inguinal hernia

7-19. A 35-year-old man presents with a 0.3-cm flat light brown lesion on his left forearm. The lesion is excised, and microscopy reveals nests of round nevus cells within the lower epidermis at the dermal-epidermal junction. There is no "fusion" present of adjacent nests of nevus cells. Cytologic atypia is not present, nor are nevus cells seen in the superficial or deep dermis. Which of the following is the most likely diagnosis?

a. Compound nevus
b. Dysplastic nevus
c. Halo nevus
d. Junctional nevus
e. Spitz nevus

7-20. A 2-month-old girl presents with a soft, high-pitched, mewing cry and is found to have microcephaly, low-set ears and hypertelorism, and several congenital heart defects. Which of the following abnormal karyotypes is most likely to be associated with these clinical signs?

a. 46,XX,4p⁻
b. 46,XX,5p⁻
c. 46,XX,13q⁻
d. 46,XX,15q⁻
e. 46,XX,17p⁻

7-21. A 56-year-old man is admitted to the emergency room after ingesting a large dose of aspirin, most of which is still within the vascular system. The patient is diaphoretic and tachypneic and has the following blood gases: pH of 7.5, P_{CO_2} of 17 mmHg, and bicarbonate of 13 mmol/L.

Aspirin has a pK of 3.5 and when it is in the un-ionized state will rapidly cross the blood-brain barrier. Which of the following treatment options would be most deleterious to this patient?

a. Breathing supplemental oxygen
b. Infusing bicarbonate
c. Decreasing alveolar ventilation
d. Increasing fluid volume
e. Administering activated charcoal

7-22. Your patient reports he spent two weeks on a desert island as part of a television survival show. It rained and was cool the last 5 days, and he developed a cough. He is now in the ER with a productive cough that produces rusty and bloodstained sputum. He also complains of significant pleural pain. You suspect a pneumococcal lobar pneumonia. From this CT scan at the T4 level, which lung lobe (indicated by the asterisk) is involved with the pneumonia?

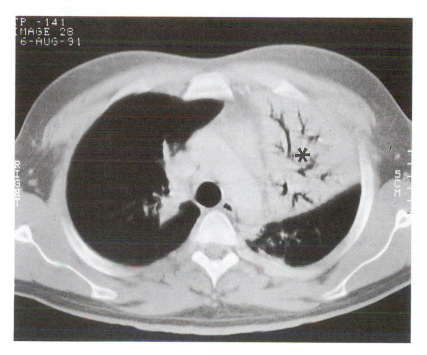

a. Right upper lobe
b. Right middle lobe
c. Right lower lobe
d. Left upper lobe
e. Left lower lobe

7-23. A 76-year-old woman with an 8-year history of CHF that has been well controlled with digoxin and furosemide develops recurrence of dyspnea on exertion. On physical examination, she has sinus tachycardia, rales at the base of both lungs, and 4+ pitting edema of the lower extremities. Which of the following agents could be added to her therapeutic regimen?

a. Dobutamine
b. Hydralazine
c. Minoxidil
d. Prazosin
e. Enalapril

7-24. A newborn infant presented with disseminated vesicular lesions and seemed not to thrive. Herpes simplex virus was suspected, and laboratory confirmation was desired to justify antiviral chemotherapy. The most sensitive test for the diagnosis of herpes simplex (HSV) meningitis in a newborn infant is which of the following?

a. Cerebrospinal fluid (CSF) protein analysis
b. HSV culture
c. HSV IgG antibody
d. HSV polymerase chain reaction
e. Tzanck smear

7-25. A 34-year-old patient with chronic schizophrenia is hospitalized on a chronic ward of a psychiatric hospital and is on an appropriate dose of antipsychotic medication. He frequently shouts in the halls, disrupting activities and annoying the other patients. The best behavioral strategy for this patient would be

a. Psychological counseling
b. Contingency management
c. Stimulus control
d. Role-play therapy
e. Modeling

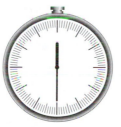

You Should Have Completed Approximately 25 Questions and Have 30 Minutes Remaining.

7-26. A patient with severe arthritis will be placed on long-term therapy with indomethacin. All other factors being equal, which of the following drugs is the most likely choice to administer as an add-on (adjunct) to prevent gastric ulcers caused by this NSAID?

a. Celecoxib
b. Cimetidine
c. Diphenhydramine
d. Misoprostol
e. Sumatriptan

7-27. A patient has steatorrhea due to pancreatic insufficiency secondary to cystic fibrosis. The most reasonable and usually effective drug for managing the symptoms and consequences is which of the following?

a. Atorvastatin (statin-type cholesterol-lowering drug)
b. Cimetidine (or an alternative, e.g., famotidine)
c. Bile salts
d. Metoclopramide
e. Pancrelipase

7-28. A medical student presents to the emergency room with a 2-day history of severe vomiting and orthostatic hypotension. What kind of metabolic abnormalities are most likely in this patient?

a. Hypokalemia, hypochloremia, and metabolic acidosis
b. Hyperkalemia, hyperchloremia, and metabolic alkalosis
c. Normal serum electrolytes and metabolic acidosis
d. Normal serum electrolytes and metabolic alkalosis
e. Hypokalemic, hypochloremic, metabolic alkalosis

7-29. A child stops making developmental progress at age 2 years and develops coarse facial features with thick mucous drainage. Skeletal deformities appear over the next year, and the child regresses to a vegetative state by age 10 years. The child's urine tests positive for glycosaminoglycans that include which of the following molecules?

a. Collagen
b. γ-aminobutyric acid
c. Heparan sulfate
d. Glycogen
e. Fibrillin

7-30. Joe is a 75-year-old man who is right-handed and was told in the past by his internist that he had an irregular heartbeat. Unfortunately, Joe decided that he didn't wish to learn anything further about this condition, so he didn't return to this physician, and it remained untreated. One morning, he awoke to find that his face drooped on the right side and that he couldn't move his right arm or right leg. When he tried to call an ambulance for help, he had a great deal of difficulty communicating with the operator because his speech was slurred, nonfluent, and missing some pronouns. The call was traced by the police; an ambulance arrived at his house and took him to an emergency room. A neurologist was called to see Joe in the emergency room. When he listened to Joe's heart, he detected an irregular heartbeat. It was very difficult to understand Joe's speech because it was halting, with a tendency to repeat the same phrases over and over. He had a great deal of difficulty repeating specific sentences given to him by the neurologist, but he was able to follow simple commands such as "Touch your right ear with your left hand." His mouth drooped on the right when he attempted to smile, but his forehead remained symmetric when he wrinkled it. He couldn't move his right arm at all, but he was able to wiggle his right leg a little bit.

What kind of language problem does Joe have?

a. Dysarthria
b. Wernicke's aphasia
c. Broca's aphasia
d. Alexia
e. Pure word deafness

7-31. A 50-year-old woman at very high risk of breast cancer is given tamoxifen for prophylaxis. This drug does which of the following?

a. Blocks estrogen receptors in breast tissue
b. Blocks estrogen receptors in the endometrium
c. Increases the risk of osteoporosis
d. Raises serum LDL cholesterol and total cholesterol, lowers HDL
e. Reduces the risk of thromboembolic disorders

7-32. A 79-year-old patient is brought to your office by his wife because he "keeps running into things" on his right side. His wife also states that he seems to ignore objects on his right. You test his vision in each eye and determine that your patient cannot see anything in the right visual fields of both eyes. You order a head MRI because you suspect which of the following?

a. A pituitary tumor compressing his optic chiasm
b. A tumor in the medial wall of the right orbit compressing the optic nerve
c. An aneurysm of the left middle cerebral artery compressing the left optic tract
d. A tumor in the middle cranial fossa compressing the right optic tract
e. A tumor in the occipital visual cortex

7-33. A 19-year-old being treated for leukemia develops a fever. You give several agents that will cover bacterial, viral, and fungal infections. Two days later, he develops acute renal failure. Which of the following drugs was most likely responsible?

a. Acyclovir
b. Amphotericin B
c. Ceftazidime
d. Penicillin G
e. Vancomycin

7-34. You are working in a research laboratory that is studying the adult form of Tay-Sachs disease. Your group is trying to develop a pharmacological approach to prevent the symptoms of that disorder. Your focus would most likely be drugs that do which of the following?

a. Stimulate ganglioside GM2 production
b. Stimulate synthesis of GM2 by the rough endoplasmic reticulum
c. Stimulate hexosaminidase production
d. Stimulate transport of ganglioside GM2 to the lysosome
e. Remove mannose-6-phosphate from hexosaminidase

7-35. A 45-year-old woman has chest pain for which a cardiac cause has been ruled out. Her esophageal motility study shows pressure waves of a very high amplitude lasting 2 to 3 s. The most likely diagnosis is

a. Esophageal web
b. Esophageal spasm
c. Achalasia
d. GERD (gastroesophageal reflux disease)
e. T-E (tracheoesophageal) fistula

7-36. A 25-year-old woman presents with the new onset of severe intermittent pain in her fingers that developed shortly after she recovered from mycoplasma pneumonia. She states the pain occurs when she goes outside in the cold, at which time her fingers turn white and then become numb. Laboratory evaluation finds the presence of an IgM autoantibody that is directed against the I-antigen found on the surface of her red blood cells. Based on these clinical findings, the diagnosis of Raynaud's phenomenon is made. Which of the following disorders is most likely present in this individual?

a. Cold autoimmune hemolytic anemia
b. Isoimmune hemolytic anemia
c. Paroxysmal cold hemoglobinuria
d. Paroxysmal nocturnal hemoglobinuria
e. Warm autoimmune hemolytic anemia

7-37. We take a blood sample from a patient (baseline) and then administer Drug A intravenously. We take additional blood samples periodically thereafter and measure drug concentration in each sample. We repeat the experiment, this time giving the same drug orally. If we then plot the logarithm of drug concentration vs. time, the *slope* of the resulting curve provides information about which of the following for Drug A?

a. Area under the curve (AUC)
b. Bioavailability
c. Elimination rate constant
d. Extraction ratio
e. Volume of distribution

7-38. Two siblings, ages 2 and 4, experienced fever, rhinitis, and pharyngitis that resulted in laryngotracheo bronchitis. Both had harsh cough and hoarseness. Which virus is the leading cause of the croup syndrome and, when infecting mammalian cells in culture, will hemabsorb red blood cells?

a. Adenovirus
b. Group B coxsackievirus
c. Parainfluenza virus
d. Rhinovirus
e. Rotavirus

7-39. Your patient is a firefighter who attempted to extinguish a car fire. She had a leak in her protective air mask. She develops cyanide poisoning from the combustion of plastic. Aside from rendering symptomatic, supportive care, which of the following might be administered to combat the cyanide poisoning?

a. Ammonium chloride
b. Deferoxamine
c. Dimercaprol (BAL; British anti-Lewisite)
d. Mannitol
e. Pralidoxime
f. Sodium thiosulfate

7-40. A 44-year-old woman experienced excruciating pain emanating from her left leg. It was concluded that she was suffering from a disorder of unknown etiology for which drug treatment proved ineffective. A decision was made to surgically cut the pathway mediating pain from the left leg to the brain. Which of the structures shown in the figure below was cut by the neurosurgeon?

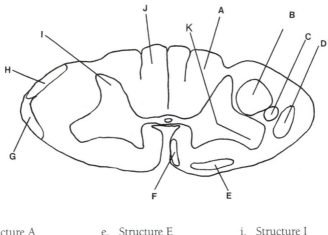

a. Structure A
b. Structure B
c. Structure C
d. Structure D

e. Structure E
f. Structure F
g. Structure G
h. Structure H

i. Structure I
j. Structure J
k. Structure K

7-41. A 28-year-old woman at 24 weeks of gestation of her first pregnancy has the following laboratory data: increased serum total thyroxine; normal free thyroxine; decreased resin triiodothyronine uptake; normal free thyroxine index; and normal thyroid-stimulating hormone. Which of the following is the best clinical interpretation of these laboratory findings?

a. Euthyroid individual with increased thyroid-binding globulin
b. Euthyroid individual with decreased thyroid-binding globulin
c. Hyperthyroid individual with decreased thyroid-binding globulin
d. Hypothyroid individual with decreased thyroid-binding globulin
e. Hypothyroid individual with increased thyroid-binding globulin

7-42. A 23-year-old woman is seen for weakness and amenorrhea. She is clinically hypothyroid. A CT scan of the pituitary shows an expanded sella with a large cystic component with calcifications. The most likely diagnosis is

a. Pituitary macroadenoma
b. Empty sella syndrome
c. Craniopharyngioma
d. Optic glioma
e. Hypothalamic hamartoma

7-43. A 72-year-old woman with emphysema presents to the emergency room with fatigue and respiratory distress. Which of the following sets of arterial blood gas values would represent her condition and reflect a shift of the hemoglobin oxygen dissociation curve to the right?

a. pH 7.05, bicarbonate 15 mM, P_{CO_2} 60, P_{O_2} 88
b. pH 7.15, bicarbonate 10 mM, P_{CO_2} 30, P_{O_2} 88
c. pH 7.25, bicarbonate 15 mM, P_{CO_2} 30, P_{O_2} 88
d. pH 7.40, bicarbonate 24 mM, P_{CO_2} 60, P_{O_2} 88
e. pH 7.45, bicarbonate 15 mM, P_{CO_2} 60, P_{O_2} 88

7-44. A 45-year-old man presents with fever, chronic diarrhea, and weight loss. He is found to have multiple pain and swelling of his joints (migratory polyarthritis) and generalized lymphadenopathy. Physical examination reveals skin hyperpigmentation. A biopsy from his small intestines reveals the presence of macrophages in the lamina propria that contain PAS-positive cytoplasm. Which of the following is the most likely diagnosis?

a. Abetalipoproteinemia
b. Crohn's disease
c. Hartnup disease
d. Nontropical sprue
e. Whipple's disease

7-45. A 54-year-old man develops a thrombus in his left anterior descending coronary artery. The area of myocardium supplied by this vessel is irreversibly injured. The thrombus is destroyed by the infusion of streptokinase, which is a plasminogen activator, and the injured area is reperfused. The patient, however, develops an arrhythmia and dies. An electron microscopic (EM) picture taken of the irreversibly injured myocardium reveals the presence of large, dark, irregular amorphic densities within mitochondria. What are these abnormal structures?

a. Apoptotic bodies
b. Flocculent densities
c. Myelin figures
d. Psammoma bodies
e. Russell bodies

7-46. A 57-year-old man undergoes resection of the distal 100 cm of the terminal ileum as part of treatment for Crohn's disease. The patient likely will develop malabsorption of which of the following?

a. Iron
b. Folate
c. Lactose
d. Bile salts
e. Protein

7-47. A 68-year-old woman suffered from an infectious disorder for several weeks. Following recovery from this disorder, she experienced some loss of taste and an increase in salivation, together with pain spasms in the region of the pharynx, which extended into the ear. She also experienced some bradycardia and cardiac arrhythmia, as well as deviation of the uvula to the unaffected side.

Which of the following cranial nerves was most directly involved in this deficit?

a. Cranial nerve VII
b. Cranial nerve IX
c. Cranial nerve X
d. Cranial nerve XI
e. Cranial nerve XII

7-48. An obstetrician sees a pregnant patient who was exposed to rubella virus in the eighteenth week of pregnancy. She does not remember getting a rubella vaccination. Which of the following represents the best immediate course of action?

a. Administer rubella immune globulin
b. Administer rubella vaccine
c. Order a rubella antibody titer to determine immune status
d. Reassure the patient because rubella is not a problem until after the thirtieth week
e. Terminate the pregnancy

7-49. A 52-year-old man is brought to the emergency room with severe chest pain. Angiography demonstrates a severe coronary occlusion. A thrombolytic agent is administered to re-establish perfusion. Which of the following does the thrombolytic agent activate?

a. Heparin
b. Plasminogen
c. Thrombin
d. Kininogen
e. Prothrombin

7-50. A 68-year-old man who worked for many years in the asbestos indus-try presents with weight loss and increasing chest pain. Examination of his sputum finds very rare asbestos bodies, while a CT scan shows a large mass involving the apical surface of his left lung. Surgery is performed and gross examination finds a lesion similar in appearance to that seen in the associated gross photograph of a sagittal section of the lung. Sections from this mass examined by electron microscopy reveal tumor cells with long microvilli on their surface. Which of the following is the most likely diagnosis?

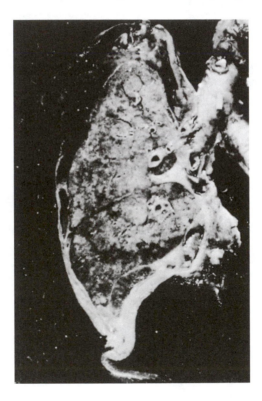

a. Malignant mesothelioma
b. Malignant thymoma
c. Metastatic malignant melanoma
d. Poorly differentiated adenocarcinoma
e. Small-cell carcinoma

BLOCK 8

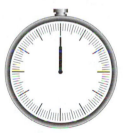

YOU HAVE *60* MINUTES TO COMPLETE *50* QUESTIONS.

Questions

8-1. A 40-year-old woman with a history of sinusitis and asthma since childhood presents to the emergency room with status asthmaticus and hypercapnic respiratory failure. She requires immediate intubation and mechanical ventilation and is treated with nebulized albuterol and IV methylprednisolone every 6 h. After muscle relaxation, on a control rate of 15 breaths/min and a tidal volume of 500 mL, the following values are obtained: $P_{A}CO_2 = 44$ mmHg, $F_{E}CO_2 = 2.8\%$.

Her $F_{A}CO_2$ is approximately

a. 0.40
b. 0.45
c. 0.50
d. 0.55
e. 0.60

8-2. A 50-year-old man presents with headaches, vomiting, and weakness of his left side. Physical examination reveals his right eye to be pointing "down and out" along with ptosis of his right eyelid. His right pupil is fixed and dilated and does not respond to accommodation. Marked weakness is found in his left arm and leg. Swelling of the optic disk (papilledema) is found during examination of his retina. Which of the following is most likely present in this individual?

a. Aneurysm of the vertebrobasilar artery
b. Arteriovenous malformation involving the anterior cerebral artery
c. Subfalcine herniation
d. Tonsillar herniation
e. Uncal herniation

8-3. A 55-year-old man who is being treated for adenocarcinoma of the lung is admitted to a hospital because of a temperature of 38.9°C (102°F), chest pain, and a dry cough. Sputum is collected. Gram stain of the sputum is unremarkable, and culture reveals many small, gram-negative rods able to grow only on a charcoal yeast extract agar. This organism most likely is which of the following?

a. *Chlamydia trachomatis*
b. *Klebsiella pneumoniae*
c. *Legionella pneumophila*
d. *M. pneumoniae*
e. *S. aureus*

8-4. A 28-year-old man with AIDS presents with moderate proteinuria and hypertension. Histologic sections of the kidney reveal the combination of normal-appearing glomeruli and occasional glomeruli that have deposits of hyaline material. No increased cellularity or necrosis is noted in the abnormal glomeruli. Additionally, there is cystic dilation of the renal tubules, some of which are filled with proteinaceous material. Electron microscopy reveals focal fusion of podocytes, and immunofluorescence examination finds granular IgM/C3 deposits. Which of the following is the most likely diagnosis?

a. Diffuse proliferative glomerulonephritis (DPGN)
b. Focal segmental glomerulonephritis (FSGN)
c. Focal segmental glomerulosclerosis (FSGS)
d. Membranous glomerulopathy (MGN)
e. Minimal change disease (MCD)

8-5. A patient presents in the Emergency Department in great distress and with the following signs and symptoms:

- bizarre behavior, delirium
- facial flushing
- clear lungs, no wheezing, rales, etc.
- high heart rate
- absence of bowel sounds
- distended abdomen, full bladder
- hot, dry skin
- absence of lacrimal, salivary secretions
- very high fever
- dilated pupils that do not respond to light

Identify the drug class that was responsible.

a. AChE inhibitors
b. α-adrenergic blockers
c. Antimuscarinics
d. β-adrenergic blockers
e. Parasympathomimetics (muscarinic agonists)
f. Peripherally acting (neuronal) catecholamine depletors

8-6. A 10-year-old girl with type I diabetes develops a neuropathy limited to sensory neurons with free nerve endings. Quantitative sensory testing will reveal higher-than-normal thresholds for the detection of which of the following?

a. Fine touch
b. Vibration
c. Pressure
d. Temperature
e. Muscle length

8-7. A 27-year-old woman with systemic lupus erythematosus complains of fatigue of a few days' duration. On physical examination, she is pale and her spleen tip is palpable. On laboratory examination, her hemoglobin is 7 g/dL and she has spherocytosis on the peripheral blood smear. Which test can make the diagnosis in the case?

a. Factor VIII assay
b. von Willebrand's factor protein
c. Direct Coombs' test
d. Vitamin B_{12} absorption test
e. Prothrombin time

8-8. A woman diagnosed with breast cancer is undergoing antineoplastic chemotherapy and develops severe nausea before chemotherapy begins. Behavioral conditioning results in anticipatory nausea in patients receiving chemotherapy in

a. Two-thirds of these patients
b. The more hopeful and optimistic patients
c. Patients high in chronic anxiety
d. The more gregarious patients
e. The less inhibited patients

8-9. A 60-year-old male suffered from excruciating pain on the left side of his face. Since drug therapy was found to be ineffective in alleviating the pain, it was decided that surgery was indicated. Which of the following structures would be surgically cut or destroyed in order to alleviate the pain?

a. First-order descending sensory fibers contained in the ipsilateral spinal tract of cranial nerve V
b. Neurons in the ventral posterolateral nucleus of the thalamus
c. Cells contained in the main sensory nucleus of the trigeminal nerve
d. Substantia gelatinosa
e. Midbrain periaqueductal gray

8-10. A 5-year-old boy presents with clumsiness, a waddling gait, and difficulty climbing steps. Physical examination reveals that this boy uses his arms and shoulder muscles to rise from the floor or a chair. Additionally, his calves appear to be somewhat larger than normal. Which of the following is the most likely diagnosis?

a. Inclusion body myositis
b. Werdnig-Hoffmann disease
c. Polymyositis
d. Duchenne's muscular dystrophy
e. Myotonic dystrophy

8-11. A 72-year-old male with diabetes mellitus is evaluated in the emergency room because of lethargy, disorientation, and long, deep breaths (Kussmaul respirations). Initial chemistries on venous blood demonstrate high glucose at 380 mg/dL (normal up to 120) and a pH of 7.3. Recalling the normal bicarbonate (22 to 28 mM) and P_{CO_2} (33 to 45 mmHg) values, which of the following additional test results would be consistent with the man's pH and breathing pattern?

a. A bicarbonate of 5 mM and P_{CO_2} of 10 mmHg
b. A bicarbonate of 15 mM and P_{CO_2} of 30 mmHg
c. A bicarbonate of 15 mM and P_{CO_2} of 40 mmHg
d. A bicarbonate of 20 mM and P_{CO_2} of 45 mmHg
e. A bicarbonate of 25 mM and P_{CO_2} of 50 mmHg

8-12. A 42-year-old man complains of fatigue and enlarged glands in the neck, both axillae, and the left groin. His blood count shows a lymphocytosis. The lymphocytes are monoclonal B cells that show CD5 antigen. On peripheral smear "smudge" cells are present and genetic studies show trisomy 12. What is the likely disorder?

a. Burkitt's lymphoma
b. Follicular diffuse lymphoma
c. Multiple myeloma
d. Chronic lymphocytic leukemia
e. Waldenström's macroglobulinemia

8-13. A 20-year-old woman presents with a 5-day history of fatigue, low-grade fever, and sore throat. Physical examination reveals bilateral enlarged, tender cervical lymph nodes, an exudative tonsillitis, and an enlarged spleen. A complete blood cell count reveals the hemoglobin and platelet counts to be within normal limits. The total white blood cell count is increased to 9200 cells/μL. Examination of the peripheral blood reveals the presence of atypical mononuclear cells with abundant cytoplasm. These cells have peripheral condensation of the cytoplasm, which gives them a "ballerina skirt" appearance. Which of the following laboratory findings is most likely to be present in this individual?

   a. Aggregates of mononuclear cells with cytoplasmic Birbeck granules in the liver
   b. Elevated levels of delta-ALA in the urine
   c. Group A streptococcus in cultures from the tonsillar exudate
   d. Heterophil antibodies in the serum
   e. M spike in the gamma region of a serum protein electrophoresis

8-14. A 29-year-old farmer develops a headache and becomes dizzy after working on a tractor in his barn. His wife suspects carbon monoxide poisoning and brings him to the emergency room where he complains of dizziness, lightheadedness, headache, and nausea. Arterial blood gas measurements reveal an elevated carboxyhemoglobin level. The patient does not appear to be in respiratory distress and denies dyspnea. The absence of respiratory signs and symptoms associated with carbon monoxide poisoning occurs because

   a. Blood flow to the carotid body is decreased
   b. Arterial oxygen content is normal
   c. Cerebrospinal fluid pH is normal
   d. Central chemoreceptors are depressed
   e. Arterial oxygen tension is normal

8-15. A family routinely consumed unpasteurized milk, claiming "better taste." Several members experienced a sudden onset of crampy abdominal pain, fever, and a bloody, profane diarrhea. *C. jejuni* was isolated and identified from all patients. The treatment of choice for this type of enterocolitis is which of the following?

   a. Ampicillin
   b. *Campylobacter* antitoxin
   c. Ciprofloxacin
   d. Erythromycin
   e. Pepto-Bismol

8-16. An active adolescent girl badly bruised her vulva on the horizontal bar of her brother's bicycle during an accident. Blood extended from 3 in below her umbilicus to just anterior to her anus, but did not pass into her thigh. Which anatomical layers most likely explain the distribution of extravasated blood?

a. Superficial membranous fascia and deep perineal fascia
b. Superficial membranous fascia and transversalis fascia
c. Dartos fascia and the perineal membrane
d. Superficial membranous fascia and the perineal membrane
e. Deep perineal fascia and inferior fascia of the pelvic diaphragm

8-17. A 56-year-old woman presents with a small mass on her left shoulder. She states that she has lost about 15 pounds over the past several months and has had trouble falling asleep at night because of "heartburn." She states that her last menstrual period was 10 years ago, and she denies any vaginal bleeding. Physical examination finds a solitary enlarged lymph node over her left clavicle. The lymph node measures 1.5 cm in greatest dimension, and a biopsy from this enlarged node reveals numerous malignant cells that are similar in appearance to those seen in the picture below. Which of the following abnormalities is most likely to be associated with this metastatic lesion?

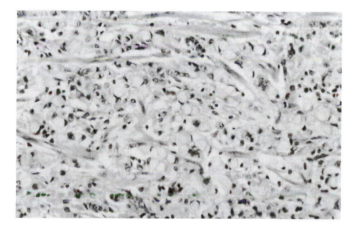

a. A breast carcinoma having a "peau d'orange" appearance
b. A skin carcinoma having a "rodent ulcer" appearance
c. Cystosarcoma phyllodes of the breast
d. Linitis plastica of the stomach
e. Sarcoma botryoides of the vagina

8-18. A patient with a history of cirrhosis and small-cell lung cancer comes to the office for routine bloodwork, which reveals a sodium of 120. Which laboratory test is most useful in determining which of these two diseases is the cause of the hyponatremia?

a. Serum osmolarity
b. Serum creatinine
c. Urine osmolarity
d. Urine sodium
e. Serum vasopressin

8-19. A patient receives a single injection of succinylcholine to facilitate an endoscopic procedure. The dose is correct for the vast majority of patients, and normally effects of this drug abate spontaneously over a couple of minutes. This gentleman remains apneic for an extraordinarily long time. A genetically based aberrant cholinesterase is eventually determined to be the cause. What would we administer if we were concerned about this unusually lengthy drug response?

a. Atropine
b. Bethanechol
c. Neostigmine
d. Nothing
e. Physostigmine
f. Tubocurarine

8-20. A 67-year-old male with a history of alcohol abuse presents to the emergency room with severe epigastric pain, hypotension, abdominal distension, and diarrhea with steatorrhea. Serum amylase and lipase are found to be greater than normal, leading to a diagnosis of pancreatitis. The steatorrhea can be accounted for by a decrease in the intraluminal concentration of which pancreatic enzyme?

a. Amylase
b. Trypsin
c. Chymotrypsin
d. Lipase
e. Colipase

8-21. Mike was a 35-year-old man who had had optic neuritis (an inflammation of the optic nerve causing blurred vision) several years before. He was told that he had a 50% chance of eventually developing multiple sclerosis (MS), a degenerative disease of the CNS white matter. One day he noticed that he had double vision and felt weak on his right side. Although he noted that the symptoms were becoming steadily worse throughout the day, he attributed this to stress from his job as a stockbroker, and in order to relax he decided to take a drive in his car. While he was driving, his vision became steadily worse. As he was about to pull over to the side of the road, he saw two trees on the right side of the road. Uncertain which was the actual image, he attempted to place his right foot on the brake pedal. Mike suddenly realized that he was unable to lift his right leg, and his car collided with the tree. A pedestrian on the side of the road called the EMS, and Mike was brought to a nearby emergency room.

A neurologist was called to see Mike because the emergency room physicians thought he might have had a stroke, despite his young age. The neurologist spoke to Mike, then examined him. He found that his left eye was deviated to the left and down. When he attempted to look to his right, his right eye moved normally, but his left eye was unable to move farther to the right than the midline. His left pupil was dilated and did not contract to light from a penlight. His left eyelid drooped, and he had difficulty raising it. In addition, the right side of his mouth remained motionless when he attempted to smile, but his forehead was symmetric when he raised his eyebrows. Mike's right arm and leg were markedly weak. The neurologist told Mike that he wasn't certain that this was necessarily a stroke, but admitted him to the hospital for observation and tests.

A lesion in which of the following nerves caused Mike's double vision?

a. Optic nerve
b. Oculomotor nerve
c. Cervical sympathetic fibers
d. Trochlear nerve
e. Abducens nerve

8-22. A 54-year-old male alcoholic presents with the sudden onset of severe, constant epigastric pain that radiates to his midback. Further evaluation finds fever, steatorrhea, and discoloration around his flank and umbilicus. Laboratory tests find elevated serum levels of amylase and lipase. Which of the following is the most likely diagnosis?

a. Acute appendicitis
b. Acute cholangitis
c. Acute cholecystitis
d. Acute diverticulitis
e. Acute pancreatitis

8-23. You have a patient with severe postoperative pain who is not getting adequate analgesia from usually effective doses of morphine. The physician orders an immediate switch to a high dose of pentazocine. Which of the following is the most likely outcome?

a. Abrupt, added respiratory depression
b. Acute development of physical dependence
c. Coma
d. Seizures
e. Worsening of pain

8-24. As a result of calcification of the internal carotid artery, which impinged upon the lateral half of the right optic nerve prior to its entrance to the brain, a 68-year-old woman experienced certain visual deficits. Which is the most likely visual deficit?

a. Total blindness of the right eye
b. Right nasal hemianopsia
c. Right homonymous hemianopsia
d. Right bitemporal hemianopsia
e. Right upper homonymous quadrantanopia

8-25. A 74-year-old male presents to the office with trouble urinating for 1 week. The force of the urinary stream is reduced, but there is no difficulty starting the stream. There is no pain. What is the problem?

a. Decreased detrusor contractility
b. Detrusor instability
c. Detrusor failure
d. Acute urinary obstruction
e. Chronic urinary obstruction

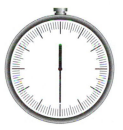

YOU SHOULD HAVE COMPLETED APPROXIMATELY
25 QUESTIONS AND HAVE 30 MINUTES REMAINING.

8-26. A 15-year-old boy has a long history of school problems and is labeled as hyperactive. His tissues are puffy, giving his face a "coarse" appearance. His IQ tests have declined recently and are now markedly below normal. Laboratory studies demonstrate normal amounts of sphingolipids in fibroblast cultures with increased amounts of glycosaminoglycans in urine. Which of the following enzyme deficiencies might explain the boy's phenotype?

a. Hexosaminidase A
b. Glucocerebrosidase
c. α-L-iduronidase
d. α-galactocerebrosidase
e. β-gangliosidase A

8-27. A 27-year-old, 6-ft-tall woman presents in the emergency room with a pneumothorax but is febrile. On physical examination it is noted that she has scoliosis, pectus excavatum, ectopia lentis, and myopia. Her musculoskeletal exam reveals long upper and lower extremities, including the fingers and toes, and an overall gangly, lanky appearance. Her armspan (6 ft, 3 in.) noticeably exceeds her height. She has very flexible fingers and a narrow face as well as a narrow mouth with overcrowded teeth. There are stretch marks across her buttocks. Which part of the cardiovascular system would be most often affected in this syndrome?

a. Middle cerebral artery
b. Basilar artery
c. Aorta
d. Lymphatic vessels
e. Superior vena cava

8-28. A 39-year-old pregnant woman requires heparin for prophylaxis of thromboembolism. What is the mechanism of action of heparin?

a. Increase in the plasma level of Factor IX
b. Inhibition of thrombin and early coagulation steps
c. Inhibition of synthesis of prothrombin and coagulation Factors VII, IX, and X
d. Inhibition of platelet aggregation in vitro
e. Activation of plasminogen
f. Binding of Ca^{2+} ion cofactor in some coagulation steps

8-29. A 2-year-old child has a high fever and is irritable. He has a stiff neck. Gram stain smear of spinal fluid reveals gram-negative, small pleomorphic coccobacillary organisms. What is the most appropriate procedure to follow in order to reach an etiological diagnosis?

a. Culture the spinal fluid in chocolate agar and identify the organism by growth factors
b. Culture the spinal fluid in mannitol-salt agar
c. Perform a catalase test of the isolated organism
d. Perform a coagulase test with the isolate
e. Perform a latex agglutination test to detect the specific antibody in the spinal fluid

8-30. A patient on long-term warfarin therapy arrives at the clinic for her weekly prothrombin time measurement. Her INR is dangerously prolonged, and the physical exam reveals petechial hemorrhages. She's had episodes of long-lasting epistaxis over the last 2 days. Aside from stopping the warfarin (and admitting the patient for follow-up), which of the following should be administered?

a. Aminocaproic acid
b. Epoetin alfa
c. Ferrous sulfate
d. Phytonadione
e. Protamine sulfate

8-31. A teenage girl presents in the emergency room with paroxysms of dyspnea, cough, and wheezing. Her parents indicate that she has had these "attacks" during the past winter, and that they have worsened and become more frequent during the spring allergy season. Which of the following cell types is correctly matched to a function it may perform in this patient's disease?

a. Alveolar macrophages, enhanced mucociliary transport
b. Plasma cells, bronchoconstriction
c. Eosinophils, bronchodilation
d. Goblet cells, hyposecretion
e. Mast cells, edema

8-32. A 59-year-old patient receiving chemotherapy with the anthracycline Adriamycin develops severe heart failure. Sections from an endocardial biopsy specimen reveal vacuolization of the endoplasmic reticulum of the myocytes. Adriamycin therapy most frequently causes what type of cardiomyopathy?

a. Dilated cardiomyopathy
b. Hyperplastic cardiomyopathy
c. Hypertrophic cardiomyopathy
d. Obliterative cardiomyopathy
e. Restrictive cardiomyopathy

8-33. A 26-year-old patient with asthma is receiving montelukast. Which of the following is the main mechanism by which this drug works?

a. Enhanced release of epinephrine from the adrenal medulla
b. Increased airway adrenergic receptor responsiveness to catecholamines
c. Inhibition of cAMP breakdown via phosphodiesterase inhibition
d. Prevention of antigen-antibody reactions that lead to mast cell mediator release
e. Stimulation of ventilatory rates (CNS effect in brain's medulla)
f. Suppression of inflammatory processes

8-34. A 75-year-old woman presents with a pruritic vulvar lesion. Physical examination reveals an irregular white, rough area involving her vulva. Which one of the following histologic changes is most consistent with the diagnosis of lichen sclerosis?

a. Atrophy of the epidermis with dermal fibrosis
b. Atypia of the epidermis with dysplasia
c. Hyperplasia of the epidermis with hyperkeratosis
d. Invasion of the epidermis by individual malignant cells
e. Loss of pigment in the basal layers of the epidermis

8-35. A 67-year-old woman with a history of venous thromboembolism is placed on warfarin (Coumadin) prophylactically. Bleeding can occur if the blood concentration of Coumadin becomes too high. Should bleeding occur, it can be prevented by the administration of

a. Aspirin
b. Heparin
c. tPA (tissue plasminogen activator)
d. Vitamin K
e. Fibrinogen

8-36. An African American infant presents with prominent forehead, bowing of the limbs, broad and tender wrists, swellings at the costochondral junctions of the ribs, and irritability. Which of the following treatments are recommended?

a. Lotions containing retinoic acid
b. Diet of baby food containing leafy vegetables
c. Diet of baby food containing liver and ground beef
d. Milk and sunlight exposure
e. Removal of eggs from diet

8-37. A middle-aged woman describes flushing, severe headaches, and a feeling that her heart is "going to explode" when she gets excited. At the beginning of a physical examination her blood pressure (130/85) is not significantly above normal. However, on palpation of her upper left quadrant, the examining physician notices the onset of sympathetic signs. Her blood pressure (200/135) is abnormally high. A subsequent CT scan confirms the suspected tumor of the left adrenal gland. The patient is scheduled for surgery.

The symptoms that the patient correlated with the onset of excitement were due to nervous stimulation of the adrenal glands. The adrenal medulla receives its innervation from which of the following?

a. Preganglionic sympathetic nerves
b. Postsynaptic sympathetic nerves
c. Preganglionic parasympathetic nerves
d. Postganglionic parasympathetic nerves
e. Somatic nerves

8-38. A 41-year-old man presents with slowly progressive diarrhea along with a dark discoloration of the skin of his neck ("necklace" dermatitis). Mental status evaluation finds changes suggestive of early dementia. Laboratory evaluation finds increased urinary 5-hydroxyindole acetic acid, and further work-up finds a 4-cm tumor in the distal small intestines. Sections of this tumor were interpreted by the pathologist as being consistent with a carcinoid tumor. In this individual, the tumor produced serotonin from tryptophan and subsequently caused a deficiency of tryptophan. This in turn led to a deficiency of niacin, which produced the clinical signs of dermatitis, diarrhea, and dementia. Which of the following is the most likely diagnosis?

a. Beriberi
b. Marasmus
c. Pellagra
d. Rickets
e. Scurvy

8-39. A 45-year-old man complains of upper abdominal discomfort, backache, and some weight loss for several months. Recently, he developed jaundice, although he did not notice it, but his friend did and mentioned it to him. On examination, his abdomen is scaphoid and nontender and no organs or masses are palpable. His laboratory findings show increased direct bilirubin, normal indirect bilirubin, and markedly elevated alkaline phosphatase. His urine shows increased bilirubin and decreased urobilinogen. This pattern is consistent with which illness?

a. Carcinoma of the head of the pancreas
b. Gilbert's syndrome
c. Hemolytic anemia
d. Intrahepatic cholestasis
e. Amyloidosis

8-40. A 23-year-old woman presents with a 0.4-cm firm brown lesion on her upper right thigh. Histologic sections from this lesion reveal an irregular area in the upper dermis that is composed of a mixture of fibroblasts, histiocytes, stromal cells, and capillaries. The majority of cells in this mixture are fibroblasts. The overlying epidermis reveals hyperplasia of the basal layers. Which of the following is the most likely diagnosis?

a. Dermatofibroma
b. Dermatofibrosarcoma protuberans
c. Fibroxanthoma
d. Pyogenic granuloma
e. Sclerosing hemangioma

8-41. A patient with undiagnosed coronary artery disease is given a medication. Shortly thereafter she develops intense tightness and "crushing discomfort" of her chest. An EKG reveals ST-segment changes indicative of acute myocardial ischemia. The patient suffered acute myocardial ischemia and angina pectoris. Which of the following drugs is most likely to have caused this reaction?

a. Clozapine
b. Pentazocine
c. Phenytoin
d. Sumatriptan
e. Zolpidem

8-42. A 16-year-old girl is seen in your office for primary amenorrhea. Your exam reveals a webbed neck, shieldlike chest, widely spaced nipples, and short stature. There is no breast development. You suspect Turner's syndrome (gonadal dysgenesis).

The preferred screening test for Turner's syndrome is

a. Karyotype
b. Testosterone
c. Estradiol
d. FSH
e. LH

8-43. A patient is being treated with an antibiotic for a vancomycin-resistant enterococcal infection. They consume an over-the-counter medication containing ephedrine and develop a significant spike of blood pressure that leads to a pounding headache. They are transported to the hospital. As part of the work-up, blood tests indicate some bone marrow suppression. Which of the following antibiotics is most likely associated with this clinical picture?

a. Azithromycin
b. Ciprofloxacin
c. Erythromycin estolate
d. Gentamicin
e. Linezolid

8-44. A 25-year-old man presents because of a recurrent rash on the sun-exposed areas of his face and arms. He has recently moved to the United States from South Africa, where he has lived all of his life. He states that he has always been sensitive to the light and he says that his face will break out in a rash if he stays in the sun too long. He notes that sometimes alcohol ingestion will make these episodes worse. Pertinent medical history includes episodes of neuropsychiatric changes, including hallucinations and manic-depressive episodes. Physical examination reveals multiple fluid-filled vesicles and bullae on his face and forearms. Laboratory examination reveals elevated levels of delta-aminolevulinic acid and porphobilinogen in the urine. This individual's disorder results from the abnormal synthesis of which one of the following substances?

a. Globin
b. Heme
c. Immunoglobulin
d. Spectrin
e. Transferrin

8-45. A newborn girl is found to have marked swelling of the dorsal areas of her feet along with a broad (webbed) neck, a broad chest, and a heart murmur that is due to coarctation of the aorta. Her physician suspects a chromosomal disorder and orders a karyotype. Which of the results pictured below is most likely?

a. Result A
b. Result B
c. Result C
d. Result D

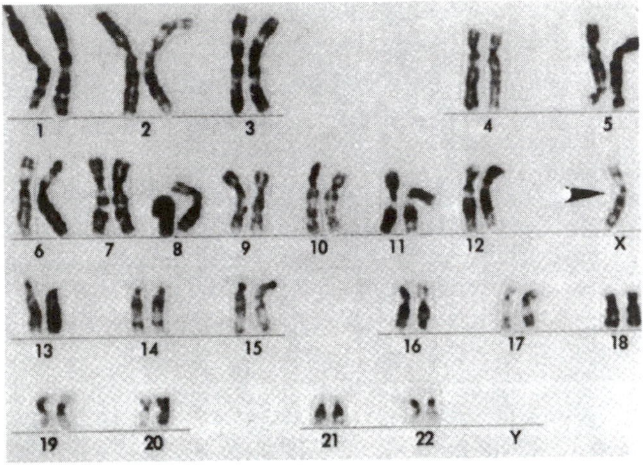

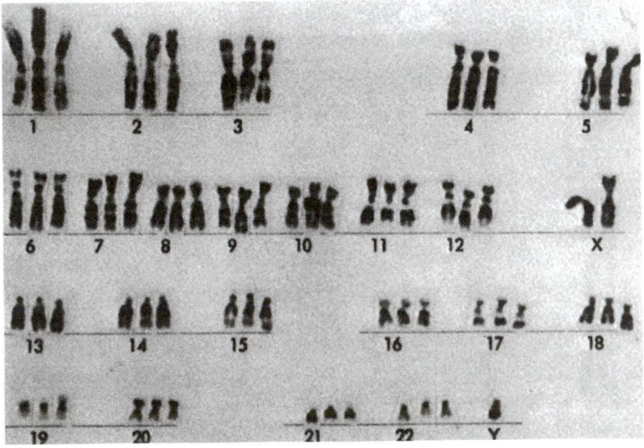

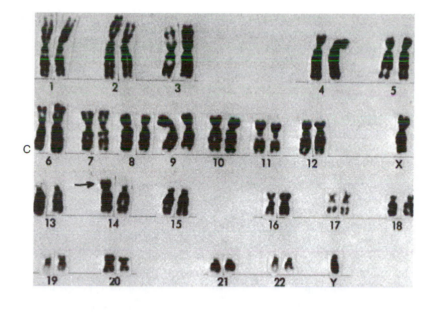

C

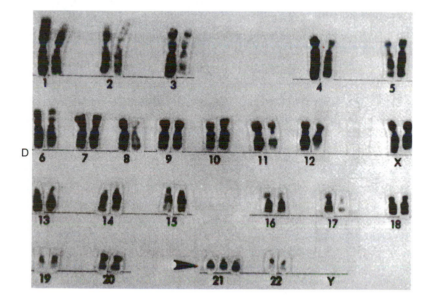

D

8-46. The daughter of a 65-year-old man describes her father as having changed from an active, vivacious, caring person to one who occasionally has trouble learning new facts, has very little motivation to do any activity, and rarely expresses feelings or emotions for his grandchildren whom he has adored. The area of the brain most apt to be involved in this type of behavior change is the

a. Hypothalamus
b. Reticular activating system
c. Heteromodal association areas
d. Limbic system
e. Unimodal association areas

8-47. A 9-year-old girl is brought to your pediatric office by her mother because the girl has been complaining about how sore her throat is, and the mother has noticed that she has started to snore loudly at night. You examine the girl's mouth and oral pharynx and you immediately discover the likely source of the problem, extremely enlarged palatine tonsils. You suggest surgical removal of the tonsils, but you do explain that there is a small risk of the surgery, which may result in which of the following?

a. Loss in the ability to taste salt in the anterior two-thirds of the tongue
b. Loss in the ability to protrude her tongue, thus limiting her ability to lick an ice cream cone
c. Weakness in the ability to open her mouth fully when eating an apple due to damage to the innervation to the lateral pterygoid muscle
d. Loss in the ability to taste in the posterior one-third of the tongue and perhaps some difficulty in swallowing
e. Weakened ability to move her jaw from side to side because of loss in innervation of the medial pterygoid muscle

8-48. A patient has acute gout. The physician initially thinks about prescribing just one or two oral doses of colchicine, 12 h apart, but then decides otherwise. The main reason for avoiding colchicine, even with a very short oral course, is the development of which of the following?

a. Bone marrow suppression
b. Bronchospasm
c. GI distress that is almost as bad as the acute gout discomfort
d. Hepatotoxicity
e. One or two oral doses seldom relieve gout pain
f. Refractoriness/tolerance with just a dose or two

8-49. A 29-year-old man uses secobarbital to satisfy his addiction to barbiturates. During the past week, he is imprisoned and is not able to obtain the drug. He is brought to the prison medical ward because of the onset of severe anxiety, increased sensitivity to light, dizziness, and generalized tremors. On physical examination, he is hyperreflexic. Which of the following agents should he be given to diminish his withdrawal symptoms?

a. Buspirone
b. Chloral hydrate
c. Chlorpromazine
d. Diazepam
e. Trazodone

8-50. A 72-year-old man presents with increasing fatigue. Physical examination reveals an elderly man in no apparent distress (NAD). He is found to have multiple enlarged, nontender lymph nodes along with an enlarged liver and spleen. Laboratory examination of his peripheral blood reveals a normocytic normochromic anemia, a slightly decreased platelet count, and a leukocyte count of 72,000 cells/μL. An example of his peripheral blood is seen in the picture below. Which of the following is the most likely diagnosis?

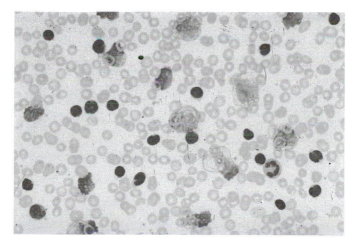

a. Acute lymphoblastic leukemia
b. Atypical lymphocytosis
c. Chronic lymphocytic leukemia
d. Immunoblastic lymphoma
e. Prolymphocytic leukemia

BLOCK 1

Answers

1-1. The answer is c. (*Cotran, pp 352–353. Mandell, pp 2746–2755.*) In the approximate center of the photomicrograph is the classic refractile, double-walled spherule of the deep fungus *Coccidioides immitis*, which is several times the diameter of the largest inflammatory cell nearby. Coccidioidomycosis is endemic in California, Arizona, New Mexico, and parts of Nevada, Utah, and Texas, where it resides in the arid soils and is contracted by direct inhalation of airborne dust. If inhaled, it produces a primary pulmonary infection that is usually benign and self-limiting in immunologically competent persons, often with several days of fever and upper respiratory flulike symptoms. However, certain ethnic groups, such as some African Americans, Asians, and Filipinos, are at risk of developing a potentially lethal disseminated form of the disease that can involve the central nervous system. If the large, double-walled spherule containing numerous endospores can be demonstrated outside the lungs (e.g., in a skin biopsy), this is evidence of dissemination. Antibodies of high titers are detectable by means of complement fixation studies in patients undergoing spontaneous recovery. Amphotericin B is usually reserved for treating high-risk and disseminated infection. The cultured mycelia of the organism on Sabouraud's agar present a hazard for laboratory workers.

1-2. The answer is c. (*Cotran, pp 769–773. Rubin, pp 1315–1316.*) Three malignant tumors of the salivary glands are adenoid cystic carcinoma, mucoepidermoid carcinoma, and acinic cell carcinoma. Adenoid cystic carcinomas form tubular or cribriform patterns histologically and have a tendency to invade along perineural spaces, especially the facial nerve. This involvement can produce Bell's palsy, which is characterized by flattening of one side of the face. Mucoepidermoid carcinomas consist of a mixture of squamous epithelial cells and mucus-secreting cells. The mucus-secreting cells of a mucoepidermoid carcinoma can demonstrate intracellular mucin with a special mucicarmine stain. Acinic cell carcinomas contain glands with cleared or vacuolated epithelial cells. Finally, a mixture of epithelial structures and mesenchyme-like stroma is seen with pleomorphic adenomas, while papillary folds composed of a double layer of oncocytic cells is characteristic of Warthin's tumors.

1-3. The answer is d. (*Moore and Persaud, Developing, pp 16–21.*) In man, the time required for the progression from spermatogonium to motile spermatozoon is about two months (61 to 64 days). Spermatogenesis, the process by which spermatogonia undergo mitotic division to produce primary spermatocytes, occurs at 1°C (2°F) below normal body temperature. Subsequent meiotic divisions produce secondary spermatocytes with a bivalent haploid chromosome number and then spermatids with a monovalent haploid chromosome number. The maturation of the spermatid, spermiogenesis, results in spermatozoa. Morphologically, adult spermatozoa are moved to the epididymis, where they become fully motile.

1-4. The answer is c. (*Waxman, 24/e, pp 162–163.*) A noncommunicating hydrocephalus is the result of an obstruction of one of the channels connecting one ventricle to the next, or the outflow of the fourth ventricle through its foramina, resulting in an enlargement of one or more of the ventricles. In the choices given for this question, the interventricular foramen, connecting the lateral with the third ventricle, is the only possible correct answer. A blockade of the interventricular foramen would lead to an enlargement of the lateral ventricle.

1-5. The answer is a. (*Brooks, p 273. Levinson, pp 165–166. Murray— 2002, pp 329–330. Ryan, p 479.*) While the essential information (i.e., the evidence that the child in question was scratched by a cat) is missing, the clinical presentation points to a number of diseases, including cat-scratch disease (CSD). Until recently, the etiologic agent of CSD was unknown. Evidence indicated that it was a pleomorphic, rod-shaped bacterium that had been named *Afipia*. It was best demonstrated in the affected lymph node by a silver impregnation stain. However, it now appears that *Afipia* causes relatively few cases of CSD and that the free-living rickettsia primarily responsible is *Rochalimaea henselae,* which has recently been renamed *Bartonella henselae.*

1-6. The answer is d. (*Craig, pp 52–53; Hardman, pp 26–27; Katzung, pp 45–46.*) Here is how you solve the problem. Note: It's easy to be misled by inconsistent use of units of measurement (mcg vs. mg, mL vs. L), so be sure you convert units as necessary.

First calculate the drug's elimination rate constant:

$$k_e = 0.693/t_{1/2} \qquad \text{or}$$

$$k_e = 0.693/0.5 \text{ h} = 1.386/\text{h}$$

Then calculate the clearance:

$$Cl = k_e \cdot V_d \qquad \text{or}$$

$$Cl = 1.386/\text{h} \cdot 45 \text{ L, which equals } 62.37 \text{ L/h, or } 62,370 \text{ mL/h}$$

Recall that $C_{ave} = (F/Cl) \cdot (\text{Dose}/\tau)$, where τ represents the dosing interval (given as 4 h).

Rearrange to solve for the dose.

$$\text{Dose} = (C_{ave} \cdot Cl \cdot \tau)/F, \text{ or}$$

$$\text{Dose} = [(2 \text{ mcg/mL}) \cdot (62,370 \text{ mL/h}) \cdot 4 \text{ h}]/1.0$$

Thus, Dose = 499,000 mcg, or 499 mg (close enough to 500 mg).

1-7. The answer is b. (*Levinson, pp 384, 386, 392.*) During a secondary antibody response—the second exposure to the same antigen—IgG predominates. It makes up about 85% of the immunoglobulin in adult serum. IgG opsonizes bacteria and neutralizes viruses.

1-8. The answer is b. (*Murray-Harper's, pp 326–333. Scriver, pp 3–45. Sack, pp 3–29.*) Before DNA replication can actually begin, unwinding protein must open segments along the DNA double helix. A defective unwinding protein slows the overall rate of DNA synthesis, but does not alter the size of replicated DNA fragments. Defects in DNA synthesis or transcription may produce a phenotype of accelerated aging, as in Cockayne's syndrome [216400 (usually defective in a transcription factor)]. After unwinding, DNA-directed RNA polymerase (primase) catalyzes the synthesis of a complementary RNA primer of approximately 50 to 100 bases on each DNA strand. Then DNA-directed DNA polymerase III adds deoxyribonucleotides to the 3′ end of the primer RNA, which replicates a segment of DNA, the Okazaki fragment. DNA polymerase I then removes the primer RNA and adds deoxyribonucleotides to fill the gaps between adjacent Okazaki fragments. The fragments are finally joined together by DNA ligase to create a continuous DNA chain.

1-9. The answer is c. (*Guyton, pp 134–136. Boron, pp 499–562, 579–582.*) Conduction abnormalities can produce first-degree, second-degree, or third-degree heart block. In a second-degree heart block a P wave is not always followed by a QRS complex as in trace C, where the second P wave is not followed by a QRS complex. In a first-degree heart block, trace D, the interval between the beginning of the P wave and the beginning of the QRS complex (the PR interval) is longer than normal (greater than 0.2 seconds). In a third-degree heart block, conduction between the atria and ventricles is completely blocked so the atrial beats (represented by the P waves) and the ventricular beats (represented by the QRS complex) are completely dissociated.

1-10. The answer is a. (*Greenberg, pp 168–187.*) The nerves innervating the knee and hip exit the spinal cord between L4 and S1. Typical characteristics of a peripheral neuropathy include muscle weakness directed in a more pronounced manner upon the proximal muscles. Depression of tendon reflexes is generally not seen, and muscle wasting might occur only at a very late stage of the disease. Damage to the neuromuscular junction, such as myasthenia gravis, produces a different constellation of deficits. These include muscle fatigue and weakness that is fluctuating. This disorder also typically affects cranial nerves. In addition, the spinal segments indicated (T8–L3) are not associated with the muscle groups in question. Damage to the ventral horn would produce an LMN (flaccid) paralysis, which is not characteristic of the muscle weakness of this patient. Likewise, damage to the lateral funiculus would produce a UMN (spastic) paralysis, and dorsal horn damage would produce sensory deficits as well as affect muscle tone. In addition, the spinal segments indicated in this last choice (e) do not relate to the muscle groups affected in the patient.

1-11. The answer is c. (*Damjanov, pp 1536–1541. Cotran, pp 732–734. Rubin, pp 637–639.*) The segmented or beaded, often dumbbell-shaped bodies are ferruginous bodies that are probably asbestos fibers coated with iron and protein. The term ferruginous body is applied to other inhaled fibers that become iron-coated; however, in a patient with interstitial lung fibrosis or pleural plaques, ferruginous bodies are probably asbestos bodies. The type of asbestos mainly used in America is chrysotile, mined in Canada, and it is much less likely to cause mesothelioma or lung cancer than is crocidolite (blue asbestos), which has limited use and is mined in South Africa. Cigarette smoking potentiates the relatively mild carcinogenic effect of asbestos. In contrast, laminated spherical (Schaumann) bodies are found in granulomas of sarcoid and chronic berylliosis, while *Candida* species histologically may show elongated chains of yeast without hyphae (pseudohyphae), and silica particles are very small and are birefringent.

1-12. The answer is e. *(Murray-Harper's, pp 434–473. Scriver, pp 4029–4240. Sack, pp 121–138.)* The major problem in myasthenia gravis is a marked reduction of acetylcholine receptors on the motor endplate where cranial nerves form a neuromuscular junction with muscles. In these patients, autoantibodies against the acetylcholine receptors effectively reduce receptor numbers. Normally, acetylcholine molecules released by the nerve terminal bind to receptors on the muscle endplate, resulting in a stimulation of contraction by depolarizing the muscle membrane. The condition is improved with drugs that inhibit acetylcholinesterase.

1-13. The answer is d. *(Afifi, pp 513–519. Nolte, pp 46–51.)* The constellation of neurological signs seen in this child is characteristic of the Dandy-Walker syndrome. It involves the presence of hydrocephalus and damage to the cerebellar vermis. The other choices constitute developmental disorders affecting other regions of the CNS, such as the spinal cord or cerebral cortex, which do not produce the syndromes in this case.

1-14. The answer is d. *(Craig, p 94; Hardman, pp 137, 146, 242, 249; Katzung, pp 81, 84, 146, 189.)* Whether you memorize that yohimbine is a selective α_2 antagonist is up to you, but you should know what the main effects of an α_2 antagonist are. That, of course, depends on knowing what α_2 receptors—at least in the peripheral autonomic nervous system—do. Recall that the preponderance of physiologically important α_2 receptors are located on adrenergic nerve terminals or adrenergic nerve "endings." When stimulated by a suitable agonist, the response is a turning-off of further norepinephrine release. Because norepinephrine is the neurotransmitter released from adrenergic nerves and it is an excellent α agonist, the pre-synaptic $α_2$ receptors upon which norepinephrine acts serve as the main physiologic mechanism for regulating neurotransmitter release.

So, when we activate those receptors with yohimbine, we enhance overall activity of the sympathetic nervous system by interfering with nor-epinephrine's ability to turn-off its own release. Of the responses listed, only hypertension (owing to the vasoconstrictor effects of norepinephrine on postsynaptic α-adrenergic receptors) occurs as a result of yohimbine (or of norepinephrine excess).

1-15. The answer is a. (*Coe, pp 1042–1052. Cotran, pp 1225–1227. Greenspan, pp 326–329. Braunwald, pp 1237–1239.*) The correct diagnosis is Paget's disease, also known as osteitis deformans because of its deforming capabilities (e.g., skull or femoral head enlargement). In this disease the serum calcium is normal, but there is an increase in osteoclastic activity (osteolytic lesions and elevated 24-hour urine hydroxyproline) and an increase in osteoblastic activity (elevated osteocalcin and alkaline phosphatase). Patients with Paget's disease exhibit a marked increase in osteoid, and the bone actually enlarges. The osteoid is never normally mineralized in this disease. In this patient, the bone scan shows significant uptake of labeled bisphosphonates, which are incorporated into newly formed osteoid during bone formation. Her proximal femur is enlarged and no longer fits properly into the acetabulum, which results in the hip pain.

There are a number of useful biochemical markers of bone metabolism. Osteoclasts synthesize tartrate-resistant acid phosphatase so that increased osteoclastic activity is reflected in increased serum levels of tartrate-resistant acid phosphatase. Bone resorption fragments of type I collagen and noncollagenous proteins increase as bone matrix is resorbed. Hydroxyproline is a good urinary marker of bone metabolism because hydroxyproline is released and excreted in the urine as collagen is broken down. The presence of pyridinoline cross-links, which are involved in the bundling of type I collagen, is used for measurement of bone resorption. Those cross-links are released only during degradation of mineralized collagen fibrils as occurs in bone resorption. Usually, pyridinoline cross-links are measured by immunoassay over a 24-hour period to detect excess bone resorption and collagen breakdown in disorders such as Paget's disease.

Markers of bone formation include osteocalcin, alkaline phosphatase, and the extension peptides of type I collagen. Osteocalcin is a vitamin

K–dependent GLA (γ-carboxyglutamic acid) protein that is synthesized by osteoblasts and secreted into the serum in an unchanged state. Serum concentrations of osteocalcin are, therefore, directly related to osteoblastic activity. It is a more specific marker than the marker alkaline phosphatase, because other organs, such as the liver and kidney, produce that enzyme.

Radiologic methods such as conventional x-ray can be used to detect osteoporosis, but only after patients have lost 30 to 50% of their bone mass. Dual-beam photon absorptiometry allows a much more accurate diagnosis of loss of bone mass.

1-16. The answer is a. (*Brooks, pp 304, 305. Levinson, p 167. Murray— 2002, pp 407–408. Ryan, p 478.*) All the listed diseases except Q fever are tick-borne. The rickettsia *C. burnetii* causes Q fever, and humans are usually infected by aerosol of a sporelike form shed in milk, urine, feces, or placenta of infected sheep, cattle, or goats. Lyme disease is caused by a spirochete, *Borrelia burgdorferi*, and produces the characteristic lesion erythema chronicum migrans (ECM). The etiologic agent of Rocky Mountain spotted fever is *R. rickettsia*. It usually produces a rash that begins in the extremities and then involves the trunk. Two human forms of ehrlichiosis can occur: human monocytic ehrlichiosis (HME), caused by *E. chaffeensis*, and human granulocytic ehrlichiosis (HGE), caused by an as yet unnamed *Ehrlichia*. Ehrlichiosis was previously recognized only as a veterinary pathogen. HME infection is transmitted by the brown dog tick and *A. americanum*. HGE infection is transmitted by *I. scapularis*, the same tick that transmits Lyme disease. Both infections cause fever and leukopenia. A rash rarely occurs. *E. chaffeensis* infects monocytes, and HGE infects granulocytes; both organisms produce inclusion bodies called *morulae*. *Francisella tularensis* is a small, gram-negative, nonmotile coccobacillus. Humans most commonly acquire the organism after contact with the tissues or body fluid of an infected mammal or the bite of an infected tick.

1-17. The answer is c. (*Murray, pp 145–152. Scriver, pp 1521–1552. Sack, pp 121–138.*) The child has symptoms of glycogen storage disease. Glycogen is a glucose polymer with linear regions linked through the C1 aldehyde of one glucose to the C4 alcohol of the next (α-1,4-glucoside linkage). There are also branches from the linear glycogen polymer that have α-1,6-glucoside linkages. Glycogen is synthesized during times of carbohydrate and energy surplus, but must be degraded during fasting to provide energy. Separate enzymes for breakdown include phosphylases (α-1,4-glucosidases) that cleave linear regions of glycogen and debranching enzymes (α-1,6-glucosidases) that cleave branch points. Glucose-6-phosphatase is needed in the liver to liberate free glucose from glucose-6-phosphate, providing fuel for other organs. There is no glucose-6-phosphatase in muscle, and muscle glycogenolysis provides energy just for muscle with production of lactate. Deficiencies of more than eight enzymes involved in glycogenolysis, including those mentioned, can produce glycogen storage disease.

1-18. The answer is c. *(Craig, pp 324–326; Hardman, pp 546–548; Katzung, pp 499, 505, 511–512.)* Pentazocine is a mixed agonist-antagonist on opioid receptors. When a partial agonist, such as pentazocine, displaces a full agonist, such as methadone, the receptor is less activated; this leads to withdrawal syndrome in an opioid-dependent person.

1-19. The answer is d. *(Moore and Dalley, pp 669–670, 810.)* The large arrows indicate the proximal humeral epiphyseal plate. The young girl was only 11 and still growing. The epiphyseal plates show up on x-rays as radiolucent cartilage and should not be confused with a fracture. The epiphysis is located at the anatomic neck of the humerus but is not discoid-shaped like many epiphyseal plates in long bones. This plate is tent-shaped, which is why it is not clearly visible all the way across the proximal humerus.

1-20. The answer is e. *(Craig, p 154; Hardman, pp 810–811; Katzung, pp 205–207.)* Digitalis inhibits the sarcolemmal Na^+, K^+-ATPase ("sodium pump"). This reduces the active (ATP-dependent) extrusion of intracellular Na^+. The excess intracellular Na^+ competes with intracellular Ca^{2+} for sites on a sarcolemmal 2Na-Ca exchange diffusion carrier. The net result is a rise of free $[Ca^{2+}]_i$ and greater actin-myosin interactions (i.e., an increased inotropic state).

1-21. The answer is a. *(Braunwald, pp 494, 617.)* AFP is secreted by nonseminoma GCT, whereas β-hCG is seen in both nonseminoma and seminoma. Approximately 70% of persons with nonseminoma GCT have elevated AFP levels. It is specific to nonseminoma GCT. Human chorionic gonadotropin (hCG) is secreted by both nonseminoma and seminoma GCTs. The half-life of αFP is 5 to 7 days. Monoclonal immunoglobulin is produced in multiple myeloma; carcinoembryonic antigen (CEA) in adeno-carcinomas of the colon, pancreas, breast, and lung; lactate dehydrongenase (LDH) in lymphoma and Ewing's sarcoma; and, CD30 in Hodgkin's disease.

I-22. The answer is c. (*Craig, p 246; Hardman, pp 702–704; Katzung, p 250.*) Thiazides and thiazide-like diuretics (e.g., chlorthalidone, metola-zone) may elevate blood glucose levels and cause frank hyperglycemia. The loop diuretics may do the same.

Several mechanisms have been proposed to explain the effect: decreased release of insulin from the pancreas, increased glycogenolysis and decreased glucogenesis, and a reduction in the conversion of proinsulin to insulin.

[You might want to recall that diazoxide (mainly used as a parenteral drug for prompt lowering of elevated blood pressure) can be used, orally, to raise blood glucose levels in some hypoglycemic states. It is, chemically, a thiazide but is not a diuretic.]

I-23. The answer is b. (*Kandel, pp 82–83, 700–704.*) In a peripheral neu-ropathy, there may be damage to either the myelin or the axon directly, although more often there is damage to the myelin. Because of myelin (or axonal) damage, there is a reduction (or loss) of conduction velocity. The disorder may affect both sensory and motor components of the peripheral nerve, thereby causing dysfunction in both the sensory and the motor processes associated with that nerve. Because there is peripheral neuronal damage, the motor loss will be reflected in a weakness, paralysis, or reflex activity associated with the affected muscle, as well as impairment of sen-sation.

I-24. The answer is d. (*Guyton, pp 74, 816, 968–970. Boron, pp 1244–1245.*) Phosphocreatine is rapidly converted to ATP in muscle. When the meta-bolic demands exceed the rate at which ATP can be generated by aerobic metabolism or glycolysis, phosphocreatine can supply the necessary ATP for a brief period of time. An increase in the concentration of phosphocre-atine in muscle may increase the amount of ATP that can be produced and therefore enhance performance.

I-25. The answer is a. (*Cotran, p 1272. McKenzie, p 194. Alberts, pp 1299–1300.*) The satellite cells in the skeletal muscle fiber proliferate and recon-stitute the damaged part of the myofibers. They are supportive cells for maintenance of muscle and a source of new myofibers after injury or after increased load. There is no dedifferentiation of myocytes into myoblasts (answer b), and fusion of damaged myofibers to form new myotubes (answer c). Hypertrophy, not hyperplasia (answer d), occurs in existing myofibers in response to increased load on the muscle as occurs during exercise and in the response of muscle to damage. Proliferation of fibroblasts (answer e) may occur in the damaged area but leads to fibrosis, not repair of skeletal muscle. The multinucleate organization of skeletal muscle is derived developmentally by fusion and not by amitosis (failure of cytokinesis after DNA synthesis). Mitotic activity is terminated after fusion occurs. In the development of skeletal muscle, myoblasts of mesodermal origin undergo cell proliferation. Myocyte cell division ceases soon after birth. Myoblasts, which are mononucleate cells, fuse with each other end to end to form myotubes. This process requires cell recognition between myoblasts, alignment, and subsequent fusion.

1-26. The answer is d. (*Cotran, pp 589–591. Rubin, pp 583–584.*) Most tumors involving the heart are secondary to metastases, most commonly from bronchogenic carcinoma or breast carcinoma, and they usually involve the pericardium. Primary tumors of the heart are quite rare; the most common in the adult is the myxoma. These tumors occur most often in the left atrium, and if pedunculated they may interfere with the mitral valve by a "ball valve" effect. Histologically they are composed of stellate cells in a loose myxoid background. In contrast, rhabdomyomas are the most common primary cardiac tumors in infants and children and often occur in association with tuberous sclerosis. Histologically, so-called spider cells may be seen. Papillary fibroelastomas usually are incidental lesions found at the time of autopsy and are probably hamartomas rather than true neoplasms.

1-27. The answer is b. (*Brooks, pp 545–548. Levinson, pp 306–307. Murray— 2002, pp 651–654. Ryan, pp 672–676.*) H. capsulatum infection is highest in the United States, especially in the Ohio and Mississippi river valleys. Numerous outbreaks have resulted from exposure of many persons to inocula of conidia. These occur when the organism is disturbed from its natural habitat, soil mixed with bird feces or bat guano. Feces provides an excellent culture for fungal growth to occur. Some 80 to 90% of residents in certain endemic areas may have positive skin tests. Histoplasmosis is not transmissible from person to person.

I-28. The answer is d. (*Cotran, pp 864–867. Chandrasoma, pp 643–645.*) Several clinical syndromes may develop after exposure to any of the viruses that cause hepatitis, including asymptomatic hepatitis, acute hepatitis, fulminant hepatitis, chronic hepatitis, and the carrier state. Asymptomatic infection in individuals is documented by serologic abnormalities only. Liver biopsies in patients with acute hepatitis, either the anicteric phase or the icteric phase, reveal focal necrosis of hepatocytes (forming Councilman bodies) and lobular disarray resulting from ballooning degeneration of the hepatocytes. These changes are nonspecific, but the additional finding of fatty change is suggestive of hepatitis C virus (HCV) infection. Clinically, acute viral hepatitis is classified into three phases. During the prodrome phase, patients may develop symptoms that include anorexia, nausea and vomiting, headaches, photophobia, and myalgia. An unusual symptom associated with acute viral hepatitis is altered olfaction and taste, especially the loss of taste for coffee and cigarettes. The next phase, the icteric phase, involves jaundice produced by increased bilirubin. Patients may also develop light stools and dark urine (due to disrupted bile flow) and ecchymoses (due to decreased vitamin K). The final phase is the convalescence phase. Fulminant hepatitis refers to massive necrosis and is seen in about 1% of patients with either hepatitis B or C, but very rarely with hepatitis A infection. The biggest risk for fulminant hepatitis is coinfection with both hepatitis B and D. Chronic hepatitis is defined as elevated serum liver enzymes for longer than 6 months. Patients may be either symptomatic or asymptomatic.

I-29. The answer is a. (*Murray, pp 358–373, 498–513. Scriver, pp 5559–5628. Sack, pp 1–40.*) The decreased amount of AAT protein, its abnormal mobility, and the engorgement of liver ER suggest a mutant AAT that is inefficiently transported from the ER to serum. Since other serum protein abnormalities were not mentioned, general deficiencies of protein synthesis arising from defective energy metabolism or defective signal recognition particles are unlikely. A mutation affecting the N-terminal methionine of AAT or its signal sequence should drastically decrease its synthesis and import to the ER lumen. This would not explain the engorgement of liver ER. The usual binding of the signal recognition particle to the signal sequence of AAT, followed by import into the ER lumen, seems intact. An altered amino acid necessary for signal peptidase cleavage of the signal sequence of AAT might be invoked, but a general deficiency of the signal peptidase should disrupt many secreted proteins and be an embryonic lethal mutation. AAT deficiency (107400) is a well-characterized autosomal dominant disease with common ZZ, SZ, and SS genotypes that can cause childhood liver disease and adult emphysema. The Z and S mutations alter AAT conformation and interfere with its secretion from ER to serum. Lack of AAT protection from proteases in lung is thought to cause the thinning of alveolar walls and dysfunctional "air sacs" of emphysema. The figure below illustrates how changes in the DNA code can effect protein products.

1-30. The answer is a. *(Guyton, pp 655–656.)* Ataxia, dysmetria, and an intention tremor all are classic findings in a patient with a lesion involving the cerebellum. Affected persons also exhibit adiadochokinesia, which is a loss of ability to accomplish a swift succession of oscillatory movements, such as moving a finger rapidly up and down. These symptoms all result from destruction of the normal feedback mechanisms that are coordinated in the cerebellum.

1-31. The answer is a. *(Baum, pp 297–301.)* Progressive muscle relaxation, or a reasonable variation, can serve as a powerful therapeutic technique for treating generalized anxiety, insomnia, headaches, neck tension, and mild forms of agitated depression. It has also effectively been used to reduce pain, the side effects of cancer chemotherapy, nausea, and mild hypertension, preferably before pharmacologic intervention. Relaxation therapy is based on the premise and observation that muscle tension is a physiologic response to anxiety and stress. There is a significant reduction in experienced anxiety if tense muscles can be relaxed. Muscle relaxation also can change the physiologic activation process. The Jacobson relaxation procedure involves tensing selected muscles for about 10 seconds, and then completely relaxing them and noticing the difference in sensation. Eventually, the patient is able to relax particular muscle groups from their present level of tension. Other effective methods of relaxation include systematic deep breathing, transcendental meditation, and yoga.

I-32. The answer is d. (*Braunwald, p 826.*) Acute osteomyelitis shows bacteria, polymorphonuclear leukocytes, and congested and thrombosed blood vessels. Its course is not prolonged, as is the course of chronic osteomyelitis. Necrotic bone, presence of granulation and fibrous tissues, very few bacteria, and the absence of living osteocytes characterize chronic osteomyelitis.

I-33 The answer is e. (*Cotran, pp 1138–1140. Rubin, pp 1166–1167.*) Goiter is a general clinical term that is used to describe any enlargement of the thyroid. Most patients with goiter are euthyroid (nonfunctional goiter), as hyperthyroidism (toxic goiter) is relatively rare. In the early stages of goiter formation, there is diffuse hyperplasia of the small thyroid follicles, which histologically resembles the changes of Graves' disease. This early stage is called a diffuse nontoxic goiter or simple goiter. The thyroid gland then undergoes repeated episodes of involution and hyperplasia. Over time this produces an enlarged multinodular goiter that histologically consists of multiple nodules, some of which consist of colloid-filled enlarged follicles and others of which show hyperplasia of small follicles lined by active epithelium. There are also areas of fibrosis, hemorrhage, calcification, and cystic degeneration. The last stage of goiter formation consists of nodules composed primarily of enlarged colloid-filled follicles. This stage is called a colloid goiter.

In contrast to the histologic appearance of multinodular or colloid goiter, diffuse toxic goiter (Graves' disease) is characterized by hyperplasia of the follicular cells with scalloping of colloid at the margin of follicles, while Hashimoto's thyroiditis has a marked lymphoplasmacytic infiltrate with lymphoid follicles and scattered oxyphilic (Hürthle) cells.

I-34. The answer is b. (*McPhee, p 360.*) The goal for improving the symptoms of GERD is to increase or maintain the LES pressure. High-protein meals generally increase LES pressure and should be encouraged. Fats, chocolate, and alcohol decrease LES pressure and these foods should be avoided. Carbohydrate content does not affect motility.

I-35. The answer is d. (*Behrman, pp 577–578, 1358–1359. Damjanov, pp 1473–1483. Cotran, pp 471–473. Ravel, pp 549–550.*) Hyaline membrane disease (HMD), which accounts for 20% of all deaths in the first 28 days of life, is basically a disease of premature infants; most affected infants weigh 1000 to 1500 g. Contributing factors in the development of HMD include diabetes in the mother (maternal diabetes with increased glucose causes increased fetal secretion of insulin, which inhibits the effects of steroids such as lung maturation and production of surfactant) and cesarean section. Infants who develop HMD appear normal at birth, but within minutes to hours their respirations become labored. Grossly the lungs are a mottled, red-purple color, while microscopically there are hyaline membranes in air spaces, similar to those of ARDS.

Two defects have been identified in infants with HMD. One is a deficiency of pulmonary surfactant. Surfactant, a lipid consisting of dipalmitoyl phosphatidylcholine, reduces the surface tension in air-fluid interfaces by getting between the molecules in the liquid and reducing their attraction to each other. This reduces the tendency for the alveoli to collapse after birth on expiration. Synthesis of surfactant increases throughout fetal development, but becomes maximal at 34 to 36 weeks. With a deficiency of surfactant, the lungs tend to collapse on expiration (atelectasis) and become stiff. The other defect is increased pulmonary epithelial permeability. This accounts for the protein-rich edema fluid in the alveoli and also for the formation of hyaline membranes. The most reliable test to determine pulmonary maturity is the ratio of lecithin to sphingomyelin (L/S), both of which are phospholipids. The production of lecithin (phosphatidylcholine) begins at 5 months of gestation, but secretion begins at 7 months of gestation, and levels rise sharply at 34 to 36 weeks of gestation. The level of sphingomyelin does not change during this time. An L/S ratio of about 2 indicates fetal maturity, 1.2 indicates a possible risk, and below 1 indicates a definite risk.

Mild cases of HMD can be treated with oxygen, while moderate cases can be treated with continuous positive airway pressure (CPAP). Severe cases may need to be treated with a ventilator with the administration of artificial surfactant.

1-36. The answer is c. (*Craig, pp 464–465; Hardman, pp 666, 670; Katzung, pp 328–329, 332.*) Given the severity of symptoms and the speed with which they are worsening, the only appropriate approach is to start the patient on an daily oral steroid until symptom control is deemed adequate and sufficiently long-lasting. At that time, carefully tapering the oral steroid and starting the inhaled agent (beclomethasone, triamcinolone, others) might be appropriate.

Although corticosteroid therapy, per se, is the correct approach, beginning the therapy change by adding an inhaled steroid (rather than starting oral treatment) would not be suitable. Inhaled steroids are efficacious, but it takes roughly 2 or more weeks of continued use until meaningful control of airway inflammation and symptoms develops. Given the nature of the patient's rapidly worsening symptoms, we do not have the luxury of time. (As noted in the paragraph above, however, it would be very reasonable to add an inhaled steroid to the sympathomimetic regimen after we have good control with an oral drug such as prednisone.)

Cromolyn would not be a good choice. The onset of this inhaled drug is slow, too, and it will be of little benefit with the quickly worsening asthma attacks. It might be considered as a prophylactic measure sometime later (after the current situation is well under control), and it would probably be suitable as an add-on only if we can determine that the asthma attacks are largely due to atopy (allergic responses).

Theophylline is not a good choice. Although it may have some prophylactic value, it will be of little benefit should acute attacks continue, as they are likely to do for a while. Other reasons why theophylline is not a good choice are its low therapeutic index (or margin of safety), the prevalence of side effects (CNS and cardiovascular stimulation), and the need for frequent blood testing to help guide dosing adjustments. Overall, theophylline and other methylxanthines are becoming passé.

Doubling the albuterol dose is a poor approach. The continuation of asthma attacks—indeed, the apparent worsening—may be due to at least two issues: (1) continued and perhaps worsening airway inflammation, which will not be suppressed with any sympathomimetic; and (2) potential airway tolerance to the actions of the adrenergic agent. Doubling the dose may briefly overcome the tolerance, but tolerance to the increased dose eventually would develop too. Moreover, increasing the dose of this "selective" β_2 agonist would likely be associated with adverse cardiovascular stimulation, because preferential β_2 activation is lost with increased dosages; the lost selectivity implies increased β_1 stimulation.

Switching from albuterol to salmeterol would be a poor choice. This slow- and long-acting adrenergic agonist is useful for prophylaxis (for some patients), but it will be of little help for this boy, given his frequent and worsening attacks. The salmeterol would be largely useless should an acute attack occur again. Even if we started therapy with salmeterol and instructed the patient to keep his albuterol inhaler and use it to abort attacks, we would be doing nothing beneficial for the underlying pathophysiologic problem: the airway inflammation.

1-37. The answer is e. *(Brooks, pp 562–563. Levinson, pp 318–319. Murray— 2002, pp 701–703. Ryan, pp 745–748.)* G. lamblia is the only common protozoan found in the duodenum and jejenum. Tropozoites are commonly found in the duodenum and do not penetrate the tissues. Four nucleii cysts (infective stage) can remain viable for up to four months. Excystation is via digestive enzymes. The mechanical irritation to tissues leads to diarrhea, with increased fat and mucus in the foul-smelling stool. Malabsorption syndrome (vitamin A and fats) leads to weight loss, anorexia, electrolyte imbalance, and abdominal cramps. Children and immunocompromised individuals are most significantly affected. Giardiasis should be considered in the differential diagnosis of any "traveler's diarrhea."

1-38. The answer is d. *(Hardman, p 468; Katzung, pp 271, 483, 492–494, 991.)* This patient has what is almost certainly the serotonin syndrome. The triptan "adds" serotonin to the circulation, and its neuronal reuptake will be blocked by fluoxetine (or sertraline, others), which is classified as a selective serotonin reuptake inhibitor (SSRI) antidepressant. When sumatriptan (or other triptans used for migraine) is added, rapid accumulation of serotonin and/or the triptan in the brain can occur. The other drugs listed are not likely to interact—at least not in the way described here.

1-39. The answer is b. *(Cotran, p 465. Rubin, pp 217, 865.)* Failure of the metanephric diverticulum to develop normally leads to bilateral renal agenesis, which in turn leads to a constellation of symptoms called Potter's syndrome (sequence). The kidneys are important for the circulation of amniotic fluid. The fetus swallows amniotic fluid (about 400 mL/day), and then absorbs it in the respiratory and digestive tracts. Waste products cross the placental membrane and enter maternal blood in the intervillous space. Excess water is excreted by the fetal kidneys into the amniotic fluid. Developmental abnormalities that impair fetal swallowing of amniotic fluid, such as esophageal atresia or severe anomalies of the CNS, lead to polyhydramnios (too much amniotic fluid), while agenesis of the kidneys or urinary obstruction leads to oligohydramnios (too little amniotic fluid). The oligohydramnios leads to characteristic facial features that include wide-set eyes; low-set, floppy ears; and a broad, flat nose.

In contrast to absence of the kidneys, absence of the thymus is seen with DiGeorge's syndrome, and congenital biliary atresia is a cause of neonatal jaundice. Urinary bladder exstrophy results from persistence of the cloacal membrane, while multicystic dysplasia of the kidney (MCDK) is the most common cause of an abdominal mass in a newborn. Most cases of unilateral MCDK involute spontaneously.

1-40. The answer is d. (*Boron, pp 603, 616–621.*) Surfactant is composed of a lipid called dipalmitoylphosphatidylcholine and a variety of proteins. It reduces the surface tension (increases the compliance) of the lung and makes it easier for the lung to expand, thereby reducing the work of breathing. Without surfactant, the respiratory muscles may not be able to produce adequate ventilation, leading to hypercapnia and hypoxia. The increase in compliance results in an increase in FRC. The patient's acid-base status will improve and bicarbonate will return toward normal. Bronchiole smooth muscle tone may have contributed to the ventilatory difficulties of the patient but the inability of NO to improve her condition indicates that the primary problem was not related to airway constriction.

1-41. The answer is b. (*Siegel, pp 326–333.*) Excitatory amino acids and, in particular, the glutamate family of compounds have long been thought to play an important role in epileptiform activity. Epileptiform activity typically includes AMPA-receptor activation. However, as the seizure becomes more intense, there is increased involvement of NMDA receptors. This is evidenced by the facts that NMDA antagonists can reduce the intensity and length of the seizure activity and that, following removal of human epileptic hippocampal tissue, there is an up-regulation of both AMPA and NMDA receptors. Metabotropic glutamate receptors have been shown to be present in the retina but have not yet been demonstrated to be present in regions of the brain that are typically epileptogenic. GABA and glycine are inhibitory transmitters; therefore, seizures would logically block such receptor activation. There has been no substantive evidence concerning the role of cortical nicotinic receptors in epilepsy.

1-42. The answer is c. (*Damjanov, pp 2630–2634. Cotran, pp 1248–1251.*) Pannus is the name given to describe the classic destructive joint lesion found in individuals with rheumatoid arthritis. This lesion is characterized by proliferation of the synovium (hyperplasia) along with numerous chronic inflammatory cells. The thickened synovial membrane may develop villous projections, which can destroy the joint cartilage. Nodular collections of lymphocytes resembling follicles are characteristically seen along with numerous plasma cells. Palisades of proliferating cells may surround areas of necrosis. This latter histologic appearance can be seen in subcutaneous nodules (rheumatoid nodules), but rheumatoid arthritis most frequently affects the small joints of the hands and feet. Larger joints are involved later. In contrast to a pannus, gummas are seen with syphilis, while tophi are found with gout. Finally, eburnation describes the "polished" appearance of the bone affected by degenerative joint disease, while spondylosis refers to a degenerative process of the vertebrae that can compress the spinal cord and its nerve roots.

1-43. The answer is d. *(Parslow, pp 326–327, 739.)* GVHD occurs due to attack by the graft against the recipient. There are three requirements for GVHD rejection: (1) histocompatibility differences between the graft (donor) and host (recipient), (2) immunocompetent graft cells, and (3) immunodeficient host cell. Immunocompetent graft cells may be "passenger" lymphocytes or major cells transplanted and must be present in the graft. Prevention of GVHD is essential, as there is no adequate treatment once it is established.

1-44. The answer is c. *(Braunwald, pp 348, 350–351, 656, 658, 666, 2019.)* Normal hematocrit for a woman is 37 to 47%. The most likely cause of the anemia is renal failure leading to decreased production of the kidney-derived red blood cell growth factor, erythropoietin (answers a and b). In the initial stages of renal failure the kidneys will increase their production of erythropoietin, but as renal damage continues, the cells that produce this factor are destroyed. Therefore, there are initially increased levels of reticulocytes (immature red blood cells) in the bloodstream, but this is later reversed, as in the anemia of renal disease, low production of reticulocytes is a hallmark of the disease. Although the patient may have decreased estrogen levels, estrogen decreases hematocrit (answers d and e). Also, women who are pregnant (third trimester) can have slightly decreased hematocrits [37 + 6 (third trimester pregnant women) vs. 40 + 6 (adult women) and 42 + 6 (postmenopausal women)]. However, this patient had a negative pregnancy test. Administration of recombinant erythropoietin (EPO) is the preferred treatment for anemia caused by advanced renal disease. Generally, EPO is administered if the hematocrit is less than 30%.

Erythropoietin is synthesized by the peritubular (interstitial) cells of the kidney cortex, stimulates the differentiation of cells from the erythrocyte colony–forming units (E-CFUs), and stimulates the differentiation and release of reticulocytes from the bone marrow. Colony-forming units (CFUs) are distinct cell lineages derived from pluripotential stem cells in the bone marrow.

I-45. The answer is a. (*Cotran, p 637. Henry, pp 628–636, 650–651.*) Platelet aggregation refers to platelets binding to other platelets. One mechanism for this involves fibrinogen, which can act as a molecular bridge between adjacent platelets by binding to GpIIb and GpIIIa receptors on the surface of platelets. Abnormalities of platelet aggregation (aggregation defects or primary wave defects) include Glanzmann's thrombasthenia and afibrinogenemia. Patients with Glanzmann's thrombasthenia have a deficiency of GpIIb-IIIa and defective platelet aggregation. Patients with low or no fibrinogen levels characteristically have prolonged PT, PTT, and TT values: in fact, they are so prolonged they are unmeasurable.

In contrast to platelet aggregation, platelet secretion refers to the secretion of the contents of two types of granules within the platelet cytoplasm. α granules contain fibrinogen, fibronectin, and platelet-derived growth factor, while dense bodies contain ADP, ionized calcium, histamine, epinephrine, and serotonin. Decreased platelet secretion (activation defects) is seen with deficiencies of these granules; these diseases are called storage pool defects. They can involve either α granules (gray platelet syndrome) or dense bodies (Chédiak-Higashi syndrome, Wiskott-Aldrich syndrome, or TAR). Wiskott-Aldrich syndrome is an X-linked disorder that is characterized by eczema, thrombocytopenia (small platelets), and immunodeficiency consisting of decreased levels of IgM and progressive loss of T cell function. These patients have recurrent infections with bacteria, viruses, and fungi. TAR refers to the combination of thrombocytopenia and absent radii.

I-46. The answer is e. (*Katzung, pp 1034–1036.*) You've all done the experiment: mix vinegar and baking soda (sodium bicarbonate) and one product is CO_2. This gas is formed when sodium bicarbonate—still used as a lay remedy for heartburn and other acid-related GI disturbances—reacts with HCl.

Normally intragastric pressure is kept in check when the gastroesophageal sphincter opens. However, when pressure can't be relieved quickly enough, or adequately, the stomach will distend. In the presence of ulcers the lesions can be stretched mechanically, favoring further damage that can lead to acute bleeding. Even in the absence of ulcers, any weakness of the gastric wall can lead to gastric rupture. (This ostensibly bizarre outcome, leading to bleeding or rupture, has been documented.)

None of the other antacids listed, whether alone or in combination, lead to production of CO_2 or any other gas that might lead to the outcome described in the scenario.

1-47. The answer is a. (*Murray, pp 249–263. Scriver, pp 1971–2006. Sack, pp 121–138.*) Lack of the enzyme homogentisate oxidase causes the accumulation of homogentisic acid, a metabolite in the pathway of degradation of phenylalanine and tyrosine. Homogentisate, like tyrosine, contains a phenol group. It is excreted in the urine, where it oxidizes and is polymerized to a dark substance upon standing. Under normal conditions, phenylalanine is degraded to tyrosine, which is broken down through a series of steps to fumarate and acetoacetate. The dark pigment melanin is another end product of this pathway. Deficiency of homogentisate oxidase is called alkaptonuria (black urine), a mild disease discovered by Sir Archibald Garrod, the pioneer of biochemical genetics. Garrod's geneticist colleague, William Bateson, recognized that alkaptonuria, like nearly all enzyme deficiencies, exhibits autosomal recessive inheritance.

1-48. The answer is d. (*Braunwald, pp 1265–1266.*) The patient's longstanding history of hypertension and EKG findings are most consistent with left ventricular hypertrophy. The large voltage described may also be seen as a normal variant in a young person or in a well-trained athlete. A tall R wave in V_1 with right axis deviation is consistent with *right* ventricular hypertrophy, that, for example, would be seen in a patient with severe lung disease or pulmonary stenosis. A bundle branch block is not related to voltage or left ventricular thickness, but rather a conduction abnormality within the His bundle. ST segment elevation in most leads is consistent with a diagnosis of pericarditis. Note that the repolarization changes associated with left ventricular hypertrophy will involve ST *depression* and T wave inversions. This pattern is described as repolarization changes or "strain" and it is associated with the high voltage caused by left ventricular hypertrophy. Q-T interval prolongation is consistent with several drug effects and to long-standing hypertension.

1-49. The answer is e. *(Baum, pp 153–155.)* Nancy Frazer-Smith (University of Montreal) conducted a controlled experimental study involving 500 patients with heart disease who were very stressed. For half of the group, she designed an experimental program with the hypothesis that life-stress often precedes myocardial infarction (MI) and recurrent heart attacks. The experimental group received regular telephone follow-up to monitor their stress status and home visits by the project nurse to assess the causes of increased distress and to work with the patients to help resolve and reduce the high level of stress through counseling, emotional support, and stress reduction therapy. The control group received the best traditional medical care. After a year, the behavioral intervention resulted in a reduction of cardiac deaths by 50%. Furthermore, the reduced death rate persisted for six months after the program ended. Reduction of MI reoccurrences persisted for seven years after the program. It was concluded that the stress reduction program provided needed social and emotional support to reduce stress, depression, and feelings of helplessness and distress, thus reducing physiologic arousal and its damaging effects on the cardiovascular system. An additional conclusion, perhaps of equal importance, was the need for individualized tailoring of prevention and intervention for each patient.

1-50. The answer is a. *(Cotran, pp 1098–1101. Rubin, pp 1034–1035.)* Fibrocystic change of the breast is one of the most common features seen in the female breast. It is most likely associated with an endocrine imbalance that causes an abnormality of the normal monthly cyclic events within the breast. These fibrocystic changes are subdivided into nonproliferative and proliferative changes. Nonproliferative changes include fibrosis of the stroma and cystic dilation of the terminal ducts, which when large may form blue-domed cysts. A common feature of the ducts in nonproliferative changes is apocrine metaplasia, which refers to epithelial cells with abundant eosinophilic cytoplasm with apical snouts. Proliferative changes include epithelial hyperplasia of the ducts. This hyperplastic epithelium may form papillary structures (papillomatosis when pronounced) or may be quite abnormal (atypical hyperplasia). Two benign, but clinically important, forms of proliferative fibrocystic change include sclerosing adenosis and radial scar. Both of these may be mistaken histologically for infiltrating ductal carcinoma, but the presence of myoepithelial cells is a helpful sign that points to the benign nature of the proliferation. Sclerosing adenosis is a disease of the terminal lobules that is typically seen in patients 35 to 45 years old. It produces a firm mass, most often located in the upper outer quadrant. Microscopically there is florid proliferation of small ductal structures in a fibrous stroma, which on low power is stellate in appearance and somewhat maintains the normal lobular architecture. A radial scar refers to ductal proliferation around a central fibrotic area.

BLOCK 2

Answers

2-1. The answer is e. (*Boron, pp 641, 648–649. Guyton, pp 360–363.*) The patient's condition is caused by a decrease in the serum concentration of ionized calcium (Ca^{2+}), which increases nerve and muscle excitability, leading to spontaneous axonal discharges and muscle contractions. Decreased Ca^{2+} concentration can result from a respiratory alkalosis because the H^+ that dissociates from plasma proteins in the presence of a high pH is replaced by Ca^{2+}. Although both a P_aCO_2 of 30 mmHg and a P_aCO_2 of 15 mmHg are consistent with respiratory alkalosis, only the combination of a P_aCO_2 of 20 mmHg and a HCO_3^- of 20 mM, produces an alkaline pH (7.6). The combination of a P_aCO_2 of 30 mmHg and a HCO_3^- of 15 mM is caused by a metabolic acidosis.

2-2. The answer is b. (*Moore and Dalley, pp 621, 626.*) The medial meniscus is attached to the medial collateral ligament. It is relatively immovable and, therefore, unable to evade damage such as occurred in this case. The medial meniscus is clearly not attached to the popliteus muscle or to the anterior cruciate ligament.

2-3. The answer is b. (*Craig, p 773; Hardman, pp 1705–1706; Katzung, p 706.*) The most common side effect of the newer sulfonylureas (glyburide, glipizide, glimeperide) is hypoglycemia, and the relative incidence is higher than with any of the other drugs listed.

Normally insulin release peaks in response to a meal. That occurs even when there is a relative insulin deficiency (type 2 diabetes mellitus). Our hypothetical meal-skipping patient essentially fasts all day. His blood glucose levels will tend to fall as the meal-free interval progresses, and during this time physiologic insulin release would be relatively low. However, the newer sulfonylureas—glyburide, glipizide, glimeperide—act by causing insulin release, whether one has eaten or fasted. Thus, the hypoglycemic effect of the drug will enhance the tendency for hypoglycemia that accompanies fasting or that occurs with increased physical activity. This is likely to apply even in the presence of insulin resistance, which is common.

Acarbose is an α-glucosidase inhibitor. The main effect of that drug is a slowed rate of carbohydrate absorption from the gut. This blunts the insulin response to rising blood glucose levels. Because acarbose's effects center on inhibiting dietary carbohydrate absorption, the drug's effects will not occur in the absence of those foodstuffs. Indeed, effects are better when the drug is taken with or right before meals, and it seems to be more efficacious as the amount of carbohydrate in the meal increases.

Metformin does not directly increase or decrease insulin secretion. In contrast with the sulfonylureas, which are correctly classified as hypoglycemic drugs (i.e., they drive blood glucose levels down), the biguanides are *antihyperglycemic*, tending instead to keep blood glucose levels from going up.

Pioglitazone (a thiazolidinedione, or "glitazone" for short) sensitizes parenchymal cells (mainly adipocytes) to insulin and so reduces insulin resistance. (The glitazones apparently activate a nuclear peroxisomal proliferator-activated receptor, PPAR-γ, that participates in the cellular response to insulin.)

Because of the insulin-dependency of their actions, the intensity of the effects of a glitazone increase when insulin levels are high (e.g., postprandial) and diminish as insulin levels fall (e.g., fasting). Regardless, and unless a glitazone is prescribed with insulin or a sulfonylurea (common), the incidence of drug-induced hypoglycemia is very low.

Repaglinide, a meglitinide, seems to trigger pancreatic insulin release in the presence of sufficient (and high) blood glucose levels. However, when blood glucose levels are sufficiently low (as can occur during fasting or meal-skipping), that effect wanes and so the drug is not likely to cause or worsen hypoglycemia.

2-4. The answer is d. *(Craig, pp 37, 559; Hardman, pp 1163, 1250, 1279, 1303; Katzung, p 1123.)* Rifampin induces cytochrome P450 enzymes, which causes a significant increase in elimination of drugs, such as oral contraceptives, anticoagulants, ketoconazole, cyclosporine, and chloramphenicol. It also promotes urinary excretion of methadone, which may precipitate withdrawal.

2-5. The answer is c. *(Casals, pp 1476–1483.)* If the brother has a child with cystic fibrosis, and then he must be a carrier of the cystic fibrotic gene, meaning there is a 50% chance that the husband is a CF carrier. Congenital absence of the ejaculatory ducts is increased in carriers of CF. If the ejaculatory ducts are absent, then there should be no sperm from the vas deferens (normally 0.5 mL of the semen volume) and no products of the seminal vesicles (normally 2.0 mL of the semen volume). The seminal vesicle is responsible for fructose normally present in the ejaculate. Prostatic secretions are normally slightly acidic. The normal physical of the husband rules out hypospadias, bilateral cryptorchidism, and hydrocele.

2-6. The answer is e. (*Levinson, pp 286–294, 461.*) A male patient with the presentation as outlined in question 2-6 (fatigue, weight loss, and lymphadenopathy) must be tested for antibodies to HIV. While other antibody tests may be relevant after the primary diagnosis, they must be considered after HIV is ruled out. Certainly, infectious mononucleosis is a possibility, but its occurrence in this age group is not as frequent as HIV. Patients are tested first by an ELISA screening test. If this test is positive (X2), then a confirmatory western blot is performed. A western blot separates the immune response into antibody production for specific components of the virus, that is, envelope, gag, and so forth. The following table shows the various bands that could be seen on a widely used western blot and their identification by specific antigen source. There are at least three schemes for interpreting western blots. Assuming technical competence in the laboratory, one of the more common reasons for falsely positive ELISAs and western blots is an influenza vaccination within the past few months. A rare patient may have antibody to the cell line used to grow virus. Unlike Lyme disease, there is no reported cross-reactivity with Epstein-Barr virus (EBV) or HTLV. There appears to be no naturally occurring antibody to retroviruses.

Antigen	Source
gp 160	Env gene product
gp 120	Env fragment
gp 41	Transmembrane fragment
gp 31	
gp 51	Pol gene product
p 66	
p 24	Core protein (gag)

Abbreviations: gp, glycoprotein; p, protein; env, envelope; pol, polymerase.

2-7. The answer is b. (*Cotran, pp 67–69.*) Complement assays can be used clinically to help determine the causes and pathomechanisms of certain diseases. For example, activation of the complement cascade can produce local deposition of C3, which can be seen with special histologic techniques. If a patient has widespread activation of the complement system, then serum assays of C3 levels might be decreased. In particular, activation of the classic complement pathway decreases levels of the early complement components, namely C1, C4, and C2. In contrast, activation of the alternate complement pathway, which bypasses these early complement components, decreases levels of C3, but the levels of the early factors (C2 and C4) are normal. An example of a disorder associated with the activation of the alternate complement system is IgA nephropathy (Berger's disease), which is characterized by the deposition of IgA in the mesangium of the glomeruli.

2-8. The answer is a. (*Braunwald, pp 1733–1734.*) The most serious consequences of chronic hepatitis B and C infections are hepatoma and cirrhosis. Complications of cirrhosis may occur, resulting in liver failure. Chronic hepatitis is not a risk factor for adenoma, cholangitis, lymphoma, or hemochromatosis.

2-9. The answer is d. (*Craig, pp 639, 653; Hardman, pp 1386, 1443; Katzung, pp 539, 919.*) Filgrastim, also known as granulocyte colony-stimulating factor (GCSF), enhances neutrophil production. One use, therefore, is to prevent neutropenia and infection associated with bone marrow depression from cancer chemotherapy. (Hint: Look at the generic name, filgrastim: *granulocyte stimulating*.)

The drug lacks antiemetic effects, potentiates the chemotherapeutic actions of no drug, has no effect on the gastric mucosa or on doxorubicin-mediated cardiotoxicity.

2-10. The answer is e. (*Kandel, pp 879–880.*) The carotid sinus reflex involves several neuronal elements. The afferent side of the reflex begins with stretch receptors in the walls of the carotid sinus. These receptors signal pressure as a result of stretch of the low-capacitance vessel. This causes an afferent volley of action potentials to pass along the glossopharyngeal nerve into the medulla, where the fibers synapse with neurons in the solitary nucleus. These neurons, in turn, synapse upon neurons in the dorsal motor nucleus (and nucleus ambiguus) of the vagus nerve whose axons innervate the heart. Activation of this reflex results in a decrease in heart rate and force of contraction. As a consequence of the decrease in cardiac output, there is an ensuing decrease in blood pressure as well.

2-11. The answer is a. (*Craig, pp 64, 66t, 68; Hardman, pp 1862–1865; Katzung, pp 974–975, 977–979.*) Arsenic is a constituent of fungicides, herbicides, and pesticides. Symptoms of acute toxicity include tightness in the throat, difficulty in swallowing, and stomach pains. Projectile vomiting and severe diarrhea can lead to hypovolemic shock, significant electrolyte derangements, and death. Chronic poisoning may cause peripheral neuritis, anemia, skin keratosis, and capillary dilation leading to hypotension. Dimercaprol [British anti-Lewisite (BAL)] is the main antidote used for arsenic poisoning.

2-12. The answer is e. (*Murray, pp 38–39, 535–539. Scriver, pp 1667–1724. Sack, pp 121–138.*) Collagen has an unusual amino acid composition in that approximately one-third of collagen molecules are glycine. The amino acid proline is also present in a much greater amount than in other proteins. In addition, two somewhat unusual amino acids, 4-hydroxyproline and 5-hydroxylysine, are found in collagen. Hydroxyproline and hydroxylysine per se are not incorporated during the synthesis of collagen. Proline and lysine are hydroxylated by specific hydroxylases after collagen is synthesized. A reducing agent such as ascorbate (vitamin C) is needed for the hydroxylation reaction to occur. In its absence, the disease known as scurvy occurs. Only proline or lysine residues located on the amino side of glycine residues are hydroxylated. Because hydroxylation of proline and lysine occurs after collagen is synthesized, addition of labeled hydroxyproline to the tissue culture will not result in labeled collagen.

2-13. The answer is d. (*Levinson, pp 155–157. Ryan, pp 434–437.*) The serologic diagnosis of Lyme disease is fraught with difficulty. Enzyme immunoassay (EIA) may be insensitive in the early stages of disease and may lack specificity in advanced stages. Western blot analysis of the antibody is the confirmatory test for Lyme disease, but it, too, is not 100% sensitive and specific. The western blot test detects antibodies to proteins and glycoproteins of *Borrelia burgdorferi*. Not all of these proteins are specific for the organism. For example, antibodies to Gp66 may reflect a cross-reaction, as many gram-negative bacteria have similar glycoproteins. For this reason, a western blot showing only antibodies to Gp66 is thought to be a nonspecific immune response.

2-14. The answer is c. (*Cotran, pp 1155–1157. Wilson, pp 573–576.*) Excess aldosterone secretion may be due to an abnormality of the adrenal gland (primary aldosteronism) or an abnormality of excess renin secretion (secondary aldosteronism). Causes of primary hyperaldosteronism (Conn's syndrome), which is independent of the renin-angiotensin-aldosterone (RAA) system, include adrenal cortical adenomas (most commonly), hyperplastic adrenal glands, and adrenal cortical carcinomas. These diseases are associated with decreased levels of renin. The signs of primary hyperaldosteronism include weakness, hypertension, polydipsia, and polyuria. The underlying physiologic abnormalities include increased serum sodium and decreased serum potassium, the latter due to excessive potassium loss by the kidneys, which together with the loss of hydrogen ions produces a hypokalemic alkalosis. The elevated level of serum sodium causes expansion of the intravascular volume. In contrast to Conn's syndrome, secondary hyperaldosteronism results from conditions causing increased levels of renin, such as renal ischemia, edematous states, and Bartter's syndrome. Causes of renal ischemia include renal artery stenosis and malignant nephrosclerosis, while Bartter's syndrome results from renal juxtaglomerular cell hyperplasia.

2-15. The answer is a. (*Damjanov, pp 1013–1018. Ravel, pp 438–441.*) Cryptosporidiosis is caused by *Cryptosporidium parvum*, a very small protozoa (2–4 μm) that attaches to colonic surface epithelial cells. It typically produces profuse, watery, nonbloody diarrhea in immunosuppressed patients (AIDS). Outbreaks in Wisconsin in rainy years are due to water run-off from dairy farms. The organism is best visualized with an acid-fast stain. In contrast, infection with the fish tapeworm *D. latum* can cause a deficiency of vitamin B_{12}, while infection with *E. vermicularis* can cause anal pruritus. In children with anal pruritus, the "Scotch tape" test can be used to help identify perianal eggs. *Enterobius* worms often attach themselves to the fecal mucosa and contiguous regions, and they can even be a cause of acute appendicitis. Finally, two tests used in the diagnosis of malabsorption include quantitative fecal fat determination (steatorrhea) and D-xylose absorption. The latter test can help to define the cause of the malabsorption. It is most likely to be abnormal with sprue-type diseases.

2-16. The answer is e. (*Scriver, pp 3827–3876. Sack, pp 97–158.*) The physician is obligated to describe a patient's disease accurately in the medical record and to share such records with legally entitled entities, such as health insurance companies. Although care should be exercised that records containing confidential information are not shared inappropriately, there was no such breach of confidentiality in this case. If the physician had declined further care without appropriate notice, then this would be a breach of ongoing care. However, insurance companies and managed care plans have excluded patients because of prior conditions or excessive expenses (i.e., capitation limits). This does constitute discrimination, but application of the Americans with Disabilities Act to patients with genetic diseases is not yet routine. These dilemmas will grow dramatically with the increasing ability to test for genetic diseases and predispositions. Although the administration of exogenous normal enzyme (enzyme therapy) or transplantation to provide a cellular source of normal enzyme has been successful in correcting lysosomal deficiencies, the enzymes fail to cross the blood-brain barrier in sufficient amounts to remit neurological symptoms in patients with lipidoses. This form of enzyme therapy has the advantage of targeting the defective organelle via the mannose-6-phosphate residues on the enzyme. It is very expensive but effective in lipidoses that have few neurological symptoms, such as Gaucher's disease (230800).

2-17. The answer is b. (*Braunwald, pp 2034–2035, 2184–2187.*) This patient may have multiple endocrine neoplasia syndrome-1, which presents with pituitary tumors, pancreatic tumors, and hyperparathyroidism. With the history of severe peptic ulcer disease (possible Zollinger-Ellison syndrome) and family history of pituitary tumors, one must suspect MEN-1. A serum calcium will be useful in diagnosing potential hyperparathyroidism. Calcitonin and urinary metanephrines are elevated and characteristic of MEN-2. Serum ferritin and fasting blood sugar would be elevated in hemochromatosis.

2-18. The answer is c. (*Baum, pp 182–185.*) The most immediate effect of cigarette smoking is damage to the respiratory tract's mucus and cilia. Damaged mucus and cilia have a reduced ability to trap invading organisms, dust, and other foreign particles. As a result, the work of other agents of the immune system will be increased. Initially, low levels of tobacco smoke and nicotine have a stimulatory effect on lymphocytes, but then shift to an inhibitory effect at higher doses. Smoking stimulates macrophages at first, but later they are destroyed. The other options listed in the question also occur, but not as rapidly as the mucociliary damage.

2-19. The answer is d. (*Moore and Dalley, p 1090–1092.*) A tumor that impinges on and compresses the optic chiasm will produce tunnel vision (bitemporal heteronymous hemianopsia). The reason for this pattern of blindness is that the lens projects reversed and inverted lateral visual fields onto the nasal portions of the retina. The pathways from the nasal retinas cross in the optic chiasm. This decussation collects both right and left visual fields. Thus, nerve fibers from the right nasal retina and left temporal retina, e.g., are collected into the left optic tract for projection to the left lateral geniculate body and then to the left occipital cortex. Injury to a lateral portion of the chiasm produces ipsilateral nasal hemianopsia, the loss of the nasal field from one eye. A lesion of the optic nerve would produce complete blindness of that eye, whereas a lesion to the optic tract produces contralateral homonymous hemianopsia, complete loss of the contralateral visual field. See figure below.

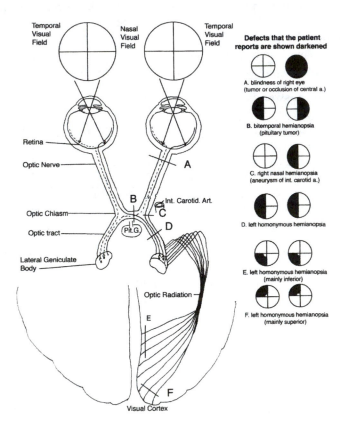

2-20. The answer is e. (*Guyton, pp 98–99. Boron, pp 244–245, 524–557.*) Phospholamban is a protein contained within the SR that inhibits the activity of the SR calcium pump. Inactivation of phospholamban results in an increase in calcium sequestration by the SR. Increasing the concentration of calcium within the SR increases the force of the ventricular contraction.

2-21. The answer is a. (*Craig, pp 113–115; Hardman, pp 260, 1834–1837; Katzung, pp 151–152.*) The secretion of aqueous humor occurs in response to activating β-adrenergic receptors located on ciliary epithelia. β-adrenergic antagonists decrease secretory activity and lower intraocular pressure. Muscarinic agents induce contraction in the circular pupillary constrictor muscles. Ciliary muscle contraction facilitates opening of the trabecular meshwork, leading to better outflow of aqueous humor. α-adrenergic agonists cause contraction of the radially oriented pupillary dilator muscles.

2-22. The answer is d. (*Murray—2003, pp 1271–1272. Ryan, pp 614–615.*) HIV RT PCR, a nucleic acid amplification test for HIV RNA, has recently been shown to be the most valuable test for (a) monitoring a patient's progress during triple drug therapy and (b) determining the chances of pro-

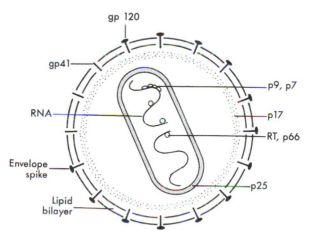

The location of the envelope glycoproteins (gp 120 and gp 124) is shown, as are the major viral core proteins (p25, p17, p9, and p7). The core protein, p17, is found outside the viral nucleoid and forms the matrix of the virion. RT indicates reverse transcriptase.

gression to AIDS. A viral load of 100,000 to 750,000 copies per mL significantly increases the chance of progression to AIDS within five years. The other tests listed do not accurately predict progression to AIDS. The figure on page 209 shows the basic structure of HIV, including the enzyme reverse transcriptase.

2-23. The answer is a. (*Cotran, pp 159–160. Damjanov, pp 293–294.*) The mucopolysaccharidoses (MPSs) result from deficiencies of specific enzymes involved in the breakdown of glycosaminoglycans (GAGs), which are also called MPSs. The seven major types of GAGs are hyaluronic acid, chondroitin sulfate, keratin sulfate, dermatan sulfate, heparan sulfate, and heparin. The MPSs are characterized by accumulation of partially degraded GAGs in multiple organs, including the liver, spleen, heart, and blood vessels. Accumulations of GAGs within leukocytes produce Alder-Reilly bodies, while accumulations within neurons can produce zebra bodies. The MPSs are also characterized by the excretion of excess acid mucopolysaccharides in the urine, a finding that helps to differentiate the MPSs from the mucolipidoses. Most of the MPSs are associated with coarse facial features, clouding of corneas, joint stiffness, and mental retardation. The characteristic appearance of patients with type IH MPS (Hurler's syndrome), which results from a deficiency of alpha-1-iduronidase, has been described as "gargoylism." These patients excrete excess dermatan sulfate and heparan sulfate, both of which are mucopolysaccharides, in the urine. Type II MPS (Hunter's syndrome) is the only MPS that has an X-linked recessive type of inheritance. These patients have a much milder disease than Hurler's syndrome patients, but they also secrete dermatan sulfate and heparan sulfate in the urine. Type IV MPS, known as Morquio's syndrome, is characterized by short stature, aortic valvular disease, and normal intelligence. These patients are prone to development of subluxation of the spine, which can produce quadriplegia. They secrete keratan sulfate in the urine.

In contrast to the MPSs, the mucolipidoses (MLs) are characterized by abnormalities affecting both the MPSs and the sphingolipidoses (SLs). Similar to the MPSs, the MLs involve abnormal bone development (dysostosis), while similar to some of the SLs, cherry-red maculae and peripheral demyelination are also seen. The MLs, however, unlike the MPSs, do not involve excessive urinary excretion of acid MPSs. The metabolism of the carbohydrates in glycoproteins and glycolipids is abnormal in the MLs and results in excess accumulation of oligosaccharides. There are three main types of MLs: type I is sialidosis, type II is inclusion cell (I cell) disease, and type III is pseudo-Hurler's disease. Patients with type II ML lack the enzyme N-acetylglucosamine phosphotransferase, which catalyzes the first step in the formation of mannose-6-phosphate. Many lysosomal enzymes in these patients, such as acid hydrolases (which includes glycoprotein and ganglioside sialidases), do not reach the cellular lysosomes and are instead secreted into the plasma. The name I cell originated from the finding of cytoplasmic granular inclusions in affected patients' fibroblasts when cultured in vitro and observed under a phase-contrast microscope. These cytoplasmic inclusions are lysosomes that are swollen with many different types of contents. I cell disease is a slowly progressive disease that starts at birth and is fatal in childhood. Treatment is symptomatic only.

2-24. The answer is d. (*Cotran, pp 1221–1222. Rubin, pp 1352–1353.*) Osteogenesis imperfecta (OI), or brittle bone disease, constitutes a group of disorders often inherited as autosomal dominant traits and caused by genetic mutations involving the synthesis of type I collagen, which comprises about 90% of the osteoid, or bone matrix. Very early perinatal death and multiple fractures occur in OI type II, which is often autosomal recessive. The major variant of OI, type I, is compatible with survival; after the perinatal period fractures occur in addition to other signs of defective collagen synthesis such as thin, translucent, blue scleras; laxity of joint ligaments; deafness from otosclerosis; and abnormal teeth. A hereditary defect in osteoclastic function with decreased bone resorption and bone overgrowth, which sometimes narrows or obliterates the marrow cavity, is characteristic of osteopetrosis, or marble bone disease. Osteomalacia is seen in adults due to vitamin D deficiency, while osteitis deformans is Paget's disease of bone.

2-25. The answer is c. (*Gilroy, pp 590–591. Afifi, pp 131–132.*) Cranial nerve IX, the glossopharyngeal nerve, innervates the skeletal muscles of the pharynx. The motor component involved arises from the nucleus ambiguus of the medulla. This cranial nerve also contains afferents, a component of which arises from the superior ganglion. These sensory neurons convey somatosensory sensation, including pain afferents that ultimately synapse in the spinal trigeminal nucleus. The motor component of the glossopharyngeal nerve mediating swallowing and coughing constitutes a special visceral efferent (because it is derived from a visceral arch), and the sensory component conveying pain is referred to as a general somatic afferent fiber.

2-26. The answer is c. (*Cotran, pp 846–847, 853–855. Rubin, pp 796–798.*) Cirrhosis refers to fibrosis of the liver that involves both central veins and portal triads. This fibrosis is the result of liver cell necrosis and regenerative hepatic nodules. These nodules consist of hyperplastic hepatocytes with enlarged, atypical nuclei, irregular hepatic plates, and distorted vasculature. There is distortion of the normal lobular architecture. These changes diffusely involve the entire liver; they are not focal. It is thought that the fibrosis is the result of fibril-forming collagens that are released by Ito cells, which are fat-containing lipocytes found within the space of Disse of the liver. They normally participate in the metabolism and storage of vitamin A, but they can secrete collagen in the fibrotic (cirrhotic) liver. Normally types I and III collagens (interstitial types) are found in the portal areas and occasionally in the space of Disse or around central veins. In cirrhosis, types I and III collagens are deposited throughout the hepatic lobule. These Ito cells are initiated by unknown factors and then are further stimulated by such factors as platelet-derived growth factor and transforming growth factor beta to secrete collagen.

In contrast to Ito cells, endothelial cells normally line the sinusoids and demarcate the extrasinusoidal space of Disse. Attached to the endothelial cells are the phagocytic Kupffer cells, which are part of the monocyte-phagocyte system. Bile ducts, and thus the epithelial cells that form them, are found in the portal triads of the liver.

2-27. The answer is b. (*Craig, pp 319–321; Hardman, pp 530–531, 536; Katzung, pp 504–505, 509.*) Unless the patient can be put on a ventilator to control blood gases (and perhaps have intracranial pressure surgically reduced), closed head injury contraindicates morphine use. Cerebral vasodilation occurs in response to expected morphine-induced ventilatory depression. That increases intracranial pressure. This is precisely what one doesn't want to do with closed head injuries (brain swelling) or with, for example, the presence of a large brain tumor—two situations in which intracranial pressure is already (likely) increased.

Parenteral morphine is a routine part of the approach to acute pulmonary edema and myocardial infarction. The drug is apt to lower blood pressure in some patients, and so there is little specific concern with respect to hypertension. Opioid abuse of recent history poses a problem: the patient may be tolerant to opioids, and so higher than usual doses of morphine may be needed to get adequate pain control and other subjective responses. However, that does not pose a risk and certainly doesn't constitute a contraindication to using the drug.

2-28. The answer is c. (*Adams, pp 246–247.*) In one form of retinitis pigmentosa, there is a genetic defect with respect to rhodopsin. The result of this defect is the production of defective opsin. As a consequence, rod cells are affected, leading to a reduced response to light. However, central vision is spared, as are cone cells. CNS neurons, such as those located in area 17, are not directly affected and vision is not totally lost.

2-29. The answer is d. (*Braunwald, pp 1879–1880, 1899–1900.*) Anti-HIV therapy is begun when any opportunitistic infection ensues in the course of this illness. The acute infection earlier was the acute HIV syndrome. Anti-HIV therapy is not started then. When the CD4 T lymphocytes decline below about 350 cells/µL and the viral load exceeds about 55,000 copies/µL in the absence of any opportunistic infection, anti-HIV therapy is started. The other answers are not reasons to start HIV therapy in a person with HIV not yet on drug treatment.

2-30. The answer is c. (*McKenzie, pp 205, 210. Junqueira, pp 166, 187, 188. Kierszenbaum, pp 30, 216. Alberts, 979–981. Kandel, pp 99–103, 1108–1109.*) Regeneration depends on the proliferation of Schwann cells, which guide sprouting axons from the proximal segment toward the target organ. The injury causes Wallerian degeneration distal to the level of injury and proximal axonal degeneration to at least the next node of Ranvier. In more severe traumatic injuries, the proximal degeneration may extend beyond the next node of Ranvier. Electrodiagnostic studies demonstrate denervation changes in the affected muscles, and in cases of reinnervation, motor unit potentials (MUPs) are present (answer a). Axonal regeneration occurs at the rate of 1 mm/day (answer b) or 1 in./month and can be monitored with an advancing Tinel's sign. The Tinel's sign is observed when tapping over nerve trunk that has been damaged or is regenerating following trauma causes a sensation of tingling and pins in its distribution up to the site of regeneration. A nerve trunk will regenerate about 1 mm/day (see transport rates discussed in the next paragraph). If this sign is absent, there is a poor prognosis. The endoneurial tubes remain intact (answer d), and, therefore, recovery is complete, with axons reinnervating their original motor and sensory targets.

The process of response to injury is referred to as *Wallerian degeneration*. Axonal regeneration occurs in neurons if the perikarya survive following damage. The segment distal (answer e) to the wound, including the myelin, is phagocytosed and removed by macrophages. The proximal segment is capable of regeneration because it remains in continuity with the perikaryon. Chromatolysis is the first step in the regeneration process, in which there is breakdown of the Nissl substance (RER, ribosomes), swelling of the perikaryon, and migration of the nucleus peripherally. Degeneration of perikarya and neuronal processes occurs when there is extensive neuronal damage. Transneuronal degeneration occurs only when there are synapses with a single damaged neuron. In the presence of inputs from multiple neurons, transneuronal degeneration does not occur.

The rate of regeneration is dependent on *axonal transport* that occurs by several different mechanisms. Slow axonal transport involves the movement of cytoskeletal elements such as actin, tubulin, and neurofilaments from the perikaryon down the axon. Slow transport occurs at a velocity of 1 to 5 mm/day. Dendritic transport occurs in a manner similar to that of slow axonal transport. In contrast to slow axonal transport, rapid anterograde (away from the perikaryon) transport and retrograde (toward the perikaryon) transport occur at rates of 200 to 300 mm/day. Membrane-bound organelles, such as newly formed secretory vesicles and mitochondria, are transported rapidly in an anterograde direction. Receptors, recycled membranes, and worn-out organelles are transported following a retrograde mechanism. Retrograde transport is also used experimentally by neuroanatomists to map connections in the CNS. Colchicine and other microtubule toxins block fast axonal transport.

2-31. The answer is b. (*Cotran, pp 1018–1024.*) Germ cell tumors of the testis often secrete enzymes or polypeptide hormones, examples of which include α-fetoprotein (AFP) and human chorionic gonadotropin (hCG). AFP is synthesized by the fetal gut, liver, and yolk sac. It may be secreted by either yolk sac tumors (endodermal sinus tumors) or embryonal carcinomas. AFP may also be secreted by liver cell carcinomas. β-hCG is a glycoprotein that is normally synthesized by placental syncytiotrophoblasts. Markedly elevated serum levels are most often associated with choriocarcinomas, which are characterized histologically by a mixture of malignant cytotrophoblasts and syncytiotrophoblasts. Mildly elevated serum levels of β-hCG may be found in patients with other types of germ cell tumors if they contain syncytiotrophoblast-like giant cells. This is found in about 10% of classic seminomas.

To summarize: markedly elevated levels of hCG are associated with choriocarcinomas, while elevated levels of AFP are most characteristic of yolk sac tumors and embryonal carcinomas. But there are many areas of overlap between tumors, and many tumors are composed of multiple types of germ cell cancers. The only definitive statement that can be made is that elevated serum levels of AFP cannot be seen in a tumor that is a pure seminoma.

2-32. The answer is c. (*Braunwald, pp 1451–1452.*) The patient most likely has a pulmonary embolism because of shortness of breath, right-sided pleuritic chest pain, a normal chest x-ray, and abnormal blood gases. A useful calculation is the assessment of alveolar oxygenation and calculating the gradient between alveolar and arterial partial pressures of the oxygen. At room air, the PA_{O2} (alveolar) can be calculated by the following formula: $PA_{O2} = 150 - 1.25 \times PA_{CO2}$. Once PA_{O2} is determined, the A-a gradient is simply the difference between the PA_{O2} and arterial PA_{O2}. In a healthy young person breathing room air, the $PA_{O2} - PA_{O2}$ is normally less than 15 mmHg; this value increases with age and may be as high as 30 mmHg in elderly patients.

2-33. The answer is d. (*Sierles, p 405. Baum, pp 60–106.*) While fearfulness, confusion, interpersonal conflict, and regression can generate stress that can have a direct effect on biologic responses, the loss of perceived control can take an even greater toll on the body. Excessive workload and job responsibility are stressful factors in terms of coronary risk, but they become even more powerful and biologically more destructive when they approach the limit of a person's capacity to control his or her own work. Whether the stress is from employment, unemployment, finance, family, disease, or other factors, the threat of loss or actual loss of control over one's being or activities appears to be the most devastating influence. Different people also have considerable variability in their responsiveness to a lack of or loss of control; this responsiveness then has a subsequent effect on their biologic processes.

2-34. The answer is e. *(Cotran, pp 1125–1127. McPhee, pp 544–548.)* Pituitary adenomas are the most common neoplasms of the pituitary gland. These benign neoplasms are classified according to the hormone or hormones that are produced by the neoplastic cells. The cell types, in order of decreasing frequency, are the following: lactotrope adenomas (which secrete prolactin), null cell adenomas (which do not secrete hormones), somatotrope adenomas (which secrete growth hormone), corticotrophic adenomas (which secrete ACTH), gonadotrope adenomas (which secrete FSH and LH), and thyrotrope cell adenomas (which secrete TSH). Prolactin-secreting tumors (lactotrope adenomas or prolactinomas) produce symptoms of hypogonadism and galactorrhea (milk secretion not associated with pregnancy). In females this hypogonadism produces amenorrhea and infertility, while in males it produces impotence and decreased libido. The same symptoms that are seen with a prolactin-secreting pituitary adenoma can also be produced by certain drugs, such as methyldopa and reserpine.

2-35. The answer is c. *(Kandel, pp 654–672, 770–777.)* The premotor areas play an important role in the programming or sequencing of responses that compose complex learned movements. They receive significant inputs for this process from the posterior parietal lobule and, in turn, signal appropriate neurons in the brainstem and spinal cord (both flexors and extensors). Lesions of the postcentral gyrus produce a somatosensory loss. Lesions of the precentral gyrus produce paralysis. Neither lesions of the prefrontal cortex nor those of the cingulate gyrus have been reported to produce apraxia.

2-36. The answer is b. *(Boron, pp 606–608, 624–625.)* Bronchospasm increases the resistance to airflow, which makes it more difficult to expel gas rapidly from the lung during expiration, so although both FEV_1 and vital capacity decreases, the percent of gas expelled in 1 s as a function of the total amount that can be expelled (the FEV_1/FVC ratio) also decreases dramatically. Obstructive disease also produces air trapping, so all static lung volumes, residual volume, functional residual capacity, and total lung capacity will increase.

2-37. The answer is a. *(Brooks, p 367. Levinson, pp 231–232. Murray—2002, p 472.)* Adenovirus type 8 is associated with epidemic keratoconjunctivitis, while adenovirus types 3 and 4 are often associated with "swimming pool conjunctivitis." There are also reports of nosocomial conjunctivitis with adenovirus. Herpes simplex virus can infect the conjunctiva and is among the most common causes of blindness in North America and Europe.

2-38. The answer is c. (*Craig, pp 356–357t; Hardman, pp 425–426; Katzung, pp 272, 360.*) Buspirone is an attractive drug for managing short-term anxiety. Among the reasons (and especially when compared with more traditional anxiolytics, such as benzodiazepines) are a lack of sedation (buspirone is not a CNS depressant) and virtually no potentiation of the effects of other CNS depressants, including alcohol; no known abuse potential (it is not regulated by the Controlled Substances Act) or tendency for development of tolerance; and no major withdrawal syndrome. One major drawback to the drug is a very slow onset of symptom relief (a week or two), and typically it takes about a month from the onset of therapy for antianxiety effects to peak. (This slow time course, obviously, does not warrant "almost daily" dosage titrations.)

You should recall that long-term benzodiazepine administration is associated with withdrawal phenomena (and, depending on the use, the syndrome can be severe). Thus, one can envisage a switch from a benzodiazepine to buspirone. Because buspirone lacks CNS depressant effects and its effects take some time to develop, one should start the buspirone several weeks before stopping the benzodiazepine and also taper the benzodiazepine dose once it's time to stop the drug.

2-39. The answer is b. (*Guyton, pp 128–130. Boron, pp 498–502.*) A stress test is conducted by asking a patient to increase his or her exercise intensity while monitoring blood pressure and the electrical activity of the heart. Ischemia occurs if the myocardial oxygen demand brought about by the increased exercise intensity is not matched by an increase in myocardial blood flow. An ischemic episode is indicated by an ST segment depression. Mean arterial blood pressure and heart rate normally rise. The presence of a diastolic murmur or conduction abnormalities in the ECG are not diagnostic of ischemic heart disease. The exercise test will also be terminated if dizziness, dyspnea, or ventricular tachycardia develop or if blood pressure falls.

2-40. The answer is d. (*Murray, pp 49–59. Scriver, pp 4571–4636. Sack, pp 3–17.*) Isozymes are multiple forms of a given enzyme that occur within a given species. Since isozymes are composed of different proteins, analysis by electrophoretic separation can be done. Lactate dehydrogenase is a tetramer composed of any combination of two different polypeptides, H and M. Thus the possible combinations are H4, H3M1, H2M2, H1M3, and M4. Although each combination is found in most tissues, M4 predominates in the liver and skeletal muscle, where as H4 is the predominant form in the heart. White and red blood cells as well as brain cells contain primarily intermediate forms. The M4 forms of the isozyme seem to have a higher affinity for pyruvate compared with the H4 form. Following a myocardial infarction, the H4 (LDH1) type of lactate dehydrogenase rises and reaches a peak approximately 36 h later. Elevated LDH1 levels may signal myocardial disease even when the total lactate dehydrogenase level is normal.

2-41. The answer is c. *(Braunwald, pp 1764–1765.)* Gastrointestinal bleeding is the single most important precipitating event of hepatic encephalopathy. It leads to an increase in ammonia and other nitrogenous substances that are absorbed. Other factors that can precipitate hepatic encephalopathy include hyperkalemia, hypernatremia, and constipation; however, constipation is a much less important precipitating event than gastrointestinal bleeding.

2-42. The answer is e. *(Cotran, pp 570–572. Rubin, pp 567–570.)* Rheumatic fever (RF) produces both acute and chronic manifestations. Chronic RF mainly produces damage to cardiac valves. The mitral valve is most commonly involved, followed by the aortic valve. The stenotic valve has the appearance of a "fish mouth" or "buttonhole." An additional finding in chronic RF is a rough portion of the endocardium of the left atrium, called a MacCallum's patch. In contrast to chronic RF, the acute lesions of rheumatic fever in the heart are characterized by the accumulation of modified tissue monocytes (called Anitschkow myocytes) around areas of fibrinoid necrosis. This entire area is called an Aschoff body. The nuclei of the Anitschkow cells are long, slender, wavy ribbons that resemble a caterpillar (hence the name "caterpillar cells"). Occasional multinucleated giant cells (Aschoff cells) may be seen. The Aschoff body, which is pathognomonic for acute rheumatic fever, may be found in any of the three layers of the heart (pancarditis). In the pericardium there is a fibrinous pericarditis, which is called a "bread and butter" pericarditis. The endocardial response in acute rheumatic fever is characterized by the formation of small friable vegetations (verrucae) along the lines of closure of the valves.

2-43. The answer is b. (*Brooks, p 267. Levinson, pp 131–132. Murray—2002, pp 356–357. Ryan, pp 324–325.*) *B. fragilis* is a constituent of normal intestinal flora and readily causes wound infections often mixed with aerobic isolates. These anaerobic, gram-negative rods are uniformly resistant to aminoglycosides and usually to penicillin as well. Reliable laboratory identification may require multiple analytical techniques. Generally, wound exudates smell bad owing to production of organic acids by such anaerobes as *B. fragilis*. Black exudates or a black pigment (heme) in the isolated colony is usually a characteristic of *Bacteroides* (*Porphyromonas*) *melaninogenicus*, not *B. fragilis*. Potent neurotoxins are synthesized by the gram-positive anaerobes such as *C. tetani* and *C. botulinum*.

2-44. The answer is c. (*Craig, pp 172–173, 816–818, 870–871; Hardman, p 919, 966; Katzung, pp 205, 1119.*) Digoxin toxicity is likely to occur within 24 to 48 h unless the digoxin dose is adjusted down. The reason is that quinidine will reduce the renal excretion of digoxin (digoxin's main elimination route).

There is no "reverse interaction"—i.e., an ability of digoxin to cause signs and symptoms of quinidine toxicity. Quinidine has no significant impact on the renal actions of any diuretics, whether these actions are expressed in terms of urine output (volume or concentration) or renal handling of electrolytes or other solutes.

Quinidine-induced digoxin toxicity may suppress cardiac contractility, but that would not be a direct effect of an interaction. Rather, it would be secondary to potential digoxin-induced arrhythmias, and it would not occur "promptly."

[Note: You may have learned that the interaction with quinidine does not apply to digitoxin, another cardiac glycoside that is eliminated mainly by hepatic metabolism. Although that is true, it is likely that you will never encounter any digitalis drug other than digoxin used clinically in the United States. Thus, whether you remember this "noninteraction" with digitoxin is up to you.]

2-45. The answer is C. (*Nolte, pp 375–387, 417–421, 538–561.*) This section is taken at the level of the posterior thalamus and, because of the oblique cut, also includes parts of the midbrain and pons. The pulvinar (A), a very large nucleus situated at this level of the thalamus, projects extensively to wide regions of the inferior parietal lobule. The fornix (E), situated just below the corpus callosum, arises from the hippocampal formation and supplies the septal area, anterior thalamic nucleus, and mammillary bodies. The hippocampal formation (C) is associated with a number of different processes, including short-term memory and as a seizure focus during temporal lobe epilepsy. Thus, a lesion of this structure will likely produce deficits in short-term memory, and trauma to this region will result in temporal lobe epilepsy. The lateral geniculate nucleus (D), situated in the far VL aspect of the posterior thalamus, is a relay nucleus for the transmission of visual information to the cortex. Damage to this structure would result in a homonymous hemianopsia. The centromedian (CM) nucleus (B), identified by its encapsulated appearance, can be found in posterior levels of the thalamus, where it receives inputs from the brainstem reticular formation and projects to the neostriatum as well as to wide regions of the cerebral cortex.

2-46. The answer is c. (*Kierszenbaum, pp 301, 303. Braunwald, 307, 311, 313, 315, 317.*) Psoriasis is a chronic disease that affects both the epidermis and dermis of the skin. There is hyperplasia of the epidermis and abnormal microcirculation in the dermis as venules predominate in the capillaries resulting in increased extravasation of inflammatory cells. Thus, the underlying cause is the infiltration of inflammatory cells into the dermis with further migration of neutrophils into the epidermis. Those inflammatory cells release cytokines that induce an inflammatory response. There is hyperplasia of the epidermis (answer a) as keratinocytes traverse the cell cycle in a shorter period of time (answer b). Microabcesses form in the epidermis (answer d) and epithelia are avascular (answer e).

2-47. The answer is d. (*Craig, pp 136–137, 459, 464; Hardman, pp 588–590; Katzung, pp 115, 266, 319–321.*) Diphenhydramine, and most of the other older antihistamines (H_1 histamine-receptor blockers) have varying degrees of antimuscarinic (atropine-like) activity. With diphenhydramine and several others, that effect is quite intense. These antihistamines do block the bronchoconstrictor effects of both histamine (via H_1 receptors) and ACh (muscarinic), and so in those regards they can be beneficial. However, the muscarinic blocking activity also thickens airway mucus, and as was the case with the patient described in Question 294 (but by a different mechanism), this increased mucus viscosity and the tendency for mucus plugs to form can do more harm than the good provided by the other effects. If the patient chooses to take an antihistamine, they might be better off taking one of the second-generation agents (e.g., fexofenadine, loratadine, others), which lack the antimuscarinic/mucus-thickening effects caused by the older agents. If an antihistamine that can cause mucus thickening must be used, then ensuring that the patient is well hydrated is paramount.

Notes: Diphenhydramine and a very similar antihistamine, doxylamine, are also common ingredients in OTC sleep aids. Airway problems from mucus thickening may also arise, therefore, with these products.

Paradoxically (you may think), atropine is an important element in managing status asthmaticus. Why use it in this life-threatening situation, but avoid it or other antimuscarinics in ambulatory patients? When used for severe asthma, the atropine is given by inhalation. It is nebulized and given with a mucus-thinning drug plus ample "moisture"—e.g., saline—along with steroids and adrenergic bronchodilators. It is this use of drug and other adjuncts that will maximize atropine's bronchodilator actions while simultaneously and virtually eliminating all the potential problems related to mucus thickening and airway obstruction.

2-48. The answer is a. (*Ryan, pp 851–855.*) "Atypical pneumonia" is an old classification used for respiratory disease that is not lobar and is not "typical." That is, it does not include pneumonia caused by pneumococcus, *Klebsiella, Haemophilus,* or β-hemolytic streptococci that results in a typical lobular infiltrate. In recent years, the atypical pneumonias have become much more frequent than pneumococcal pneumonia. They are characterized by a slower onset with headache, joint pain, fever, and signs of an acute upper respiratory infection. There are usually no signs of acute respiratory distress, but patients report malaise and fatigue. The most common cause of atypical pneumonia is *M. pneumoniae.* A quick test for *M. pneumoniae* infection is cold agglutinins. The test may lack both sensitivity and specificity, but it is rapid and readily available compared with culture of *M. pneumoniae* or specific antibody formation.

2-49. The answer is a. (*Cotran, p 1210. Rubin, p 444.*) Fungal infections of the skin can be classified into superficial mycoses, cutaneous mycoses, and subcutaneous mycoses. The superficial mycoses are characterized by infection of the superficial layers of the skin. The most common type is pityriasis versicolor (tinea versicolor), an infection of the upper trunk that is caused by *M. furfur (Pityrosporum orbiculare)*. Clinically, there are multiple groups of macules (discolorations) with a fine peripheral scale. These macules are hyperpigmented (dark) in white-skinned races but hypopigmented (light) in dark-skinned races. These areas fluoresce yellow under a Wood's lamp. Potassium hydroxide (KOH) is used to identify fungal infections from scrapings of the skin. The KOH dissolves the keratin, and then the mycelial fungi can be seen. With tinea versicolor, KOH examination reveals a characteristic "spaghetti and meatball" appearance. The fragments of hyphae are the "spaghetti," and the round yeast cells are the "meatballs." Different types of tinea include tinea capitis, tinea corporis, tinea pedis (athlete's foot), and tinea versicolor.

2-50. The answer is a. (*Guyton, pp 686–687.*) The Klüver-Bucy syndrome is produced in animals by removal of the amygdala from both temporal lobes. The syndrome is characterized by a tendency to examine objects orally and excessive sexual behavior. The full syndrome is rarely encountered in humans but many of its characteristics are observed in patients with bilateral temporal lobe lesions produced by encephalitis or traumatic injury.

BLOCK 3

Answers

3-1. The answer is a. (*Scriver, pp 4077–5016. Sack, pp 121–144.*) Sex steroids are synthesized from cholesterol by side-chain cleavage (employing a P450 enzyme) to produce pregnenolone. Pregnenolone is then converted to testosterone in the testis, to estrogen in the ovary, and to corticosterone and aldosterone in the adrenal gland. The enzymes 3β-hydroxysteroid dehydrogenase, 21-hydroxylase, 11β-hydroxylase, and 18-hydroxylase modify pregnenolone to produce other sex and adrenal steroids. Deficiencies in adrenal 21-hydroxylase can thus lead to inadequate testosterone production in males and produce ambiguous external genitalia. Such children can also exhibit low sodium and high potassium due to deficiency of the more distal steroids corticol and aldosterone. 5α-reductase converts testosterone to dihydrotestosterone, and its deficiency produces milder degrees of hypogenitalism without salt wasting. Deficiency of the androgen receptor is called testicular feminization, producing normal looking females who may not seek medical attention until they present with infertility.

3-2. The answer is e. (*Cotran, pp 334, 369. Rubin, pp 361, 380, 406–407, 1303, 1320.*) Numerous diseases result from bacterial infections of the oral cavity. *A. israelii*, a normal inhabitant of the mouth, is a branched, filamentous gram-positive bacteria that may produce an indurated (lumpy) jaw with multiple draining fistulas or abscesses. Small yellow colonies, called sulfur granules, may be seen in the draining material. Scarlet fever, a disease of children, is caused by several strains of β-hemolytic group A streptococci (*S. pyogenes*). An erythrogenic toxin damages vascular endothelium and produces a rash on the skin and oral mucosa. The tongue in a patient with scarlet fever may be fiery red with prominent papillae (raspberry tongue) or white-coated with hyperemic papillae (strawberry tongue). Acute necrotizing ulcerative gingivitis (Vincent's angina or trench mouth) is caused by two symbiotic organisms, a fusiform bacillus and a spirochete (*B. vincentii*), the combination being termed fusospirochetosis. *C. diphtheriae* causes diphtheria, which is characterized by oral and pharyngeal pseudomembranes and a peripheral lymphocytosis. Rhinoscleroma, a chronic inflammation of the nose, is caused by *K. rhinoscleromatis* and histologically is characterized by numerous foamy macrophages, called Mikulicz cells.

3-3. The answer is b. (*Craig, pp 154, 246; Hardman, pp 703–704; Katzung, pp 208, 212, 254.*) Low K stores due to the effects of potassium-wasting diuretics such as hydrochlorothiazide increase susceptibility to cardiac glycoside toxicity. Note that in this scenario we have listed hydrochlorothiazide as the correct answer choice, but in clinical practice and when we are using a diuretic to manage edema secondary to heart failure, the best choice would be a loop diuretic: also potassium-wasting drugs.

3-4. The answer is d. (*Braunwald, p 883.*) Wasting and cachexia are caused by a bloodstream infection with *Mycobacterium avium* complex (MAC), which includes *M. avium* and *M. intracellulare*. MAC organisms occur widely in nature—soil and animals—and spread to humans. However, almost only immunosuppressed persons become infected, especially persons with AIDS who possess few CD4 lymphocytes. The other organisms do not cause wasting in AIDS persons.

3-5. The answer is b. (*Cotran, pp 433–434. Townsend, pp 346–348. Rubin, pp 334–335.*) Burns of the skin, which may involve partial thickness or the full thickness of the skin, are classified as being first-, second-, or third-degree burns. The first two are partial-thickness burns, while third-degree burns are full-thickness burns. First-degree burns, such as with a sunburn, are mild and heal without scarring. Clinically, erythema is present, which is due to dilation of the capillaries in the dermis. Histologic sections of the skin would show epidermal edema and focal epithelial necrosis. Second-degree burns are classified as being either superficial partial-thickness burns or deep partial-thickness burns. The former are characterized by injury to the epidermis and superficial dermis. Clinically they have ruptured red, weeping, blisters that are painful. They usually heal in 1–3 weeks without scarring. Deep partial-thickness second-degree burns have more injury to the deeper dermis. Still there is no necrosis of the adnexal structures that are located deeper in the dermis. Clinically they are whiter and less erythematous than superficial second-degree burns. They heal after 3–4 weeks, and scarring may occur. Third-degree burns are the most severe types of burns and consist of extensive necrosis of the epidermis, dermis, and adnexal structures. Clinically these burns are typically white, brown, or black. These third-degree burns, which have a high risk of infection, heal with severe scarring and need skin grafts for treatment.

3-6. The answer is b. (*Guyton, pp 220–221. Boron, pp 441–444.*) Cardiac output can be measured by using Fick's principle, which asserts that the rate of uptake of a substance by the body (e.g., O_2 consumption in milliliters per minute) is equal to the difference between its concentrations (milliliters per liter of blood) in arterial and venous blood multiplied by the rate of blood flow (cardiac output). This principle is restricted to situations in which arterial blood is the only source of the substance measured. If oxygen consumption by the body at steady state is measured over a period of time and the difference in arterial O_2 and venous O_2 measured by sampling arterial blood and pulmonary arterial blood (which is fully mixed venous blood), cardiac output is obtained from the expression

$$CO = \frac{\dot{V}O_2}{(AO_2 - VO_2)\text{content}}$$

$$CO = \frac{280 \text{ ml/min}}{20 \text{ ml/100 ml} - 12 \text{ ml/100 ml}}$$

$$CO = 3500 \text{ ml/min} = 3.5 \text{ L/min}$$

3-7. The answer is d. (*Junqueira, pp 417–418. Sadler, pp 355–356. Moore and Persaud, Developing, pp 304, 307, 318.*) The newborn described is genotypically female and suffers from adrenogenital or congenital virilizing hyperplasia in which there is a deficiency in the pathway that leads to cortisol synthesis. The inability to synthesize cortisol in turn leads to production of high levels of ACTH and ACTH-releasing factor from the hypothalamus. The result is hypertrophy of the fetal adrenal cortex, which is a critical fetal structure that produces dehydroepiandrosterone. The excessive production of androgens by the fetal adrenal leads to masculinization of the female genitalia. Increased secretion of cortisol cannot occur because of the metabolic defect in this pathway; therefore, negative feedback control is not functional. The fetal cortex is part of maternal-feto-placental unit because the dehydroepiandrosterone is used by the placenta to produce estradiol. The fetal adrenal cortex involutes following birth, causing an overall reduction in the size of the adrenal. The adult cortex (zona glomerulosa, zona fasciculata, and zona reticularis) replaces the fetal adrenal cortex. The zona fasciculata and zona reticularis produce androgens after birth. Vasopressin [(AVP) also known as antidiuretic hormone (ADH)] is released by the posterior pituitary and regulates fluid balance. ADH increases the permeability of the collecting duct through an aquaporin-mediated mechanism. Androgen insensitivity is the cause of testicular feminization and is not a factor in the adrenogenital syndrome.

3-8. The answers is b. (*Levinson, pp 8, 53–57, 87–88. Ryan, pp 16, 232–233.*) First described in 1884 by a Danish physician, Hans Christian Gram, the Gram stain has proved to be one of the most useful diagnostic laboratory procedures in microbiology and medicine. The Gram stain procedure is characterized by the following steps: (1) *fixation* of the bacteria to the slide, (2) crystal violet (acridine dye) treatment, (3) iodine treatment, (4) *decolorization* using alcohol/acetone wash, and (4) *counterstaining* using safranin. Gram-positive bacteria have thick outer walls with no lipids, whereas gram-negative bacteria have a thin wall and an outer membrane. The difference between gram-positive and gram-negative organisms is in the cell-wall permeability to these complexes on treatment with mixtures of acetone and alcohol solvents. Thus, gram-positive bacteria retain purple iodine-dye complexes, whereas gram-negative bacteria do not retain these complexes when decolorized using an alcohol/acetone wash. If the iodine treatment step is omitted during the Gram stain process, the purple iodine-dye complexes will not form. The crystal violet will wash away during the alcohol/acetone decolorization washing step and all cells will appear *red*. Gram staining of pus or fluids along with clinical findings can guide the management of an infection before culture results are available in the clinical setting.

3-9. The answer is d. (*Murray, pp 86–101. Scriver, pp 2367–2424. Sack, pp 159–175.*) All of the poisons shown affect either electron transport or oxidative phosphorylation. Dinitrophenol is unique in that it disconnects the ordinarily tight coupling of electron transport and phosphorylation. In its presence, electron transport continues normally with no oxidative phosphorylation occurring. Instead, heat energy is generated. The same principle is utilized in a well-controlled way by brown fat to generate heat in newborn humans and cold-adapted mammals. The biological uncoupler in brown fat is a protein called thermogenin. Barbiturates, the antibiotic pie-ricidin A, the fish poison rotenone, dimercaprol, and cyanide all act by inhibiting the electron transport chain at some point.

3-10. The answer is d. *(Kandel, pp 1209–1221.)* Clinical studies of patients with major depressive disorders indicate that an intrinsic regulatory defect involving the hypothalamus underlies the disorder. It also involves the monoamine pathways. The hypothalamic modulation of neuroendocrine activity has been implicated, as have been the neurotransmitter systems of serotonin and norepinephrine. Recent evidence suggests a major role for the heritability of such neurochemical disorders. The role of behavior in stimulating or triggering such mechanisms is also being explored. While the frontal lobes, the pituitary, the hippocampus, and the corpus callosum are related to the emotions, memory, and neural communications, they do not play as major a role in the depressive disorders as does the hypo-thalamus.

3-11. The answer is b. *(Gilroy, p 337. Kandel, pp 951–953.)* Sleep apnea can occur for several reasons. One common basis is an obstruction of the airways (called *obstructive sleep apnea*). In this case, as indicated in the statement of the question, the physicians ruled out this possibility. Another possible cause involves central sleep apnea. This is due to disruption of the mechanism involving chemoreceptors in the carotid body that monitors carbon dioxide and oxygen levels in the blood. Axons in the carotid body project via the glossopharyngeal nerve (IX) to the reticular formation of the medulla. Therefore, disturbances involving the carotid body could result in central sleep apnea. Here, inappropriate signals are sent to the medullary reticular formation, which, in part, projects caudally to ventral horn sites in the spinal cord, governing such muscles as those that regulate the diaphragm and, therefore, disrupt the normal breathing process.

3-12. The answer is f. *(Craig, p 451; Hardman, p 648; Katzung, pp 260, 438.)* Tubocurarine, arguably the prototypic nondepolarizing skeletal neuromuscular blocker (competitive antagonist of the effects of ACh on skeletal muscle nicotinic receptors), differs from most of the other nonde-polarizing neuromuscular blockers (including pancuronium) because it quite effectively triggers histamine release. It is a "direct" effect on mast cells, not one involving activation of antibodies on the mast cells. This effect is not clinically significant for patients who do not have asthma, but for many who do, the bronchoconstriction can be problematic (even though the patient is intubated while they are receiving the blocker). In the absence of (released) histamine, curare and the other neuromuscular blockers would have no effect on airway smooth-muscle activity.

(Note: In addition to tubocurarine, morphine and several intravascular contrast media used in diagnostic radiology—particularly some of the iodinated compounds—also have a reputation as "histamine-releasers." Some venoms and other animal toxins also cause mast cell degranulation, a component of which is histamine release.)

Atropine causes bronchodilation by blocking muscarinic receptors on airway smooth muscle cells. Isoproterenol, the β_1/β_2 agonist, is a bronchodilator. Propranolol triggers airway smooth-muscle contraction in asthmatics, but that is due to blockade of epinephrine's agonist (bronchodilator) actions on β_2 receptors. Histamine is not involved in the responses to any of these drugs.

3-13.   The answer is e. (*Cotran, pp 164–165, 1287. Damjanov, pp 298–299.*) Almost all genes occur on chromosomes within the nucleus. There are a few genes, however, that are located within the mitochondria. These mitochondrial genes are found on mitochondrial DNA (mtDNA). These genes are all of maternal origin, possibly because ova have mitochondria within the large amount of cytoplasm while sperm do not. This maternal origin means that mothers transmit all of the mtDNA to both male and female offspring, but only the daughters transmit it further. No transmission occurs through males. This mtDNA contains genes that mainly code for oxidative phosphorylation enzymes, such as NADH dehydrogenase, cytochrome c oxidase, and ATP synthase. Symptoms of deficiencies of these enzymes occur in organs that require large amounts of ATP, such as the brain, muscle, liver, and kidneys. The mtDNA of these patients may be composed of either a mixture of mutant and normal DNA (heteroplasm) or of mutant DNA entirely (homoplasmy). The severity of these diseases correlates with the amount of mutant mtDNA that is present. One disease associated with mitochondrial inheritance is Leber hereditary optic neuropathy (LHON), which is characterized by progressive bilateral loss of central vision and usually occurs between 15 and 35 years of age. Other examples of mitochondrial inheritance include mitochondrial myopathies, which are characterized by the presence in muscle of mitochondria having abnormal sizes and shapes. These abnormal mitochondria may result in the histologic appearance of the muscle as ragged red fibers. Electron microscopy reveals the presence within large mitochondria of rectangular crystals that have a "parking lot" appearance.

3-14. The answer is b. *(Braunwald, pp 1365–1366.)* This is a rather classic presentation of acute pericarditis. The most common presentation of pericarditis or inflammation of the pericardium is chest pain, which may be quite severe. Often acute pericarditis follows a previous viral illness, which is important to elicit in the history when you are interviewing these patients because viruses are the most common cause of acute pericarditis. The classic EKG findings of acute pericarditis are diffuse ST elevation and PR depression (best seen in lead II). The crucial differential diagnosis to exclude pericarditis is acute myocardial infarction. This is best done by lack of reciprocal changes (ST depression) in any leads, which is quite common in acute myocardial injury. In acute pericarditis, the ST segment elevation involves all or almost all 12 EKG leads. If reciprocal ST depression occurs, pericarditis is not the likely diagnosis. A friction rub is very common. It is best heard if the patient is sitting up and leaning forward. It sometimes completely disappears if the patient is in the supine position. The friction rub can change frequently. The intensity and quality of the friction rub are variable. It may be very loud one day and markedly decreased the following day when you re-examine the patient. A pericardial effusion often accompanies pericardial inflammation and usually can be seen by echocardiogram. Acute myocardial infarction causes a large release of serum creatine kinase level in the blood. This is in contrast to pericarditis, which has a very small, if any creatine kinase release. This is usually not required to make the correct diagnosis, but it is important to recognize that minimal serum creatine kinase release occurs with acute pericarditis.

3-15. The answer is e. *(Boron, pp 53–54. Guyton, pp 361–363.)* The anion gap is the difference between the concentration of Na^+ and the concentration of the major plasma anions, Cl^- and HCO_3^-. The minor ions, lactate, phosphate, and sulfate, comprise the anion gap. Increases in lactate or citrate could have produced the anion gap. The low calcium favors citrate as the cause of the anion gap because citrate complexes with calcium. The high serum potassium concentration accounts for the peaked T waves seen on the EKG. Acidosis caused the shift of K^+ from the intracellular to the extracellular space. The low calcium produced relaxation of vascular smooth muscle, accounting for the low blood pressure.

3-16. The answer is E. *(Nolte, pp 52–60, 62–69, 375–394, 440–445, 507–524.)* This figure is a lateral view of the cerebral cortex. Cells in the "arm" area of the primary motor cortex (H) project their axons to the cervical level of the spinal cord and are activated at the time when a response of this limb occurs. The leg region of the left primary somatosensory cortex (A) lies immediately caudal to the central sulcus, is almost devoid of pyramidal cells, is referred to as a *granulous cortex,* and receives inputs from the right leg. Damage to this region would result in loss of vibration sensibility (as well as tactile sensation and two-point discrimination) from the right leg. Damage to the cells situated in the region of the dorsal border of the superior temporal gyrus and the adjoining area of the inferior parietal lobule (Wernicke's area; C) causes impairment in the appreciation of the meanings of written or spoken words.

The primary, secondary, and tertiary auditory receiving areas in the cortex are located mainly in the superior temporal gyrus (D). It is the final receiving area for inputs from the medial geniculate nucleus, which represents an important relay in the transmission of auditory signals to the cortex. Damage to this region of the cortex would result in some hearing loss. An additional area of the cortex governing speech (F) is called the *motor speech area,* or *Broca's area.* It is situated in the inferior aspect of the frontal lobe immediately rostral and slightly ventral to the precentral gyrus. Lesions of this region produce impairment of the ability to express words in a meaningful way or to use words correctly. The orbital frontal cortex (E) lies in a position inferior and rostral to Broca's motor speech area. This region governs higher-order intellectual functions and some aspects of emotional behavior. Damage to this region often results in personality changes and emotionality. The caudal aspect of the middle frontal gyrus (G) contains cells that, when activated, produce conjugate deviation of the eyes. This action is believed to be accomplished, in part, by virtue of descending projections to the superior colliculus, pretectal region, and horizontal gaze center of the pons. A lesion of this region would result in loss of capacity to produce voluntary horizontal movement of the eyes in one direction. Lesions of the posterior parietal lobe (B) of the nondominant hemisphere will produce a disorder of body image, referred to as *sensory neglect.* The patient will frequently fail to recognize or neglect to shave or wash those body parts. The patient may even fail to recognize the presence of a hemiparesis involving that part of the body as well. The precentral gyrus (H) constitutes the primary motor cortex. Lesions of this region produce a UMN paralysis involving a contralateral limb.

3-17. The answer is e. (*Braunwald, pp 2162–2165.*) Hypothyroid patients tend to gain weight. Prolactin-secreting tumors (prolactinomas), being located in the pituitary, might show abnormal physical examination findings at the eyes, given that the tumor typically sits on the optic chiasm or might cause galactorrhea. Early menopause is unlikely in a 22-year-old. Resistance to LH and FSH would have prohibited this patient from ever having menses. This leaves excessive exercise as the only remaining plausible cause in this patient.

3-18. The answer is c. (*Cotran, pp 739, 945, 951. Rubin, pp 890–892.*) Type I rapidly progressive glomerulonephritis reveals linear staining of IgG and C3 along the glomerular basement membrane, this being a classic type II hypersensitivity reaction. The majority of these patients are found to have Goodpasture's syndrome, which is characterized by the presence of autoantibodies against the noncollagenous portion of type IV collagen. Patients with Goodpasture's syndrome are usually males age 20 to 40. The lungs and kidneys are most often involved with this disease. Pulmonary hemorrhage produces hemoptysis and renal involvement produces hematuria; the chronic hemorrhage leads to anemia. Treatment is plasmapheresis or plasma exchange to remove autoantibodies from serum.

None of the other possible answers for this question have linear immunofluorescence patterns. Alport's syndrome is characterized clinically by recurrent hematuria, progressive hearing impairment, and ocular abnormalities, such as cataracts and dislocated lens. Henoch-Schönlein glomerulonephritis is a cause of focal segmental glomerulonephritis, and deposits may be found within the mesangial matrix. Finally, Wegener's granulomatosis, a disorder that is characterized by acute necrotizing granulomas of the respiratory tract along with focal necrotizing vasculitis, is a cause of type III rapidly progressive glomerulonephritis (pauci-immune crescentic GN).

3-19. The answer is c. (*Young, pp 329–331. McKenzie, pp 352–356. Junqueira, p 235.*) The cell marked with a star is a Leydig cell (i.e., interstitial cell) and is regulated by luteinizing hormone (LH), also known as interstitial cell–stimulating hormone (ICSH), secreted by gonadotrophs in the anterior pituitary. Leydig cells are located between seminiferous tubules and are responsible for the production of testosterone. The photomicrograph is from the human testis. The star delineates a cluster of Leydig cells, found between the seminferous tubules. The Leydig cells normally synthesize and release testosterone in response to ICSH/LH (interstitial cell–stimulating hormone/ luteinizing hormone) that is produced by gonadotrophs in the anterior pituitary. Leydig cell tumors develop in males between 20 and 60 years of age and produce androgens, estrogens, and sometimes glucocorticoids. Calcitonin is synthesized by C cells in the thyroid (answer a). Progesterone (answer b) is synthesized by corpora lutea under the influence of LH. FSH (follicle-stimulating hormone) plays a key physiological role in both males (spermatogenesis) and females (regulation of follicular growth) and is produced and released by gonadotrophs in the anterior pituitary (answer d). FSH stimulates the maturation of ovarian follicles. FSH treatment of humans results in development of more than the usual number of mature follicles and an increased number of mature gametes. FSH is also critical for sperm production. It supports the function of Sertoli cells, which serve a nutritive role in sperm cell maturation. Parathyroid hormone (answer e) is synthesized and released from the principal cells of the parathyroid gland.

Sertoli cells (asterisks, *) function in a nutritive and supportive role somewhat analogous to the glial cells of the CNS. The Sertoli cells produce inhibin, which feeds back on the anterior pituitary and hypothalamus to regulate FSH release. Testosterone is modified by binding to androgen-binding protein (ABP), which is synthesized by the Sertoli cells. The testosterone is necessary for the maintenance of spermatogenesis as well as the male ducts and accessory glands. ABP is regulated by FSH, testosterone, and inhibin. Sertoli cells have extensive tight (occluding) junctions between them that form the blood-testis barrier. Sertoli cells communicate with adjacent cells through gap junctions and extend from outside the blood-testis barrier (basal portion) to luminal to the blood-testis barrier (apical portion). During spermatogenesis, derivatives of spermatocytes cross from the basal to the adluminal compartment across the zonula occludens between adjacent Sertoli cells. Each Sertoli cell is, therefore, associated with multiple spermatogenic cells.

The testis is composed of seminiferous tubules containing a number of spermatogenic cells undergoing spermatogenesis and spermiogenesis. The cells labeled with the arrowheads are spermatogonia, the derivatives of the embryonic primordial germ cells. These cells comprise the basal layer and undergo mitosis (spermatocytogenesis) to form primary sper-matocytes, which have distinctive clumped or coarse chromatin (marked by arrows). Secondary spermatocytes are formed during the first meiotic division and exist for only a short period of time because there is no lag period before entry into the second meiotic division that results in the formation of spermatids. The spermatids begin as round structures and elongate with the formation of the flagellum. This last part of seminifer-ous tubule function is the differentiation of sperm from spermatocytes (spermiogenesis) and is complete with the release of mature sperm into the lumen of the tubule.

3-20. The answer is a. (*Craig, p 479; Hardman, pp 55, 1010–1011; Katzung, pp 1086–1087, 1128–1129, 1119.*) Cimetidine differs (signifi-cantly) from the other H_2 blockers, famotidine, nizatidine, and ranitidine, in that it is a very effective inhibitor of the hepatic mixed function oxidase (P450) drug-metabolizing enzyme systems. The alternatives have no sig-nificant P450-inhibiting activity, nor do they cause side effects as frequent or as problematic as those caused by cimetidine, especially at high doses. The outcome of P450 inhibition, of course, is reduced hepatic clearance of the interactants, leading to excessive serum concentrations and effects if their dosages are not reduced properly. The examples cited in the ques-tion—phenytoin, warfarin, quinidine, and theophylline—are among the most important interactants with cimetidine. They, and other interactants such as lidocaine, have rather low margins of safety, so even slight increases in serum levels may be enough to cause toxicity. Given the fact that the alternative H_2 blockers don't inhibit the P450 system, there's no rational reason or excuse for prescribing cimetidine to patients on multiple drug therapy (and in this case, the patient should have been warned about self-medicating with it).

Omeprazole and the related proton pump inhibitors participate in no clinically significant interactions with the drugs noted here, or others.

3-21. The answer is b. (*Mandell, pp 1685–1691. Rubin, pp 361–364. Cotran, p 333.*) The cytopathic effect of viruses is often a clue to the diag-nosis of the type of infection that is present. There are several types of her-pesviruses, which are relatively large, double-stranded DNA viruses. Infection by herpes simplex virus (HSV) or varicella-zoster virus (VZV) is recognized by nuclear homogenization (ground-glass nuclei), intranuclear inclusions (Cowdry type A bodies), and the formation of multinucleated cells. Herpes simplex type 2, a sexually transmitted viral disease, results in the formation of vesicles that ulcerate and cause burning, itching, and pain. These lesions heal spontaneously, but the virus remains dormant in the lumbar and sacral ganglia. Recurrent infections may occur, and transmission to the newborn during delivery is a feared complication that may be fatal to the infant. Shingles and chickenpox are caused by herpes zoster, which is identical to varicella. Cytomegalovirus (CMV) causes both the nucleus and the cytoplasm of infected cells to become enlarged. Infected cells have large, purple intranuclear inclusions surrounded by a clear halo and smaller, less prominent basophilic intracytoplasmic inclusions. Adenoviruses can produce similar inclusions, but the infected cells are not enlarged. Adenoviruses also produce characteristic smudge cells in infected respiratory epithelial cells. Human papillomavirus (HPV) infection may produce a characteristic effect that is called koilocytosis. Histologic examination reveals enlarged squamous epithelial cells that have shrunken nuclei ("raisinoid") within large cytoplasmic vacuoles. Candidiasis is the most common fungal infection of the vagina and is especially common in patients who have diabetes or take oral contraceptives. *Candida* infection causes vulvar itching and produces a white discharge. Microscopic examination of the vaginal discharge reveals yeast and pseudohyphae. *T. vaginalis*, a large, pear-shaped, flagellated protozoan, causes severe vaginal itching with dysuria. It produces a thick yellow-gray discharge.

3-22 The answer is d. (*Moore and Dalley, p 131.*) The presence of a systolic ejection-type murmur suggests that blood is becoming turbulent during contraction of the ventricles, consistent with the aortic valve stenosis. Aortic stenosis (often discovered in adults due to a congenital bicuspid aortic valve) produces a jet of blood, which in turn causes the subsequent dilation of the ascending aorta. Secondarily, the left ventricle hypertrophies in size due to the increased resistance of forcing blood through a small valve. Tetralogy of Fallot would generally be diagnosed in cyanotic newborns. Pulmonary valve stenosis is unlikely since the pulmonary trunk on this patient is normal. Atherosclerosis has nothing to do with the findings. A tricuspid valve defect would not produce a systolic murmur.

3-23. The answer is c. (*Craig, pp 738–740; Hardman, pp 850–851, 1303; Katzung, p 189.*) This is the interaction (and one that can be fatal) between sildenafil, tadalafil, or vardenafil, and organic nitrovasodilators (e.g., and perhaps especially, nitroglycerin). It occurs because both interactants cause vasodilation through a nitric oxide-cGMP-dependent mechanism, and the combination causes greater than additive effects of each agent alone. It is also an interaction that should be foremost in the mind of any physician who prescribes one of these wildly popular drugs for erectile dysfunction. For more complete comments on the mechanisms and manifestations of the interaction, check the answer to Question 213 (cardiovascular chapter).

3-24. The answer is c. (*Scriver, pp 3–45. Sack, pp 97–158.*) Males always transmit their single X chromosome to their daughters. Therefore, a daughter of a male affected with an X-linked disorder is an obligate carrier for that disorder. When the condition is X-linked recessive, as with most forms of color-blindness, the daughter is unlikely to show any phenotypic evidence that she is carrying this abnormal gene. Offspring of female carriers are of four types: (1) female carrier with one normal and one mutant allele, (2) normal female with two normal alleles, (3) affected male with a single mutant allele, and (4) normal male with a single normal allele. The chance of having an affected child is thus ¼ or 25%. If the obligate carrier female gives birth to a son, the chance of the son being color-blind is 50%.

3-25. The answer is a. (*Moore and Persaud, Developing, pp 256–259.*) Blockage of the foregut in the newborn produces projectile vomiting. Congenital hypertrophic pyloric stenosis, occurring in 0.5 to 1.0% of males and rarely in females, involves hypertrophy of the circular layer of muscle at the pylorus. This usually does not regress and must be treated surgically. During the fifth and sixth weeks of development, the lumen of the duodenum is occluded by muscle proliferation but normally recanalizes during the eighth week. Failure of recanalization results in duodenal atresia. Because this occurs distal to the hepatopancreatic ampulla, the vomitus will occasionally be stained with bile. Annular pancreas, rare in itself, seldom completely blocks the duodenum. Imperforate anus results in intestinal distention with bloating.

3-26. The answer is c. (*Brooks, pp 445–447. Levinson, pp 268–269. Murray—2002, pp 562–563. Ryan, p 591.*) Saint Louis encephalitis virus has structural and biologic characteristics in common with other Flaviviruses.

It is the most important arboviral disease in North America. Saint Louis encephalitis virus was first isolated from mosquitoes in California. Patients who contract the disease usually present with one of three clinical manifestations: febrile headache, aseptic meningitis, or clinical encephalitis.

3-27. The answer is b. (*Moore and Dalley, pp 191 and 257.*) The spleen is a large blood filled organ with a relatively thin capsule that can rupture upon sudden deceleration, causing bleeding into the peritoneal cavity. Appearing pale, the positional hypotension and tachycardia would be consistent with bleeding into the peritoneal cavity, which would lead to generalized abdominal pain, and guarding. (Answer a) Being pregnant does not cause pain. (Answer c) Peritonitis from a ruptured gallbladder would not occur in just 20 min and does not fit with the blood loss symptoms. Neither diverticulitis (answer d) nor hemorrhoids (answer e) would cause the set of symptoms listed.

3-28. The answer is d. (*Greenberg, pp 167–170.*) Multiple sclerosis is a demyelinating disease. The lesions may also involve some reactive gliosis and axonal degeneration as well. It occurs mainly in the white matter of the spinal cord and brain as well as in the optic nerve.

3-29. The answer is a. (*Murray, p 300. Scriver, pp 2537–2570. Sack, pp 97–158.*) The child has Lesch-Nyhan syndrome (308000), an X-linked recessive disorder that is caused by HGPRT enzyme deficiency. HGPRT is responsible for the salvage of purines from nucleotide degradation, and its deficiency elevates levels of PRPP, purine synthesis, and uric acid. PRPP is also elevated in glycogen storage diseases due to increased amounts of carbohydrate precursors.

3-30. The answer is d. (*Cotran, pp 97–98, 104–106.*) Growth factors are chemicals that are associated with cell growth. For example, fibroblast growth factor (FGF) can induce the growth and proliferation of fibroblasts. Additionally, one type of FGF, basic FGF, is capable of inducing all of the stages of angiogenesis (basement membrane and extracellular matrix degradation, endothelial migration, endothelial proliferation, and endothelial differentiation). The epidermal growth factor family includes epidermal growth factor (EGF) and transforming growth factor α (TGF-α). These substances can cause proliferation of many types of epithelial cells and fibroblasts. The EGF receptor is c-erb B1. Platelet-derived growth factor (PDGF), which is found in platelets, activated macrophages, endothelial cells, and smooth muscle cells, can cause migration and proliferation of fibroblasts, smooth muscle cells, and monocytes. TGF-β, produced by platelets, endothelial cells, T cells, and macrophages, is associated with fibrosis. In low concentrations it causes the synthesis and secretion of PDGF, but in high concentrations it inhibits growth due to inhibition of the expression of PDGF receptors.

3-31. The answer is e. (*Cotran, pp 618–619. Hoffman, pp 491–495.*) The thalassemia syndromes are characterized by a decreased or absent synthesis of either the α- or the α-globin chain of hemoglobin A (alpha2-beta2). α thalassemias result from reduced synthesis of α-globin chains, while β thalassemias result from reduced production of β-globin chains. The α thalassemias result from deletions of one or more of the total of four α-globin genes, while β thalassemias result from point mutations involving the β-globin gene. There are two α-globin genes on each chromosome 16, and the normal genotype is $\alpha,\alpha/$. On each chromosome either or both of the α genes can be deleted. Deletion of both genes (— —/) is called alpha thal 1. This genotype is found in individuals in Southeast Asia and the Mediterranean. In contrast, deletion of only one α gene on a chromosome (— $\alpha/$) is called alpha thal 2 and is found in Africans. The severity of α thalassemia depends on the number of α genes deleted. Deletions of only one gene (— $\alpha/\alpha,\alpha$) results in a silent carrier. These patients are completely asymptomatic and all laboratory tests are normal. This clinical state can only be inferred from examination of a pedigree. Deletion of two α genes results in alpha thal trait. There are two possibilities for deletion of two α genes: the deletions may be on the same chromosome (— —/α,α, which is called the *cis* type) or the deletions may be on different chromosomes (— $\alpha/$—α, which is called the *trans* type). The former, which is also called heterozygous alpha thal 1, is more common in Asians, while the latter, which is also called alpha thal 2, is more common in Africans. Clinically this is quite important because the offspring of parents with the *trans* deletions cannot develop H disease or hydrops. Deletion of three α genes (— —/—α) is called hemoglobin H disease. This name results from the fact that excess β chains postnatally form aggregates of β tetramers, which are called hemoglobin H. These aggregates form Heinz bodies, which can be seen with crystal blue stain. The most severe form of α thalassemia, hydrops fetalis, results from deletion of all four α genes (— —/— —) (Note that Cooley's anemia is the most severe form of β thalassemia). In hydrops fetalis, which is lethal in utero, no α chains are produced. Staining of the erythrocytes with a supravital stain demonstrates numerous intracytoplasmic inclusions within the red cells, which are aggregates of hemoglobin Bart's (gamma4).

3-32. The answer is c. (*Brooks, pp 366–369, 378–379, 384, 436–438, 512–513. Levinson, pp 225–226, 231–233. Murray—2002, pp 458, 467, 484, 494–495, 548. Ryan, pp 509–510, 564–565, 568, 579, 619.*) Varicella-zoster virus is a herpesvirus. Chickenpox is a highly contagious disease of childhood that occurs in the late winter and early spring. It is characterized by a generalized vesicular eruption with relatively insignificant systemic manifestations.

Adenovirus has been associated with adult respiratory disease among newly enlisted military troops. Crowded conditions and strenuous exercise may account for the severe infections seen in this otherwise healthy group.

Papillomavirus is one of two members of the family Papovaviridae, which includes viruses that produce human warts. These viruses are host-specific and produce benign epithelial tumors that vary in location and clinical appearance. The warts usually occur in children and young adults and are limited to the skin and mucous membranes.

Rotavirus is worldwide in distribution and has been implicated as the major etiologic agent of infantile gastroenteritis. Infection with this virus varies in its clinical presentation from asymptomatic infection to a relatively mild diarrhea to a severe and sometimes fatal dehydration. The exact mode of transmission of this infectious agent is not known. Because of severe side effects, the rotavirus vaccine has been recalled and is temporarily unavailable.

Infectious mononucleosis caused by cytomegalovirus (CMV) is clinically difficult to distinguish from that caused by Epstein-Barr virus. Lymphocytosis is usually present, with an abundance of atypical lymphocytes. CMV-induced mononucleosis should be considered in any case of mononucleosis that is heterophil-negative and in patients with fever of unknown origin.

3-33. The answer is e. (*Boron, pp 273–275. Guyton, pp 636–639.*) The Babinski reflex causes the toes to dorsiflex in response to stroking the plantar or lateral portion of the foot. It is an abnormal reflex caused by damage to the corticospinal (pyramidal) tract that travels from the cortical motor cortex through the pyramids to the spinal cord. Other signs of pyramidal tract lesions include loss of the hopping and placing reaction, the cremasteric reflex, and the abdominal scratch reflex. Damage confined to the pyramidal tract results in distal muscular weakness and loss of fine motor control. Damage to other areas of the cortical motor control system is referred to as upper motor neuron disease and produces spasticity. Damage to the basal ganglia produces a variety of signs including dystonia (striatum), ballism (subthalamic nucleus), and tremor (substantia nigra). Damaging the cerebellum causes uncoordinated movements (dysmetria).

3-34. The answer is b. *(Braunwald, pp 2149–2150.)* Testicular causes are those with a direct effect on the testicles. Alcohol directly affects the testicles, causing atrophy with inadequate sperm production. It also causes decreased plasma testosterone. Posttesticular causes are those that affect sperm transport, and pretesticular causes are those that affect the hormones that stimulate the testicles. Idiopathic causes represent those causes that are likely genetic and not elsewhere classified.

3-35 The answer is a. *(Sierles, pp 182–184. Wedding, pp 184–199.)* There are a number of ways a physician can facilitate an interview, but in this case momentary silence would be most appropriate; i.e., you should continue to listen and perhaps offer a tissue, a nod, or a simple affirmation of understanding her import, such as "I see." This would do more to support her by letting her express her feelings and not interrupt her flow of thoughts with another question or statement. Studies show that doctors tend to interrupt a patient after about 18 seconds and that crying is very upsetting to many doctors, who then feel compelled to say something—anything. Statements such as "I know how you feel" are usually inappropriate because most doctors do not know how a patient feels (unless they have had a son come home with AIDS). "Don't worry, it'll be OK" is a shallow response and does not support or help the patient, as the patient realizes that the doctor does not know that the patient will be fine. The question "Why are you so upset" is often interpreted as an accusation or inability to understand or express empathy. Saying "You know you can tell me anything" may be an attempt to reassure the patient, but it is inappropriate in a new patient who does not know that you can be told everything at this point in the relationship. The question "Are you thinking you may have AIDS?" is an inappropriate interruption and a very unlikely guess as to what may be upsetting the patient. It could be appropriate later in the interview, but only after exploring many other physical and psychological factors.

3-36. The answer is e. *(Kandel, pp 36–37. Siegel et al., pp 244–245. Gilroy, pp 370–371.)* Phenylketonuria results in severe mental retardation and is caused by a defect in the gene that provides the code for Phe hydroxylase, the enzyme that converts Phe to tyrosine. As a result of this defective gene, there is an abundance of Phe in the brain, which produces a toxic metabolite, thus interfering in brain development and maturation.

3-37. The answer is e. *(Cotran, pp 1109–1111. Rubin, pp 1041, 1044.)* Lobular carcinoma of the breast, both in situ and invasive, is an important lesion clinically because of its tendency to occur multicentrically within the same breast and also because of its association with a high frequency of disease (both ductal and lobular carcinoma) in the opposite breast. Lobular carcinoma in situ is characterized histologically by proliferation of cells of the terminal duct lobular unit, which fills and expands the lobules. Unlike the case with intraductal carcinoma, papillary and cribriform structures are not formed and neither is central necrosis present. Invasive lobular carcinoma is distinguished by its tendency to infiltrate the stroma in a single file. This pattern is not seen with invasive ductal carcinoma, which tends to cause a marked desmoplastic response, causing a scirrhous carcinoma. Infiltrating lobular carcinomas also form concentric "targets" around ducts, and they have an increased frequency of being estrogen receptor-positive.

In contrast to the histologic appearance of infiltrating lobular carcinoma, Paget's disease is characterized by infiltration of the epidermis by malignant cells with clear cytoplasm. Histologic sections of a medullary carcinoma of the breast reveal large syncytium-like sheets of pleomorphic cells surrounded by aggregates of lymphocytes, while colloid breast carcinoma shows small individual malignant cells dispersed within extracellular pools of mucin.

3-38. The answer is E. *(Afifi, pp 104–117.)* The nucleus gracilis (A) contains cells that respond to movement of the lower limb as a result of joint capsule activation. Damage to this region will result in loss of conscious proprioception associated with the leg, and, additionally, the loss of conscious proprioception will result in ataxia because this input is essential for normal ambulation to occur. The nucleus cuneatus (B) contains cells that respond to a variety of stimuli applied to the upper limb, including vibratory stimuli. One component of the descending medial longitudinal fasciculus (E) contains fibers that arise from the medial vestibular nucleus that project to cervical levels and contribute to reflex activity associated with the position of the head. The descending track of the trigeminal nerve (C) contains first-order fibers mediating pain and temperature information from the head region. Because of its lateral position in the brainstem, a surgical procedure is sometimes carried out to cut these fibers as a means of alleviating excruciating pain. Fibers of the medial lemniscus (D) arise from the contralateral dorsal column nuclei and ascend to the ventral posterolateral nucleus of the thalamus. These fibers transmit the same information noted earlier for the dorsal column nuclei, which includes two-point discrimination and conscious proprioception from the opposite side of the body.

3-39. The answer is e. *(Boron, pp 606–616, 678–682, 710.)* The reduced lung volumes indicate a restrictive lung disease. Although the amount of gas that can be expelled from the lung in 1 s will be less than normal, the increased recoil force of the lung will produce an FEV_1/FVC ratio that is close to normal. Patients with restrictive lung disease have small tidal volumes. The diffusing capacity will be reduced because the small lung volumes reduce the surface area available for gas exchange. The presence of V/Q abnormalities is indicated by the need for supplemental oxygen.

3-40. The answer is d. *(Brooks, pp 272, 613. Levinson, p 158. Murray—2002, p 424. Ryan, p 904.)* Microscopic examination can readily demonstrate clue cells (epithelial cells with *Gardnerella* bacteria attached) as pseudohyphae (*Candida*). A wet mount will be needed to demonstrate motile *Trichomonas* cells. *Candida, Trichomonas,* and bacterial vaginitis are seen most often. *S. aureus* is involved much less frequently. While *E. coli* may be a common cause of genitourinary infection, clue cells are usually absent.

3-41. The answer is b. *(Nolte, p 227.)* A principal descending component of the MLF arises from the medial vestibular nucleus, and, accordingly, this bundle is sometimes referred to as the *medial vestibulospinal tract.* The overall function of the MLF is to help coordinate changes in position or balance with the position of the head and eyes. The descending fibers of the MLF provide the anatomic substrate by which the inputs from the vestibular apparatus can influence the manner in which the head will be positioned.

It accomplishes this by modulating upper cervical neurons that innervate muscles of the neck that control the position of the head. Since the projection is to the cervical cord, it would not likely have any direct effect upon extensor reflex activity of the lower limbs. Likewise, these descending fibers do not affect any structures that would cause alterations in blood pressure. This pathway does not innervate neurons of the spinal cord that supply the upper or lower limbs. Therefore, a UMN paralysis would not be expected. In addition, these fibers do not innervate the cerebellum or mediate conscious proprioception. Only if there were damage to the cerebellum or fibers mediating this form of sensation would one expect ataxia to occur.

3-42. The answer is e. (*Craig, pp 693–694; Hardman, p 1667; Katzung, p 650.*) These findings are characteristic of what one would expect with long-term (and high dose) systemic glucocorticoid therapy (i.e., prednisone and many others, but not beclomethasone, which is given by oral inhalation and is not absorbed appreciably). Psychoses, peptic ulceration with hemorrhage (coffee-grounds stool, indicative of gastric bleeding) or without (possibly causing guaiac-positive stools), increased susceptibility to infection, edema, osteoporosis, myopathy, and hypokalemic alkalosis can occur. Other adverse reactions include cataracts, hyperglycemia, slowed lineal growth in children, and iatrogenic Cushing's syndrome.

Hydrochlorothiazide (and other thiazide and thiazide-like diuretics, such as chlorthalidone or metolazone) can increase blood glucose levels. However, they typically lower blood pressure (as evidenced by their widespread use as antihypertensives) and tend to raise, not lower, serum calcium levels (which would be inconsistent with the decreased bone density described in this man). None of the other drugs listed would cause a collection of findings consistent with what we described here.

3-43. The answer is a. (*Cotran, pp 712–716. Rubin, pp 630–633.*) Chronic obstructive pulmonary diseases (COPDs) are characterized by obstruction to airflow somewhere along the airways. These diseases may affect the bronchus, the bronchiole, or the acinus. Asthma, bronchiectasis, and chronic bronchitis affect primarily the bronchus, while emphysema affects primarily the acinus. Asthma is a pulmonary disease that is caused by excessive bronchoconstriction secondary to airways that are hyperreactive to numerous stimuli. Asthma has been divided into extrinsic and intrinsic categories. The extrinsic category includes atopic (allergic) asthma, occupational asthma, and allergic bronchopulmonary aspergillosis. The intrinsic category includes nonreaginic asthma and pharmacologic asthma. The former is related to respiratory tract infections, while the latter is often related to aspirin sensitivity. These aspirin-sensitive patients often have recurrent rhinitis and nasal polyps. In these patients the aspirin initiates an asthmatic attack by inhibiting the cyclooxygenase pathway of arachidonic acid metabolism without affecting the lipoxygenase pathway. This causes the relative excess production of the leukotrienes, which are bronchoconstrictors.

3-44. The answer is a. (*Brooks, pp 285–288. Levinson, pp 153–155. Murray—2002, pp 381–383. Ryan, pp 424–429.*) In men, the appearance of a hard chancre on the penis characteristically indicates syphilis. Even though the chancre does not appear until the infection is two or more weeks old, the VDRL test for syphilis still can be negative despite the presence of a chancre (the VDRL test may not become positive for two or three weeks after initial infection). However, a lesion suspected of being a primary syphilitic ulcer should be examined by dark-field microscopy, which can reveal motile treponemes.

3-45. The answer is d. (*McKenzie, pp 334–335. Kierszenbaum, pp 373–375. Junqueira, pp 383–384, 388, 389.*) The genetic mutation in COL4A5 leads to a defect in the α chains that comprise type IV collagen found in the lamina densa of the basement membrane in the accompanying electron micrograph of the basal lamina. The glomerular basement membrane will therefore show abnormal splitting and thinning in the lamina densa and overall thickening. The hematuria results from breakdown of the basal lamina, allowing the passage of red blood cells and eventually protein (proteinuria). The patient suffers from Alport's syndrome resulting from a mutation of the α_5 chain of type IV collagen. Remember that type IV collagen consists of three α chains forming a triple helix. The noncollagenous C-terminal (NC1) and the 7S N-terminal are particularly important for the cross-linking of type IV collagen. The cross-linking forms the scaffolding of the basement membrane necessary for the normal filtration properties of the basal lamina. Proliferation of mesangial cells and increased production of mesangial matrix are typical of later stages of Alport's syndrome when glomerulonephritis is a prominent feature of the disease.

The glomerular filtration barrier consists of the pedicel (**B**) of the podocyte (**A**), the basal lamina (**C**) synthesized by the podocyte, and the endothelial cell (**E**). The podocyte consists of a "cell body" of cytoplasm with long processes that encircle the glomerular basement membrane. The filtration slits are labeled **E**. The filtration slits are located between adjacent pedicels (foot processes of the podocytes). The remainder of the filtration barrier is formed by the glomerular basement membrane, which contains type IV collagen and heparan sulfate. At high magnification there are three distinct layers within the glomerular basement membrane: (1) an electron-dense lamina densa (type IV collagen) in the center surrounded by (2) the lamina rara externa on the glomerular side and by (3) the lamina rara interna on the capillary endothelial side.

The glomerular filtration barrier is a physical and charge barrier that exhibits selectivity based on molecular size and charge. The presence of collagen type IV in the lamina densa of the basement membrane presents a physical barrier to the passage of large proteins from the blood to the urinary space. Glycosaminoglycans, particularly heparan sulfate, produce a polyanionic charge that binds cationic molecules. The foot processes are coated with a glycoprotein called podocalyxin, which is rich in sialic acid and provides mutual repulsion to maintain the structure of the filtration slits. It also possesses a large polyanionic charge for repulsion of large anionic proteins.

3-46. The answer is c. (*Craig, pp 37, 559; Hardman, p 1279; Katzung, p 1123.*) Rifampin is an excellent example of a drug that induces the hepatic metabolism of many other drugs, thereby lowering blood levels (and effects) of its interactants. Theophylline and corticosteroids are among them. Thus, as a result of the interaction we would expect decreases—not increases—in the effects of theophylline and/or of the prednisone. Both are susceptible to the metabolizing-inducing effects of rifampin.

With the expected decline in blood levels of both the oral bronchodilator (theophylline) and the anti-inflammatory drug (prednisone), it is likely that control of the patient's asthma will be lost and symptoms will appear.

Absorbed rifampin is rapidly eliminated in the bile and undergoes enterohepatic recirculation. However, there is no reason to suspect that either the theophylline, the corticosteroid, or their combination would have effects on rifamycin elimination. Likewise, these drugs do not increase the risk of rifampin-induced hepatotoxicity, which is quite rare unless the patient is taking other hepatotoxic drugs or has pre-existing liver disease.

3-47. The answer is d. (*Cotran, pp 1145–1147. Rubin, p 1177.*) The development of a thyroid mass in a young person who gives a familial history for a similar lesion should raise high clinical suspicion of the possibility that the mass is a medullary carcinoma of the thyroid (MCT). MCT is a tumor of the parafollicular (C) cells of the thyroid and as such is associated with secretion of calcitonin. The procalcitonin is deposited in the stroma of the tumor and appears as amyloid, which stains positively with Congo red stain. The tumor cells have peripheral nuclei that give them a plasmacytoid appearance when viewed cytologically with fine-needle aspiration (FNA). Electron microscopy reveals membrane-bound dense-core neurosecretory granules in the neoplastic cells. MCT may secrete other substances in addition to calcitonin, such as ACTH, CEA, and serotonin. It is also associated with paraneoplastic syndromes, such as carcinoid syndrome (due to serotonin) and Cushing's syndrome (due to ACTH).

3-48. The answer is a. (*Craig, pp 66–67, 94, 340–341; Hardman, pp 127, 143; Katzung, pp 90, 444, 1107.*) Botulinus (botulinum) toxin prevents release of acetylcholine (from storage vesicles) by virtually all cholinergic nerves. Thus, there is no activation of any cholinergic receptors, whether nicotinic or muscarinic. Noteworthy findings, then, include an inability to activate all postganglionic neurons (sympathetic and parasympathetic), no physiologic release of epinephrine from the adrenal medulla, and flaccid skeletal muscle paralysis due to failure of ACh release from motor nerves. The cause of death is ventilatory failure because the intercostal muscles and diaphragm are nonfunctional.

Pralidoxime is a cholinesterase reactivator, an antidote for poisonings with "irreversible" cholinesterase inhibitors such as soman, sarin ("nerve gases"), and many organophosphorus insecticides. Because no ACh is being released in botulinus poisoning, "reactivation" of the enzyme that normally metabolizes the neurotransmitter is irrelevant (and ineffective).

3-49. The answer is d. (*Braunwald, p 878.*) β-Lactam antibiotics, in particular high-dose penicillin G and imipenin, are known to induce seizures especially in the presence of renal dysfunction. Acute treatment of the seizure would be the same as for any other source of seizure. Other medications could contribute to lowering seizure threshold via lowering the magnesium level (such as diuretics). The use of phenytoin should not be necessary unless recurrent events occur. The CT of the head is reasonable; however, the discontinuation of the β-lactam would be the first step.

3-50. The answer is e. (*Cotran, p 561. Henry, pp 296–300.*) The clinical diagnosis of myocardial infarction depends on correlating clinical symptoms, ECG findings, and serum cardiac enzyme changes. The classic description of the pain produced by an MI is crushing, substernal pain that may radiate down the patient's left arm. This pain may be associated with sweating, nausea, and vomiting. ECG findings associated with MI include ST segment elevation (which may return to normal), inverted T waves, and abnormal Q waves. Serum enzymes that may be elevated after an MI include troponin, CPK, SGOT (AGT), and LDH, which are increased temporally in that order. The troponin complex is made up of three protein subunits: troponin I (Tn-I), troponin T, and troponin C. There are three isoforms of Tn-I: two in skeletal muscle and one in cardiac muscle (cTn-I). cTn-I levels begin to increase 4 to 6 h after the onset of chest pain, reach maximal serum concentration in about 12 to 24 h, and remain elevated for about 3 to 10 days. CPK exists in three isoenzymes, MM, MB, and BB, where M stands for muscle and B stands for brain. Elevation of the CPK MB isoenzyme is seen following an MI. Levels begin to rise at 4 to 8 h, peak at 12 to 24 h, and return to normal in 3 to 4 days. LDH exists in five isoenzyme forms. Normally serum LDH2 is greater than LDH1, but following an MI this ratio is flipped; that is, LDH1 is greater than LDH2. LDH1 levels begin to rise at 10 to 12 h, peak at 2 to 3 days, and return to normal in 7 to 10 days.

Finally note that new cardiac markers use monoclonal antibodies directed against myoglobin, CK-MB mass assay, and cardiac troponin levels. Myoglobin is a small monomer with a rapid rise and fall in serum (narrow window) that may be used to test the effect of "clot-busting" drugs, especially with rapid serial detection.

BLOCK 4

Answers

4-1. The answer is a. *(Cotran, pp 516–518. Rubin, pp 516–517.)* Giant cell arteritis (temporal arteritis), although not a major public health problem, is an important disease to consider in the differential diagnosis of patients of middle to advanced age who present with a constellation of symptoms that may include migratory muscular and back pains (polymyalgia rheumatica), dizziness, visual disturbances, headaches, weight loss, anorexia, and tenderness over one or both of the temporal arteries. The cause of the arteritis (which may include giant cells, neutrophils, and chronic inflammatory cells) is unknown, but the dramatic response to corticosteroids suggests an immunogenic origin. The disease may involve any artery within the body, but involvement of the ophthalmic artery or arteries may lead to blindness unless steroid therapy is begun. Therefore, if temporal arteritis is suspected, the workup to document it should be expedited and should include a biopsy of the temporal artery. Frequently, the erythrocyte sedimentation rate (ESR) is markedly elevated to values of 90 or greater. Whereas tenderness, nodularity, or skin reddening over the course of one of the scalp arteries, particularly the temporal, may show the ideal portion for a biopsy, it is important to recognize that the temporal artery may be segmentally involved or not involved at all even when the disease is present.

4-2. The answer is a. *(Guyton, pp 84–86. Boron, pp 241–243.)* The ryanodine receptor or calcium release channel on the sarcoplasmic reticulum (SR) is normally opened when skeletal muscle is activated. The flow of calcium through the open ryanodine receptor binds to troponin and initiates muscle contraction. The metabolic activity accompanying muscle contraction can warm the body. If a mutation in the ryanodine receptor causes uncontrolled release of calcium from the SR, the body temperature can rise to levels that cause brain damage.

4-3. The answer is d. *(Levinson, pp 396–397.)* Allograft rejection is an acute process that occurs 11 to 14 days after placement of the allograft (grafts among genetically different individuals of the same species), in this case skin allografts, that is mediated by T cells. Most of the killing of allograft cells is carried out by cytotoxic CD8-positive T cells. B cell antibody responses, IgE, and nitric oxide do not play a role in the rejection of allografts.

4-4. The answer is b. *(Craig, pp 389–391; Hardman, pp 432–437; Katzung, pp 483–486.)* Amitriptyline is a tertiary amine tricyclic antidepressant. It functions as a norepinephrine reuptake inhibitor. Brain levels of amines are increased. This results in increased vesicular stores of norepinephrine and serotonin. Amitriptyline is a prototypical tricyclic antidepressant that has proved useful in patients with sleep and appetite disorders.

4-5. The answer is e. *(Alberts, pp 720–722, 724, 729–730, 744–745. Junqueira, pp 40, 51.)* The child is suffering from inclusion (I)–cell disease. There is an absence or deficiency of N-acetylglucosamine phosphotransferase and an absence of mannose-6-phosphate (M6P) on the lysosomal enzymes. The failure to add M6P in the cis-Golgi results in inappropriate vesicular segregation by M6P receptors in the trans–Golgi network (TGN). The default pathway is transport to the cell membrane and secretion from the cell by exocytosis for proteins lacking M6P. Lysosomal enzymes are secreted into the bloodstream, and undigested substrates build up within the cells. There is no missorting back to the Golgi (answer a). Peroxisomal enzymes, which are sorted by the presence of three specific amino acids located at the C-terminus: –Ser–Lys–Leu–COO⁻, are not affected (answer b). KDEL (answer c) is the signal used for retrieval of proteins from the Golgi back to the endoplasmic reticulum. SNAREs [soluble-N-ethylemalemide sensitive factor (NSF) attachment protein receptors] are the receptors for SNAPs [soluble-N-ethylemalemide sensitive factor (NSF) attachment proteins] and bind vesicles to membranes (answer d). Trafficking to other structures, such as the nucleus and mitochondria, is regulated by nuclear localization signals (NLSs) or an N-terminal signal peptide, respectively.

4-6. The answer is c. *(Craig, p 263; Hardman, pp 1354, 1356–1357; Katzung, p 554.)* Clopidogrel (and the somewhat older related drug, ticlopidine) decreases platelet aggregation by blocking a proaggregatory interaction between adenosine 5′-diphosphate (ADP) and a population of platelet ADP receptors. There are at least two populations of platelet ADP receptors, and both must be activated to trigger aggregation. Thus, clopidogrel is sufficient to block one of those obligatory pathways. Clopidogrel has no effect on prostaglandin synthesis.

4-7. The answer is F. (*Afifi, 118–139. Nolte, pp 230–239, 255–274, 284–307.*) The inferior vestibular nucleus (B) lies immediately medial to the inferior cerebellar peduncle (shown at C) and receives direct inputs from first-order vestibular fibers that arise from the vestibular apparatus. The medial longitudinal fasciculus (E) contains second-order vestibular fibers, the majority of which ascend in the brainstem to innervate cranial nerve nuclei III, IV, and VI. A small component of this bundle also descends to cervical levels of the spinal cord from the medial vestibular nucleus. As noted previously, the descending component of the MLF integrates vestibular signals, which help to regulate the position of the head with changes in position of the body. Damage to this structure will also affect the ascending fibers, which innervate the neurons controlling the extraocular eye muscles. Such damage would result in nystagmus. The solitary nucleus (D) receives inputs from first-order taste fibers and is thus a special visceral afferent nucleus that transmits taste signals to the ventral posteromedial nucleus of the thalamus. The solitary nucleus also receives cardiovascular inputs from cranial nerve IX and, for this reason, has properties of a general visceral afferent nucleus as well. The hypoglossal nucleus (A) innervates the muscles of the tongue, causing it to protrude outward and to the opposite side. Thus, when this nerve is damaged, the opposite (normal) nerve causes the tongue to deviate to the side of the lesion when the patient attempts to stick out his tongue.

The medial lemniscus (G) ascends to the thalamus and transmits information associated with conscious proprioception from the contralateral side of the body as a result of the decussating fibers of the medial lemniscus. This bundle constitutes a second-order neuron that arises from the dorsal column nuclei of the lower medulla. The dorsal column nuclei receive first-order signals that mediate conscious proprioception from fibers contained within the dorsal columns of the spinal cord. Damage to the medial lemniscus would result in loss of conscious proprioception on the side of the body opposite the lesion. The spinal nucleus of cranial nerve V (F) receives pain and temperature fibers from first-order trigeminal neurons that arise from the head. Damage to this region would result in loss of pain sensation from the ipsilateral side of the face. The inferior cerebellar peduncle (C) is one of two principal cerebellar afferent pathways. One major fiber group contained within the inferior cerebellar peduncle arises from brainstem structures such as the contralateral inferior olivary nucleus and reticular formation. The other groups of fibers contained within this bundle arise from the spinal cord. Of the fibers that ascend in this bundle from the spinal cord, many constitute second-order muscle spindle afferents that arise from the nucleus dorsalis of Clarke.

4-8. The answer is e. *(Baum, pp 138–148, 275–281.)* Hostility and anger are major triggers for a coronary and increased mortality rate. The Cook-Medley Hostility Inventory is a scale devised from the hostility components of the Minnesota Multiphasic Personality Inventory (MMPI) and has a high predictability of incidence of coronary heart disease and death from all causes.

The Millon Behavioral Health Inventory is a 150-item inventory assessing personality, coping styles, stress, psychosomatic correlates, and indices that predict complications or difficulties with illness. The Cohen Perceived Stress Scale contains a general distress factor, a perceived coping-ability measure, and a scale for symptoms related to depression. The Rosenman and Friedman Type A Structured Interview has a high degree of interrater agreement in categorizing people as having type A or type B personality characteristics: tense, impatient, hostile, and urgent versus relaxed, quiet, and less hostile, respectively. The Jenkins Activity Survey of type A behavior is a self-report questionnaire asking about specific type A behaviors such as hurrying a person along or setting deadlines and quotas that fit the stereotype of the coronary-prone individual. All of the tests listed can provide information on personality factors linked to coronary proneness, but the Cook-Medley Hostility Inventory is the best behavioral predictor because it yields the most accurate data on hostility.

4-9. The answer is e. *(Murray, pp 326–340. Scriver, pp 5587–5628. Sack, pp 3–29.)* Normal parents having two affected children, male and female, is suggestive of autosomal recessive inheritance. This interpretation fits with the usual inheritance of oculocutaneous albinism (203100), implying a ¼ risk for a newborn in whom signs and symptoms of albinism are not yet evident. The defect in melanin synthesis in albinism decreases the amount of this protective pigment in skin and increases the exposure of DNA in skin cells to sunlight. Ultraviolet rays from sunlight cause DNA cross-linkage between at least two bases in the same or opposite strands of DNA. Cross-linking occurs through the formation of thymine-thymine dimers. The DNA cross-links cause higher rates of mutation and skin cancer in albinism, mandating the wearing of protective clothing, sunglasses, and sunscreens by affected individuals. DNA deletions and point mutations are less common than DNA cross-links after sunlight exposure.

4-10. The answer is d. (*Cotran, pp 261–264. Chandrasoma, pp 264–268.*) The names given to tumors are based on the parenchymal component of the tumor, which consists of the proliferating neoplastic cells. In general, benign tumors are designated by using the suffix -oma attached to a name describing either the cell of origin of the tumor or the gross or microscopic appearance of the tumor. Examples of benign tumors whose names are based on their microscopic appearance include adenomas, which have a uniform proliferation of glandular epithelial cells; papillomas, which are tumors that form finger-like projections; fibromas, which are composed of a uniform proliferation of fibrous tissue; leiomyomas, which originate from smooth muscle cells and have elongated, spindle-shaped nuclei; hemangiomas, which are formed from a uniform proliferation of endothelial cells; and lipomas, which originate from adipocytes. The suffix -oma is unfortunately still applied to some tumors that are not benign. Examples of this misnaming include melanomas, lymphomas, and seminomas.

4-11. The answer is d. (*Brooks, p 201. Levinson, p 92. Murray—2002, p 211. Ryan, pp 264–266.*) Toxic shock syndrome (TSS) is a febrile illness seen predominantly, but not exclusively, in menstruating women. Clinical criteria for TSS include fever greater than 102°F (38.9°C), rash, hypotension, and abnormalities of the mucous membranes and the gastrointestinal, hepatic, muscular, cardiovascular, or central nervous system. Usually three or more systems are involved. Treatment is supportive, including the aggressive use of antistaphylococcal antibiotics. Certain types of tampons may play a role in TSS by trapping O_2 and depleting magnesium. Most people have protective antibodies to the toxic shock syndrome toxin (TSST-1).

TSS is caused by a toxin-producing strain of *S. aureus* (TSST-1). While there have been reports that *S. epidermidis* produces TSS, they have largely been discounted. Vaginal colonization with *S. aureus* is a necessary adjunct to the disease. *S. aureus* is isolated from the vaginal secretions, conjunctiva, nose, throat, cervix, and feces in 45 to 98% of cases. The organism has infrequently been isolated from the blood.

Epidemiologic investigations suggest strongly that toxic shock syndrome is related to use of tampons, in particular, use of the highly absorbent ones that can be left in for extended periods of time. An increased growth of intravaginal *S. aureus* and enhanced production of TSST-1 have been associated with the prolonged intravaginal use of these hyperabsorbent tampons and with the capacity of the materials used in them to bind magnesium. The most severe cases of TSS have been seen in association with gram-negative infection. TSST-1 may enhance endotoxin activity. Recently, group A streptococci have been reported to cause TSS.

4-12. The answer is b. (*McKenzie, p 281. Junqueira, p 366. Cotran, pp 707–711. Braunwald, pp 1491–1493.*) The patient suffers from emphysema, in which neutrophils enter the lung parenchyma and secrete elevated levels of elastase, leading to the destruction of the bronchiolar and alveolar septal elastic tissue support. The destruction of the elasticity in emphysema leads to diminished breath sounds. This is coupled with faint high-pitched rhonchi at the end of expiration and a hyperresonant percussion note. The rhonchi are adventitious (not normally present) sounds that may be high pitched, generally because of bronchospasm, or low pitched, generally because of the presence of airway secretions. Emphysema is a disease characterized by parenchymal tissue destruction and, therefore, is not associated with adventitious breath sounds. However, because most emphysema is due to cigarette smoking, there is almost always some degree of chronic bronchitis, and therefore, rhonchi can be auscultated.

There are genetic and environmental causes of emphysema. The environmental causes include smoking and air pollution, whereas deficiency in α_1-antitrypsin (antiprotease) activity is the genetic cause of the disease. The balance between normal elastase-elastin production and protease-antiprotease activity is altered in emphysema. Persons with a deficiency in α_1-antitrypsin activity lack sufficient antiprotease activity to counteract neutrophil-derived elastase. When there is an increase in the entry and activation of neutrophils in the alveolar space, more elastase is released, and elastic structures are destroyed. In smoking there is an increase in the number of neutrophils and macrophages in alveoli and increased elastase activity from neutrophils and macrophages. Those changes are coupled with a decrease in antielastase activity because of oxidants in cigarette smoke and antioxidants released from the increased numbers of neutrophils. The increased protease activity causes breakdown of the alveolar walls and dissolution of elastin in the bronchiolar walls. The loss of tethering of the bronchioles to the lung parenchyma leads to their collapse. The bronchioles, unlike the trachea and bronchi, do not contain hyaline cartilage. A relatively thick layer of smooth muscle is found in the bronchioles, but the bronchioles are tethered to the lung parenchyma by elastic tissue, which plays a key role in the stretch and recoil of the lungs during inhalation and exhalation.

4-13. The answer is d. (*Craig, pp 381–382; Hardman, pp 475–476; Katzung, pp 390–391.*) Ethosuximide is especially useful in the treatment of absence seizures. Although it may act at several sites, the principal mechanism of action is on T-type Ca currents in thalamic neurons at relevant concentrations. This action blocks the pacemaker current that effects the generation of rhythmic cortical discharge associated with an absence attack.

4-14. The answer is c. (*Kandel, pp 472–485.*) Referred pain is a phenomenon in which pain impulses, arising from primary afferent fibers from one part of the body (such as from deep visceral structures), terminate on dorsal horn projection neurons that normally receive cutaneous afferents from a different part of the body (such as the arm). In this situation, a person who is suffering a heart attack experiences pain that appears to be coming from the arm. It is the convergence of these distinctly different inputs onto the same projection neurons that provides the basis for this phenomenon. None of the other possible mechanisms listed in this question have an anatomic or physiologic basis.

4-15. The answer is c. (*Cotran, pp 129–132.*) An embolus is a detached intravascular mass that has been carried by the blood to a site other than where it was formed. Most emboli originate from thrombi (thrombotic emboli), but they can also originate from material other than thrombi (nonthrombotic emboli). Types of nonthrombotic emboli include fat emboli, air emboli, and amniotic fluid emboli. Fat emboli, which result from severe trauma and fractures of long bones, will stain positively with an oil red O stain or Sudan black stain. They can be fatal as they can damage the endothelial cells and pneumocytes within the lungs. Air emboli are seen in decompression sickness, called caisson disease or the bends, while amniotic fluid emboli are related to the rupture of uterine venous sinuses as a complication of childbirth. Amniotic fluid emboli can also lead to a fatal disease, disseminated intravascular coagulopathy (DIC), which is marked by the combination of intravascular coagulation and hemorrhages. In this setting DIC results from the high thromboplastin activity of amniotic fluid.

It is important to remember, however, that most emboli arise from thrombi (thromboemboli) that are formed in the deep veins of the lower extremities. These thrombi may embolize to the lungs and form thrombotic pulmonary emboli (venous emboli). The majority of small pulmonary emboli do no harm, but, if they are large enough, they may occlude the bifurcation of the pulmonary arteries (saddle embolus), causing sudden death. In contrast, arterial emboli most commonly originate within the heart on abnormal valves (vegetations) or mural thrombi following myocardial infarctions. If there is a patent foramen ovale, a venous embolus may cross over through the heart to the arterial circulation, producing an arterial (paradoxical) embolus.

4-16. The answer is a. (*Guyton, pp 154, 246–247. Boron, pp 431, 508–511.*) In aortic stenosis, the resistance of the aortic valve increases, making it more difficult for blood to be ejected from the heart. Because a pressure drop occurs over the stenotic aortic valve, the ventricular pressure is much larger than the aortic pressure. Although stroke volume typically decreases, leading to a decrease in pulse pressure, a normal cardiac output and arterial pressure can still be maintained by increasing heart rate. However, the increased afterload will lead to a decreased ejection fraction and increased cardiac oxygen consumption.

4-17. The answer is c. (*Craig, pp 773–774; Hardman, pp 1705–1706; Katzung, p 708.*) Metformin, classified as a biguanide, "sensitizes" peripheral cells to insulin, thereby facilitating glucose uptake and utilization, and suppresses release of glucose from the liver and into the blood. It is largely ineffective in the absence of insulin and so is approved only for type 2 diabetes (used alone or in conjunction with such other drugs as a sulfonylurea or insulin).

Most patients taking metformin lose weight. This is probably due to an appetite-suppressing effect (leading to reduced caloric intake), rather than because of a specific effect on some metabolic reaction(s) or anorexia secondary to GI side effects.

The drug seldom causes hypoglycemia. Rather than actively driving down blood glucose levels (as, say, insulin does), metformin acts as if it caps physiologic rises of glucose concentrations. (Thus, it has been described as being an *antihyperglycemic* drug, rather than a hypoglycemic agent.)

Metformin is not metabolized by the liver, but liver dysfunction is one contraindication. That's mainly because of the risks of the drug's most important adverse effect, lactic acidosis, which is rare but often fatal when it does occur: impaired liver function impairs lactate elimination and favors its accumulation to toxic levels.

However the main primary cause of the lactic acidosis is renal insufficiency (serum creatinine > 1.5 mg/dL in men, 1.4 mg/dL in women), whether caused by renal disease or by renal hypoperfusion (ischemia, as might occur with heart failure and/or hypotension).

4-18. The answer is a. (*Braunwald, pp 745–750.*) This patient likely has chronic ITP of adults on the basis of her symptoms and thrombocytopenia, and lack of anemia or abnormal renal function. In von Willebrand's disease the platelet count is normal and in splenectomy the platelet count increases by about 30%. Hemolytic-uremic syndrome occurs in infancy and childhood and these patients have hypertension and abnormal renal function. Patients with thrombotic thrombocytopenic purpura (TTP) have renal failure and anemia.

4-19. The answer is d. (*Cotran, pp 869, 875–876. Chandrasoma, pp 655–658.*) Reye's syndrome (RS) is an acute postviral illness that is seen mainly in children. It is characterized by encephalopathy, microvesicular fatty change of the liver, and widespread mitochondrial injury. Electron microscopy (EM) reveals large budding or branching mitochondria. The mitochondrial injury results in decreased activity of the citric acid cycle and urea cycle and defective β-oxidation of fats, which then leads to the accumulation of serum fatty acids. The typical patient presents several days after a viral illness with pernicious vomiting. RS is associated with hyperammonemia, elevated serum free fatty acids, and salicylate (aspirin) ingestion.

In contrast, Wilson's disease, which is related to excess copper deposition within the liver and basal ganglia of the brain, is characterized by varying liver disease and neurologic symptoms. The liver changes vary from fatty change to jaundice to cirrhosis, while the neurologic symptoms consist of a Parkinson-like movement disorder and behavioral abnormalities. A liver biopsy may reveal steatosis, Mallory bodies, necrotic hepatocytes, or cholestasis. Increased copper can be demonstrated histologically using the rhodamine stain. α_1 antitrypsin deficiency causes both liver disease and lung disease, especially panacinar emphysema. Liver biopsies reveal red blobs within the cytoplasm of hepatocytes that are PAS-positive and diastase-resistant. Dubin-Johnson syndrome is associated with conjugated hyperbilirubinemia that results from decreased hepatic excretion of conjugates of bilirubin.

4-20. The answer is d. (*Cotran, pp 286–287, 1372–1373. Rubin, pp 1563–1565.*) Retinoblastoma is the most common malignant tumor of the eye in children. Clinically, retinoblastoma may produce a white pupil (leucoria). This is seen most often in young children in the familial form of retinoblastoma, which is due to a deletion involving chromosome 13. These familial cases of retinoblastoma are frequently multiple and bilateral, although like all the sporadic, nonheritable tumors they can also be unifocal and unilateral. Histologically, rosettes of various types are frequent (similar to neuroblastoma and medulloblastoma). There is a good prognosis with early detection and treatment; spontaneous regression can occur but is rare. Retinoblastoma belongs to a group of cancers (osteosarcoma, Wilms tumor, meningioma, rhabdomyosarcoma, uveal melanoma) in which the normal cancer suppressor gene (antioncogene) is inactivated or lost, with resultant malignant change. Retinoblastoma and osteosarcoma arise after loss of the same genetic locus—hereditary mutation in the q14 band of chromosome 13.

In contrast to the histologic appearance of retinoblastoma, a proliferation of benign fibroblasts and endothelial cells, which can form a retrolental mass, is seen with retinopathy of prematurity (ROP), a cause of blindness in premature infants that is related to the therapeutic use of high concentrations of oxygen. The presence of foamy macrophages with cytoplasmic clear vacuoles is not a specific histologic finding and can be seen with several disorders. Congo red–positive stroma, however, is characteristic of medullary carcinoma of the thyroid, while spindle-shaped cells with cytoplasmic melanin is characteristic of malignant melanoma, the most common primary intraocular malignancy of adults.

4-21. The answer is b. (*Murray, pp 396–414. Scriver, pp 4517–4554. Sack, pp 245–257.*) Red cell hemolysis after drug exposure suggests a red cell enzyme defect, most easily confirmed by enzyme assay to demonstrate deficient activity. A likely diagnosis here is glucose-6-phosphate dehydrogenase (G6PD) deficiency (305900), probably the most common genetic disease (it affects 400 million people worldwide). Tropical African and Mediterranean peoples exhibit the highest prevalence because the disease, like sickle cell trait, confers resistance to malaria. DNA analysis is available to demonstrate particular alleles, but simple enzyme assay is sufficient for diagnosis. More than 400 types of abnormal G6PD alleles have been described, meaning that most affected individuals are compound heterozygotes. The phenotype of jaundice and red blood cell hemolysis with anemia is triggered by a variety of infections and drugs, including a dietary substance in fava beans. Sulfonamide and related antibiotics as well as antimalarial drugs are notorious for inducing hemolysis in G6PD-deficient individuals. G6PD deficiency exhibits X-linked recessive inheritance, explaining why male offspring but not the parents become ill when exposed to antimalarials.

4-22. The answer is c. (*Moore and Dalley, pp 846, 1085.*) The styloglossus muscle is innervated by the hypoglossal nerve, which leaves the posterior cranial fossa by way of the anterior condylar canal. In addition to the internal jugular vein, the jugular foramen contains the glossopharyngeal nerve (innervating the stylopharyngeus muscle), the vagus nerve (innervating palatal, pharyngeal, and laryngeal musculature), and the spinal accessory nerve (innervating the sternomastoid and trapezius muscles).

4-23. The answer is f. (*Craig, p 720; Hardman, p 231; Katzung, pp 135–138.*) Ritodrine, a predominantly β_2-selective adrenergic agonist, slows uterine contractions by that action. The sequence of events following binding of ritodrine to its receptor includes increased myometrial cAMP formation, activation of cAMP-dependent protein kinase, and extrusion of Ca^{2+} from smooth-muscle cells such that contractile force is reduced. There are no effects on oxytocin synthesis or release, nor on hypothalamic or pituitary function. Ritodrine's effects are not at all like those of ergot compounds (e.g., methylergonovine), which induce uterine contraction by a mechanism that involves α-adrenergic receptor activation. Be sure to understand that despite the classification of ritodrine as a "β_2-selective adrenergic agonist," or as a uterine relaxant, the drug can activate all β-adrenergic receptors and cause a host of unwanted side effects or adverse responses that include tachycardia (direct and reflexly, in response to reduced blood pressure), pulmonary edema, and myocardial ischemia. This very effective drug is contraindicated in eclampsia or severe eclampsia. In these situations the goal is to deliver the fetus (the definitive cure for eclampsia), not prolong labor.

4-24. The answer is b. *(Brooks, p 302. Levinson, p 163. Murray—2002, pp 409–410. Ryan, p 477.)* Q fever is an acute, flulike illness caused by *C. burnetii*. It is the one rickettsial disease not transmitted by the bite of a tick. *C. burnetii* is found in high concentrations in the urine, feces, and placental tissue/amniotic fluid of cattle, goats, and sheep. Transmission to humans is by aerosol inhalation of those specimens.

4-25. The answer is c. *(Sierles, pp 400–402.)* During active coping (Cannon's fight or flight) there is an increase in heart rate, cardiac output, activity of striate muscle, catecholamines, and cortisol, along with vasodilation in the muscles. Under the condition of coping effort without distress, there is an increase in catecholamines (especially norepinephrine), but with a suppression of cortisol. On the other hand, coping effort associated with negative emotions (e.g., embarrassment or feeling harassed) leads to preferential secretion of epinephrine. Attempts to cope with such stressful situations over a long period of time have important implications for health maintenance and vulnerability to disease.

4-26. The answer is D. *(Nolte, pp 277–278, 380–388, 544–561. Waxman, p 199.)* This section is taken at the level of the septum pellucidum, the anterior commissure, and the substantia innominata. While a variety of structures may show degeneration in Huntington's disease, it is generally agreed that Huntington's disease is associated with loss of GABAergic neurons situated principally in the caudate nucleus (A). Fibers from the region of the basal nucleus of Meynert located in the substantia innominata (D) (at the base of the brain in the far rostral forebrain) send a cholinergic projection to wide areas of the neocortex. Loss of these cholinergic neurons has generally been associated with the presence of Alzheimer's disease. The globus pallidus (B) receives GABAergic inputs from the neostriatum (i.e., caudate nucleus and putamen), and these inputs represent the principal afferent supply of the neostriatum to the pallidum. The septal area (E), seen at this level of the forebrain as a thin structure separated by the lateral ventricles on both sides, receives major inputs from the hippocampal formation and is a principal component of the limbic system.

4-27. The answer is a. (*Craig, pp 541–542; Hardman, pp 1227–1229; Katzung, pp 767–768.*) Aminoglycosides (gentamicin, tobramycin, others) are classic examples of ototoxic drugs, and they can affect both branches of the eighth cranial nerve.

The risks of aminoglycoside-induced ototoxicity (and nephrotoxicity) are among the reasons why it is important to keep an eye on peak and trough drug levels during therapy, adjust dosages accordingly, and avoid concomitant use of other ototoxic drugs. That is because the hearing loss is blood level–dependent (as opposed to being an idiosyncratic or allergic reaction). Aminoglycoside-induced ototoxicity is usually irreversible. The risk and severity of hearing loss from aminoglycosides are increased if they are administered with other ototoxic drugs (below).

Recall that there are two main forms of drug-induced ototoxicity. Cochlear toxicity includes hearing loss, tinnitus ("ringing in the ears"), or occasionally both. Hearing loss may also occur with loop diuretics (particularly ethacrynic acid), *cis*-platinum, and the vinca alkaloids (anticancer drugs). These drugs are intrinsically ototoxic; use one or more of them together or with an aminoglycoside and the risk of ototoxicity increases greatly.

Tinnitus (usually reversible) is typically associated with such drugs as aspirin (and, possibly, some other NSAIDs) and quinidine.

The other main form of ototoxicity is vestibular toxicity, which is typically manifest as balance and gait problems, vertigo, and nausea resulting from vestibular apparatus dysfunction.

Nephrotoxicity may develop during or after the use of an aminoglycoside. It is generally more common in the elderly when there is preexisting renal dysfunction. In most patients, renal function gradually improves after discontinuation of therapy. Aminoglycosides rarely cause neuromuscular blockade that can lead to progressive flaccid paralysis and potential fatal respiratory arrest. Hypersensitivity and dermatologic reactions occasionally occur following use of aminoglycosides.

None of the other antibiotics listed are linked to ototoxicity, whether from excessive blood levels or due to a hypersensitivity or true allergic reaction. Azithromycin (not an answer choice) is, however, another antibiotic for which there is growing evidence of a link to sudden onset hearing loss. The mechanism is unknown, and the incidence is neither dose-dependent nor predictable.

4-28. The answer is a. (*Brooks, pp 553–554. Levinson, pp 312–313. Murray— 2002, pp 667–668. Ryan, pp 665–667.*) *Aspergillus* species cause infections of the skin, eyes, and ears and "fungus ball" in the lungs. *Aspergillus* species occur only as molds (not dimorphic). They have septate hyphae that form V-shaped branches, whose walls are parallel. Septate, branching hyphae invading tissue are typically seen in biopsy. On culture, colonies with radiating chains of conidia (photo) are typical. These molds are widely spread in nature, and transmission is by airborne conidia. The organism is very opportunistic in immunocompromised individuals, and antifungal treatment may be difficult.

4-29. The answer is c. (*Craig, p 253; Hardman, pp 710–711; Katzung, pp 249–250, 254–256.*) Chlorthalidone is a thiazide-like diuretic. If maximum dosages don't yield the desired effects, there's little likelihood that switching to another thiazide or thiazide-like agent (e.g., hydrochlorothiazide, metolazone, many others) will do better. Likewise, and given the relatively "flat" dose-response relationship for these drugs, nothing good is likely to be gained by adding "yet another" agent that works in precisely the same way as the drug that has already proven inadequate. If a maximum recommended dose isn't adequate, giving more of the same or a similar drug won't be better. So, in situations such as this, it's time to switch to a drug that is intrinsically more efficacious and works via a different mechanism: a loop diuretic.

4-30. The answer is e. (*Cotran, pp 991–994. Rubin, pp 915–916.*) Renal cell carcinoma accounts for 85% of primary renal tumors and usually occurs in the sixth decade, although sometimes at a much younger age. The combination of costovertebral pain, a palpable mass, and hematuria is the classic triad of symptoms seen in about 10% of patients with renal cell carcinoma. Hematuria is often the first symptom, but it often occurs late, after invasion of the renal vein or widespread metastases, frequently to lung, bone, or brain. Histologically, renal cell carcinoma is predominantly of the clear cell type (clear cell carcinoma) with intracytoplasmic glycogen and lipid, but less often granular cells with numerous mitochondria or spindle cells occur. Grossly, the lesions are greater than 3 cm in diameter and are yellow in color (similar to tumors of the adrenal cortex; thus another name for renal cell carcinoma is hypernephroma). These tumors arise from the renal epithelial cells and thus may be classified as adenocarcinomas, but tubular formation, not glandular formation, may be present. Renal cell carcinomas may produce hormones or hormone-like substances: for example, renin (hypertension), glucocorticoids (Cushing's syndrome), and gonadotropins (feminization and masculinization). More frequently, though in only 5 to 10% of patients, polycythemia or erythrocytosis occurs owing to production of erythropoietin. Renal cell carcinoma is associated with von Hippel-Lindau syndrome, in which many patients develop bilateral renal cell carcinomas. Translocations between chromosomes 3 and 8 and between 3 and 11 have been found in some cases of familial renal cancer and in a few sporadic cases of renal cancer.

In contrast, carcinomas originating from the renal pelvis (not the cortex) arise from transitional epithelial cells and microscopically are similar to tumors arising in the urinary bladder, i.e., transitional cell carcinomas. Finally, immature tubules and abortive glomerular formation are characteristic features of nephroblastoma (Wilms' tumor).

4-31. The answer is b. (*Boron, pp 885, 890.*) Motilin is the gastrointestinal peptide hormone associated with the initiation of migrating motor complexes during the interdigestive period. The hormone stimulates increased contractions by a direct action on smooth muscle and by activation of excitatory enteric nerves. Erythromycin belongs to the group of macrolide antibiotics and also shows an ability to excite motilin-like receptors on enteric nerves and smooth muscle. As a result, a common side effect of the antibiotic is abdominal cramping and diarrhea.

4-32. The answer is e. (*Braunwald, p 1431.*) In locomotive repair shops, workers are exposed to asbestos from the brake linings. On x-ray examination, asbestos exposure causes diffuse interstitial pulmonary fibrosis that is slowly evolving and characterized by linear or irregular opacities of the lungs. Usually, about 10 years elapse since first exposure to asbestos and the development of asbestosis. Benign pleural effusions occur and these may resolve without treatment. However, pleural blebs, enlargement of the right ventricle, and increased prominence of the pulmonary vascular are not features of asbestosis on x-ray.

4-33. The answer is a. *(Craig, p 137; Hardman, pp 150–153, 158; Katzung, p 440–441.)* Skeletal muscle paralysis from curare-like drugs involves competitive blockade of skeletal muscle nicotinic receptors. We reverse that by administering an ACh esterase inhibitor (e.g., neostigmine). Of course, the increased peripheral ACh levels will not only overcome skeletal muscle blockade, but also exert expected muscarinic-activating effects of various smooth muscles (e.g., the airways), the heart, and exocrine glands. We prevent those unwanted "parasympathomimetic" effects by giving atropine (antimuscarinic) right before giving the cholinesterase inhibitor. None of the other approaches are rational or used for "reversal."

4-34. The answer is b. *(Hardman, pp 1341–1342, 1350, 1353; Katzung, pp 316, 574.)* Aspirin inhibits cyclooxygenase (I and II). In terms of clotting, the main effect will be inhibition of platelet aggregation by reduced formation of thromboxane A_2. Bleeding time will be prolonged and will remain that way until sufficient numbers of new platelets have been released into the bloodstream, because aggregation of those platelets exposed to the drug will be inhibited for the lifetime of the platelets. The APTT, which should not be affected by aspirin, is used to monitor effects and adjust the dose of heparin. The prothrombin time (and its normalized value, the INR) are used with warfarin. Platelet counts, also not affected by aspirin, are used to assess for the development of thrombocytopenic purpura, which may rarely occur during therapy with (for example), clopidogrel or ticlopidine.

4-35. The answer is c. *(Cotran, pp 190–191. Braunwald, p 274. Goldman, pp 954–956.)* The immunologic classification of acute lymphoblastic leukemia is based on the normal developmental sequence of maturation of B and T lymphocytes, which is characterized by gene rearrangement and the acquisition of surface markers. Both B and T lymphocytes originate from a common lymphoid stem cell that is characterized by the intranuclear enzyme terminal deoxynucleotidyl transferase (TdT) and the surface antigens CD34 and CD38. The first definable stage of B cell maturation occurs as the cell begins the process of producing immunoglobulin (Ig). The heavy-chain genes, which are located on chromosome 14, are first rearranged, but because this occurs before the rearrangement of the light-chain genes, complete immunoglobulin is not yet expressed on the cell surface. Instead mu heavy-chain genes are rearranged first and are found within the cytoplasm. This defines these developing cells as being pre-B cells. These cells also demonstrate surface CD10 (CALLA) and the pan–B cell markers CD19, CD20, and CD22. Next these developing B cells begin to synthesize light chains. Kappa light-chain genes are found on chromosome 2 and are rearranged first. If something goes wrong in this process, then the lambda light-chain genes on chromosome 22 are rearranged; otherwise they stay in their germline configuration. The synthesized light chains then combine with the intracytoplasmic mu heavy chains to form complete IgM, which is then transported to the surface, forming surface IgM (sIgM). These cells, which have also acquired CD21 but have lost TdT and CD10, are called immature B cells. Next these developing B cells produce IgD, which is also expressed on the cell surface (sIgD). These cells with surface IgM and IgD are called mature B cells. They are also called "virgin" B cells because these cells have not encountered any foreign antigen. (Note that all of the preceding steps occur in the bone marrow of the developing fetus.)

4-36. The answer is a. (*Adams, pp 347, 350. Kandel, pp 887–888, 898–902, 1307–1311.*) The CT scan of Louise's brain revealed a large, acute stroke of her upper pons and midbrain. Strokes of these areas often result from occlusion of the basilar artery and can produce coma or a variant of hypersomnia called *akinetic mutism* or *coma vigil.* An EEG of a patient like this shows a pattern associated with slow-wave sleep, but eye movements are preserved. It is likely that the corticospinal tracts within the pons were damaged during this very large stroke, causing the increased tone from lack of inhibition, as well as the lack of movement in Louise's arms and legs. Infarctions of perforators of the basilar artery, supplying the reticular formation of the pons, may cause coma. These perforators also supply the corticospinal tracts, causing the increased tone and weakness of Louise's legs, so a large stroke may involve both functions. Coma occurs because there is damage to the brainstem tegmentum, which is a major component of the ascending reticular activating system. Although it is not known exactly which area is precisely responsible for consciousness, lesions of this region, as well as projections from the medial regions of the midbrain reticular formation can produce coma. The two main monoaminergic systems of the reticular formation are the noradrenergic and the serotonergic systems, originating in the locus ceruleus and raphe nuclei, respectively. The mesolimbic, mesostriatal, and mesocortical dopaminergic systems are located within the ventrorostral aspect of the brainstem, but not within the reticular formation.

4-37. The answer is a. (*Cotran, pp 1160–1161. Rubin, pp 1187–1188.*) In 1855, when Thomas Addison first described primary adrenal insufficiency, the most common cause was tuberculosis of the adrenal gland. Now the majority of patients have adrenal autoantibodies and are thought to have autoimmune Addison's disease. Half of these patients have other autoimmune endocrine diseases, because autoimmune diseases affecting one organ is frequently associated with involvement of other organs. Two major patterns of polyglandular autoimmune (PGA) syndromes have been described. Patients with type I PGA syndrome have at least two of the following three diseases or abnormalities: Addison's disease, hypoparathyroidism, and mucocutaneous candidiasis. Type II PGA syndrome, also called Schmidt's syndrome, lacks hypoparathyroidism and mucocutaneous candidiasis and instead is associated with autoimmune thyroid disease (Hashimoto's thyroiditis) and type 1 diabetes mellitus. Finally, do not confuse PGA with MEN (multiple endocrine neoplasia). Hyperplasia of the parathyroid glands is seen with both type I and type II MEN, while neoplasms of the anterior pituitary are seen with type I MEN only.

4-38. The answer is d. (*Boron, pp 692, 730–731.*) Hypoventilation produces a rise in arterial P_{CO_2}, which causes a respiratory acidosis. Renal compensation for a respiratory acidosis results in an increase in bicarbonate and a decrease in chloride concentration, which results in a normal anion gap. Left heart failure is a common cause of right heart failure and of pulmonary edema but neither will produce a pure respiratory acidosis. If the pulmonary edema or reduction in cardiac output is severe enough, a metabolic acidosis could result from anaerobic metabolism.

4-39. The answer is a. (*Afifi, pp 235–252, 266–271.*) Damage to the VA, VL, dorsomedial, and anterior thalamic nuclei would most likely result in motor impairment such as a hemiparesis (because of the connections of these nuclei with the motor and premotor cortices). Damage to the dorsomedial nucleus could also be linked with neuropsychological impairment because of its connections with the prefrontal cortex and adjoining regions of the frontal lobe. The other processes mentioned in question 432 have not been shown to be related to these groups of nuclei. As noted earlier, the VA nucleus is associated with motor functions, not only in its projections to motor regions of the cerebral cortex—the premotor and prefrontal cortices—but also in the inputs that it receives from structures associated with motor functions such as the globus pallidus and substantia nigra.

4-40. The answer is c. (*Murray, pp 21–29, 40–48. Scriver, pp 3–45. Sack, pp 1–3.*) Protein electrophoresis is an important laboratory technique for investigating red cell proteins such as hemoglobin or plasma proteins such as the immunoglobulins. The proteins are dissolved in a buffer of low pH where the amino groups of amino acid side chains are positively charged, causing most proteins to migrate toward the negative electrode (anode). Red cell hemolysates are used for hemoglobin electrophoresis, plasma (blood supernatant with unhemolyzed red cells removed) for plasma proteins. Serum (blood supernatant after clotting) would not contain red cells but would contain many blood enzymes and proteins. In sickle cell anemia, the hemoglobin S contains a valine substitution for the glutamic acid at position 6 in hemoglobin A. Hemoglobin S thus loses two negative charges (loss of a glutamic acid carboxyl group on each of two β-globin chains) compared to hemoglobin A. Hemoglobin S is thus more positively charged and migrates more rapidly toward the anode than hemoglobin A. Lane B must represent the heterozygote with sickle cell trait (hemoglobins S and A), establishing lane A as the normal and lane D as the sickle cell anemia sample. The hemoglobin in lane C migrates differently from normal and hemoglobin S, as would befit an abnormal hemoglobin that is different from S. Lane E must be serum, which does not contain red blood cells.

4-41. The answer is b. (*Moore and Dalley, p 99.*) One would expect a cracked rib that allows blood from the subcostal vessels to bleed into the pleural cavity, partially collapsing the left lung, causing the shortness of breath. Blood in the pleural cavity is an irritant and causes generalized chest pain. The left-sided midback pain is from the cracked eleventh rib. Because only one lung appears to have a fluid accumulation and he is young and exercises regularly pulmonary hypertension is unlikely, especially give his physical findings and history and sudden onset of symptoms. Cardiac tamponade, which is blood within the pericardial sac, is unexpected. Neither gallbladder pain, nor an inflamed appendix would typically cause chest pain. Note: the CT of the abdomen is to rule out damage to kidneys and spleen.

4-42. The answer is c. *(Brooks, pp 562–563, 582–584, 587–590, 593–594. Levinson, pp 318–319, 323–324, 332–335, 338–340, 351–352. Murray— 2002, pp 701–703, 717–720, 731–732, 750–752, 754–757. Ryan, pp 695–696, 723–727, 746–748, 779–784, 809–813.)* All the diseases listed in the question have significant epidemiologic and clinical features. Toxoplasmosis, for example, is generally a mild, self-limiting disease; however, severe fetal disease is possible if pregnant women ingest *Toxoplasma* oocysts. Consumption of uncooked meat may result in either an acute toxoplasmosis or a chronic toxoplasmosis that is associated with serious eye disease. Most adults have antibody titers to *Toxoplasma* and thus would have a positive Sabin-Feldman dye test.

Trichinosis most often is caused by ingestion of contaminated pork products. However, eating undercooked bear, walrus, raccoon, or possum meat also may cause this disease. Symptoms of trichinosis include muscle soreness and swollen eyes.

Although giardiasis has been classically associated with travel in Russia, especially St. Petersburg (Leningrad), many cases of giardiasis caused by contaminated water have been reported in the United States as well. Diagnosis is made by detecting cysts in the stool. In some cases, diagnosis may be very difficult because of the relatively small number of cysts present. Alternatively, an enzyme immunoassay may be used to detect *Giardia* antigen in fecal samples.

Schistosomiasis is a worldwide public health problem. Control of this disease entails the elimination of the intermediate host snail and removal of streamside vegetation. Abdominal pain is a symptom of schistosomiasis.

Visceral larva migrans is an occupational disease of people who are in close contact with dogs and cats. The disease is caused by the nematodes *Toxocara canis* (dogs) and *Toxocara cati* (cats) and has been recognized in young children who have close contact with pets or who eat dirt. Symptoms include skin rash, eosinophilia, and hepatosplenomegaly.

4-43. The answer is b. *(Feldman, pp 666, 847. Berman, 578–582.)* Gastrointestinal stromal tumors (GIST) are mesenchymal tumors of the GI tract that are lumped together because of a common histologic finding of spindle-shaped tumor cells. Seventy percent of GIST occur in the stomach, most of these behaving in a benign fashion, and 30% occur in the small intestines, most of these behaving in a malignant fashion. GIST have abnormalities of KIT gene. Therapy for this type of tumor is with the tyrosine kinase inhibitor Glivec (formerly known as STI571), which is also used to treat chronic myelocytic leukemia (CML). GIST stain positively with CD117 (the KIT protein) and negatively with desmin and S-100. Spindle cell tumors that are negative for CD117 and positive for desmin are leiomyomas, which are also found in the wall of the stomach.

In contrast, MALTomas, lymphomas of mucosa-associated lymphoid tissue, are indolent B cell lymphomas that are forms of marginal zone lymphomas. They typically involve sites outside of lymph nodes, such as the gastrointestinal tract, thyroid gland, breast, skin, or lungs. Finally, chemodectomas are benign, chromaffin-negative tumors of the chemoreceptor system. Common locations are the neck (carotid body tumor) and the inner ear (glomus jugulare tumor).

4-44. The answer is e. *(Brooks, p 555. Levinson, pp 324–325. Murray— 2002, pp 669–671. Ryan, pp 685–689.)* P. carinii causes pneumonia in immunocompromised patients. Once considered a protozoan, it is not classified as a fungus. Effective chemoprophylactic regimens have resulted in a dramatic decrease in pneumonia deaths in AIDS patients. P. carinii has the morphologically distinct forms (trophozoite and cyst) described in the question. Cysts stain well with silver stain. In clinical specimens, trophozoites and cysts are present in a tight mass. P. carinii cannot be cultured. The organism is widespread in nature and does not cause disease without immunosuppression. It may represent a member of normal flora.

4-45. The answer is a. *(Boron, pp 823–824, 859. Guyton, pp 360, 873.)* Aldosterone promotes the loss of both H^+ and K^+, producing metabolic alkalosis and hypokalemia. Persistent diarrhea will cause the loss of bicarbonate from the body, resulting in metabolic acidosis. Renal failure is often accompanied by metabolic acidosis because of the inability to excrete H^+. Diabetes also causes metabolic acidosis because of the accumulation of keto acids. Hyperventilation results in a respiratory alkalosis, which is compensated for by a decreased bicarbonate concentration.

4-46. The answer is a. *(Murray, pp 102–110. Scriver, pp 1521–1552. Sack, pp 121–138.)* Glycosides are formed by condensation of the aldehyde or ketone group of a carbohydrate with a hydroxyl group of another compound. Other linked groups (aglycones) include steroids with hydroxyl groups (e.g., cardiac glycosides such as digitalis or ouabain) or other chemicals (e.g., antibiotics such as streptomycin). Sucrose (α-D-glucose-β-1 $\rightarrow$ 2-D-fructose), maltose (α-D-glucose-α-1 $\rightarrow$ 4-D-glucose), and lactose (α-D-galactose-β-1 $\rightarrow$ 4-D-glucose) are important disaccharides. Fructose is among several carbohydrate groups known as ketoses because it possesses a ketone group. The ketone group is at carbon 2 in fructose, and its alcohol group at carbon 1 (also at carbon 6) allows ketal formation to produce pyranose and furanose rings as with glucose. Most of the fructose found in the diet of North Americans is derived from the disaccharide sucrose (common table sugar). Sucrose is cleaved into equimolar amounts of glucose and fructose in the small intestine by the action of the pancreatic enzyme sucrase. Deficiency of sucrase can also cause chronic diarrhea. Hereditary fructose intolerance (229600) is caused by deficiency of the liver enzyme aldolase B, which hydrolyzes fructose-1-phosphate.

4-47. The answer is b. *(Braunwald, pp 2074–2075.)* The pattern and amount of radioiodine uptake on ^{123}I scan is fundamental to the correct diagnosis of thyrotoxicosis. Low-uptake thyrotoxicosis can occur when there is destruction of the thyroid follicles with release of thyroid hormone, such as in subacute thyroiditis, which usually presents as an exquisitely painful gland. Iodine-induced hyperthyroidism, factitious hyperthyroidism, and painless (silent) thyroiditis also cause low-uptake thyrotoxicosis.

4-48. The answer is b. *(Goldman, p 2140. Goetz, pp 416, 945, 949–950. Young & Young, pp 275, 277.)* The dominant cerebral hemisphere, usually the left side in right-handed individuals, is involved with language, speech, and calculation, while the nondominant side is involved with three-dimensional or spatial perception, perception of social cues, and nonverbal ideation, such as music and poetry. Damage to the dominant parietal lobe can produce apraxia, which is the inability to carry out learned movements. Furthermore, damage to this area can produce the Gerstmann's syndrome, which is characterized by right-left confusion, finger agnosia (problems naming and identifying fingers), agraphia (problems writing), and dyscalculia (problems with simple math calculations). In contrast to these clinical findings, Déjérine-Roussy syndrome refers to the clinical combination of contralateral loss of sensory with contralateral dysthesia (pain); Parinaud's syndrome refers to large impaired conjugate vertical gaze, pupillary abnormality, and absence of accommodation reflex due to compression of upper midbrain and pretectal areas; Wallenberg's syndrome is the lateral medullary syndrome and results from occlusion of the vertebral artery or occlusion of the posterior inferior cerebellar artery (hence its other name, PICA syndrome); and Weber's syndrome refers to the medial midbrain syndrome.

4-49. The answer is b. (*Henry, pp 612–613. Cotran, pp 662–663.*) Burkitt's lymphoma (small noncleaved non-Hodgkin's lymphoma) is characterized by a rapid proliferation of primitive lymphoid cells with thick nuclear membranes, multiple nucleoli, and intensely basophilic cytoplasm when stained with Wright's stain. The cells are often mixed with macrophages in biopsy, giving a starry sky appearance. The cytoplasmic vacuoles of the lymphoma cells contain lipid, and this would be reflected by a positive oil red O reaction. The African type of Burkitt's lymphoma is the endemic form and typically involves the maxilla or mandible, while the American type of small noncleaved NHL is nonendemic and commonly involves the abdomen, such as bowel, ovaries, or retroperitoneum. The African type is associated with Epstein-Barr virus (EBV) and a characteristic t(8;14) translocation.

4-50. The answer is a. (*Braunwald, p 1582.*) A classical scenario for poststreptococcal glomerulonephritis, which is a nephritic process with hypertension due to salt retention, hypervolemia that causes face and lower extremity swelling, and hematuria. Fewer than 5% develop nephrotic syndrome. Hypocomplementemia typically resolves after 6 to 8 weeks. A more prolonged depression should suggest membranoproliferative glomerulonephritis. In children, evolution to chronic renal failure is rare.

BLOCK 5

Answers

5-1. The answer is c. (*Moore and Dalley, p 231.*) The splenic artery originates from the celiac trunk and courses tortuously along the posterior aspect of the pancreas. The left gastric artery is a separate branch of the celiac trunk and courses along the lesser curvature of the stomach where it anastomoses with the right gastric artery, a branch of hepatic artery. The right gastro-omental (gastroepiploic) artery is a branch of the gastroduodenal artery and courses along the greater curvature of the stomach.

5-2. The answer is d. (*Cotran, pp 1045–1046, 1048–1053. Rubin, pp 980–983.*) Cervical condylomata and cervical intraepithelial neoplasia (CIN), which comprises both dysplasia and carcinoma in situ (CIS), are associated with human papillomavirus (HPV) infection. More than 50 genotypes of HPV are known at present, and condylomata acuminata are associated with types 6 to 11, while types 16 to 18 are usually present in CIN. Histologically, HPV infection is characterized by prominent perinuclear cytoplasmic vacuolization with shrunken, dark, irregular nuclei (koilocytosis). Following an abnormal Pap smear report suggesting condyloma, CIN, or possible invasive carcinoma, work-up of the patient should include colposcopy, multiple cervical punch biopsies, and endocervical curettage to distinguish among patients who have invasive cancer, CIN, or flat condylomata. In contrast, Epstein-Barr virus is a cause of infectious mononucleosis ("mono"), herpes simplex virus is a cause of "herpes," and parvovirus B19 is a cause of "fifth disease."

5-3. The answer is d. (*Baum, pp 304–306.*) There is an increased interest in self-control or self-management programs in terms of what individuals can do for themselves. Many weight loss programs have established that self-reward is the most effective tool during both posttreatment and follow-up. Self-reward acts as a contingent reinforcement for losing weight. Self-monitoring is a part of some self-management programs, but is not as effective as self-reward. Self-control procedures have been applied to other areas, such as self-management of diabetes where patients can pay attention to specific adaptive behaviors that they can control. Thus, self-reinforcement becomes a powerful cognitive-behavioral intervention.

5-4. The answer is b. *(Kandel, pp 1305–1309. Nolte, pp 120–128, 421–425.)* An arterial occlusion compromised the blood supply to the occipital lobe on the left side of the brain. Therefore, it would result in a right homonymous hemianopsia with no motor deficits (since no motor regions of the brain are affected).

5-5. The answer is e. *(Craig, pp 553–554; Hardman, p 1264; Katzung, p 749.)* This "red man" syndrome is characteristically associated with vancomycin. It is thought to be caused by histamine release. Prevention consists of a slower infusion rate and pretreatment with antihistamines.

5-6. The answer is a. *(Murray, pp 173–179. Scriver, pp 2367–2424. Sack, pp 159–175.)* Acetyl-CoA carboxylase deficiency drastically alters the ability of the patient to synthesize fatty acids. The fact that the infant was born at all is due to the body's ability to utilize fatty acids provided to it. However, all processes dependent on de novo fatty acid biosynthesis are affected. The lungs, in particular, require surfactant, a lipoprotein substance secreted by alveolar type II cells, to function properly. Surfactant lowers alveolar surface tension, facilitating gas exchange. It contains significant amounts of dipalmitoyl phosphatidylcholine. Palmitate is the major end product of de novo fatty acid synthesis. Acetyl-CoA carboxylase formation of malonyl-CoA is the first step of fatty acid synthesis. Biotin deficiency cannot be the problem because pyruvate carboxylase in gluconeogenesis is not affected. None of the other answers listed would result in all of the symptoms given.

5-7. The answer is b. *(Craig, p 614; Hardman, p 1084; Katzung, pp 871–782.)* Hemolysis is the most common and serious adverse response to primaquine. The risk is clearly highest in patients who have red cell deficiencies in glucose-6-phosphate dehydrogenase, a heritable trait and one that can be screened for before giving the drug. [This G6PD deficiency is more common in blacks, and whites with darker skin (e.g., some from certain regions of the Middle East or the Mediterranean countries).] Regardless of the results of pretreatment screening, periodic blood counts should be done, and the urine checked for unusual darkening (indicating the presence of hemoglobin from lysed red cells), during treatment.

Note: If you answered "retinopathy," you were probably thinking about chloroquine, because that adverse response (accompanied by visual changes) is associated with that "other main" antimalarial drug.

5-8. The answer is b. (*Craig, pp 650, 732; Hardman, pp 1442, 1645; Katzung, pp 688, 917, 926.*) Flutamide, one of three androgen receptor blockers used for managing prostate cancer, is used as an adjunct to leuprolide. Leuprolide acts like gonadotropin-releasing hormone (GnRH; or luteinizing hormone-releasing hormone). When leuprolide therapy is started, it stimulates release of interstitial cell–stimulating hormone from the pituitary, thereby increasing testosterone production and supporting tumor growth. It is only with continued exposure to leuprolide that GnRH receptors become desensitized, and the eventual inhibition of testosterone production (and, thereby, support of tumor growth) occurs. Flutamide, by blocking androgen receptors, prevents the potential worsening of the tumor in the early phase of leuprolide therapy when testosterone levels rise. Even when leuprolide's pituitary-desensitizing effects occur, androgens that can support prostate tumor growth will come from the adrenal gland. Their effects, too, are blocked by the flutamide.

5-9. The answer is a. (*Parslow, pp 79–80, 700–703. Levinson, pp 82, 146, 429.*) Recurrent severe infection is an indication for clinical evaluation of immune status. Live vaccines, including BCG attenuated from M. *tuberculosis,* should not be used in the evaluation of a patient's immune competence because patients with severe immunodeficiencies may develop an overwhelming infection from the vaccine. For the same reason, oral (Sabin) polio vaccine is not advisable for use in such persons.

5-10. The answer is b. (*Moore and Dalley, pp 339–341, 418–423.*) The indicated line represents the sacroiliac joint. These structures are seen bilaterally between the alae of the sacrum and the ilia. The sacroiliac ligaments might have been sprained by the trauma of the fall. The pathway for spinal nerves is through foramina of the sacrum, not through long bony canals. Similarly, the pathway for the gluteal arteries is through the greater sciatic foramen between the ilium and the sacrum. However, the bones are not contiguous at that level.

5-11. The answer is d. (*Braunwald, pp 1713, 1756–1758.*) The signs and symptoms in this patient, especially pruritus, suggest primary biliary cirrhosis (PBC), a disease that occurs predominantly in women ages 35 to 60. The slightly elevated bilirubin and the elevated alkaline phosphatase are common in cirrhosis, and in particular, elevated alkaline phosphatase occurs in PBC. However, a positive IgG antimitochondrial antibody is detected in more than 90% of patients with PBC and provides an important diagnostic finding.

5-12. The answer is a. (*Alberts, pp 872–874, 1015. Cotran, p 920. Braunwald, p 2119.*) Platelet-derived growth factor (PDGF) stimulates chemotaxis of monocytes and macrophages as well as fibroblasts to the site of a wound. PDGF also induces proliferation of vascular smooth muscle cells (answer b) to facilitate blood vessel repair and fibroblasts (answer c) to synthesize type I collagen. PDGF stimulates the formation of granulation tissue (answer d) consisting of new connective tissue and small blood vessels that form in the wound site. Type II collagen (answer e) is synthesized by chondrocytes in hyaline and elastic cartilage. Wound healing is a complex process initiated by damage to capillaries in the dermis. The clot forms through the interaction of integrins on the surface of blood platelets with fibrinogen and fibronectin. Fibrin is the primary protein that constructs the three-dimensional structure of the clot. A scar is formed as a very dense region of type I collagen fibers. Macrophages remove debris at the wound site and are also involved in the remodeling of the scar. All wound healing processes are slower in diabetics, and the presence of advanced-glycation end products (AGE) and their interaction with the receptor for AGE (RAGE) as well as the endogenous ligand for RAGE (ENRAGE) appear to contribute to inhibited healing in diabetes. AGE are produced by the nonenzymatic glycation and oxidation of proteins/lipids and alter those molecules and therefore the function and structure of tissues and organs such as the kidney (diabetic nephropathy), peripheral nerves (neuropathy), and the retina (diabetic retinopathy).

5-13. The answer is a. (*Craig pp 385–386, 389–391; Hardman, pp 453, 456–458, 466–468.*) Of the listed antidepressants, only amitriptyline, a tricyclic, causes adverse effects related to blockade of muscarinic acetylcholine receptors. Both trazodone and amitriptyline cause adverse effects related to α-adrenoreceptor blockade.

5-14. The answer is c. (*Waxman, p 94.*) The symptoms indicate that the lesion is at the level of the midbrain. The spastic paralysis, hyperreflexia, and positive Babinski reflect an upper motor neuron lesion. The corticob-ulbar and corticospinal tracts pass through the cerebral peduncles (basis pedunculi). Those originating in the right cortex will pass through the right peduncle and then cross to the contralateral side in the pyramidal decussa-tion, resulting in left-side hemiplegia. It is of interest that the lower motor neurons innervating muscles of facial expression located below the eye receive upper motor neurons (corticobulbar tract) only from the contralat-eral cortex, whereas lower motor neurons innervating facial muscles above the eye (e.g., frontalis) receive input from both sides of the cortex. This explains why only the lower portion of the left face was paralyzed. The deficit in movement of the right eye indicates damage to the ipsilateral ocu-lomotor nerve (CN III), which passes through the cerebral peduncle en route to the interpeduncular fossa. The "down and out" direction of the right eye is explained by unopposed contraction of the lateral rectus (CN VI) and superior oblique (CN IV) muscles. Because there were no sensory deficits, neither the thalamus nor sensory cortex were involved. The sen-sory tracts are arranged dorsolaterally in the midbrain and do not pass through the affected area.

5-15. The answer is e. (*Hughes, pp 348–349.*) Single parenthood has become a major health and social problem in America. One child in four (25%) in the United States lives with only one parent. Forty-seven percent of single mothers live below the poverty level, as compared with 8% of families headed by two parents. When mothers become single, their house-hold income is precipitously reduced due to loss of the spouse's income and less training and lower pay for working women. Generally, the situa-tion continues to decline, depending in part on the number of children in the family. The married poor family with children usually is able to work themselves out of poverty, while the poor single parent is not. The number of single parent men has increased from 10% to 15% in the last decade.

5-16. The answer is d. (*Parslow, pp 23–24. Levinson, pp 47, 359, 379, 399, 428.*) The acute-phase response is a primitive, nonspecific defense reac-tion, mediated by the liver, that increases innate immunity and other pro-tective functions in stressful times. It can be triggered by chronic autoimmune disorders such as rheumatoid arthritis and Crohn's disease. This response occurs when hepatocytes are exposed to IL-6 and IL-1 of TNF-α. LPS is a potent inducer of these cytokines. They are responsible for fever, somnolence, loss of appetite, and, if the response is prolonged, anemia and cachexia (wasting). A traditional assay known as the *erythro-cyte sedimentation rate* (ESR) may be used as an indicator of an acute-phase response. The ESR involves measuring the rate at which the red blood cells fall through plasma, which increases as fibrinogen concentration rises. Currently, Crohn's disease may be treated with infusions of a drug known as Infliximab which is a mouse-human chimeric antibody against human TNF-α.

5-17. The answer is a. (*Craig, p 370; Hardman, p 513; Katzung, p 454.*) This cutaneous response, called livedo reticularis, is characteristically associated with amantadine. Recall that this seldom-used antiparkinson drug probably works by releasing endogenous dopamine and blocking its neuronal reuptake. Livedo reticularis is not associated with levodopa (used alone or with carbidopa), nor with the dopamine agonists bromocriptine or pramipexole (a newer and generally preferred drug for starting treatment of mild parkinsonian signs and symptoms).

5-18. The answer is d. (*Craig, pp 182–184, 232–233; Hardman, pp 774–775; Katzung, pp 154, 171.*) Labetalol is the best choice. Given its combination of both α- and β-adrenergic (β_1 and β_2) blocking effect, it offers the best approach for managing the hypertension, the tachycardia, the resulting oxygen supply-demand imbalance that leads to both chest discomfort and the ischemic ST-changes; and the ventricular ectopy (which is probably a reflection of excessive catecholamine stimulation of β_1 receptors). If the patient is having an acute myocardial infarction, starting β-blocker therapy early is also decidedly beneficial short term and for the long run. (Most any other β blocker might be a suitable alternative, but only labetalol has the combined α/β-blocking actions that are likely to be of greatest benefit. Carvedilol has the same profile, but it is given orally and in this setting that would not be ideal because of slow onset of action.)

Aspirin will do no harm in this situation, but it will also do no good acutely unless there is ongoing platelet aggregation and coronary occlusion. Even if there were, the aspirin would do little to control heart rate, blood pressure, or the EKG changes.

Nothing in the scenario suggests this patient is volume-overloaded or suffering acute pulmonary edema. Therefore, administering the furosemide in such a situation is not appropriate. Moreover, giving it is likely to cause prompt reductions of blood volume and, along with it, of blood pressure. The latter effect is likely to lead to further—and unwanted—reflex sympathetic activation that would make matters worse.

Lidocaine might be suitable for the ventricular ectopy. However, we have identified several other important signs and symptoms that would not be relieved by this antiarrhythmic drug. As noted above, the profile of labetalol offers the greatest likelihood of managing multiple problems with one drug.

Increasing the dose of nitroglycerin (and especially giving it as a bolus) is likely to drop blood pressure acutely, triggering reflex (baroreceptor) stimulation of the heart. The usual "anti-ischemic" effects of the drug would be counteracted by such "pro-ischemic" changes as further rises of heart rate and a probable worsening of the premature ventricular beats.

Prazosin would lower blood pressure nicely. However, once again we have to worry about excessive pressure lowering, triggering the baroreceptor reflex, and worsening many of the already worrisome findings (e.g., heart rate, PVCs).

5-19. The answer is d. (*Cotran, pp 1236–1237. Rubin, pp 1384–1385.*) Osteosarcoma is the most common primary malignant bone tumor except for multiple myeloma and lymphoma. It is the most common bone cancer of children. Osteosarcomas usually arise in the metaphyses of long bones of the extremities, although they may involve any bone. They are composed of malignant anaplastic cells, which are malignant osteoblasts that secrete osteoid. There may be marked variation histologically depending on the amount of type I collagen, osteoid, and spicules of woven bone produced. Osteosarcomas produce a characteristic sunburst x-ray pattern due to calcified perpendicular striae of reactive periosteum adjacent to the tumor. They may also show periosteal elevation at an acute angle (Codman's triangle) or penetrate cortical bone with extension into the adjacent soft tissue. Two-thirds of cases are associated with mutations of the retinoblastoma (Rb) gene. Patients with retinoblastoma are at an increased risk for developing osteogenic sarcoma. In older patients, there is an association with multifocal Paget's disease of bone, radiation exposure (as in painters of radium watch dials), fibrous dysplasia, osteochondromatosis, and chondromatosis. Osteosarcomas metastasize hematogenously and usually spread to the lungs early in the course of the disease. With surgery, radiation, and chemotherapy the 5-year survival rate is now about 60%.

In contrast to the histologic appearance of osteogenic sarcoma, aneurysmal bone cysts are composed of multiple blood filled spaces that are not lined by endothelial cells. They are not true neoplasms. Fibrous dysplasia displays a haphazard arrangement of immature bony trabeculae forming "Chinese letters," while benign chondromas display lobules of hyaline cartilage with few cells. Finally, osteopetrosis is characterized clinically by thick bone trabeculae with osteoclasts that lack a normal ruffled border.

5-20. The answer is d. (*McPhee, pp 128–132. Braunwald, pp 674–680.*) Pernicious anemia, a megaloblastic anemia, results from a complex cascade of events that is autoimmune in origin. Antibodies against gastric parietal cell components and intrinsic factor are common, and antibody-generating B lymphocytes are found in the gastric mucosa. The signs of vitamin cobalamin (B_{12}) deficiency are delayed by the liver storage of cobalamin, provided that the patient's intake has previously been normal. Cobalamin deficiency is almost always due to malabsorption. Normal diets usually provide adequate intake of cobalamin; however, in vegetarians the intake is inadequate. Persons suffering from pernicious anemia can develop very low hemoglobin levels, as low as 4 g/dL, unlike other anemias. The Schilling test will be abnormal. Multiple neurologic findings (due to demyelination at first and then axonal degeneration) include numbness and paresthesias, weakness, ataxia, difficulties with mentation, and abnormal deep tendon reflexes, and pathological reflexes, high output failure, and sallow color are consistent with pernicious anemia. In autoimmune hemolysis, the Coombs' test is positive. These patients require treatment with cobalamin, which reverses the anemia and the neurologic abnormalities. Folate treatment alone fails to reverse neurologic abnormaties of cobalamin deficiency.

5-21. The answer is e. (*Guyton, pp 360, 377.*) The rise in H^+ and fall in HCO_3^- that occurs in type I (distal) renal tubular acidosis (RTA) does not increase the anion gap because the decrease in HCO_3^- is accompanied by an increase in Cl. The failure of the distal nephron H^+ ATPase causes a reduction in net acid excretion and a reduced H^+ secretion, which causes less ammonium to be excreted in the urine. The low HCO_3^- in the glomerular filtrate reduces Na^+ reabsorption by Na-H exchanger and therefore more Na^+ is delivered to the distal nephron. The increased Na^+ delivery results in salt wasting and a secondary hyperaldosteronism which, in turn, causes K^+ concentration to fall.

5-22. The answer is c. *(Afifi, pp 91–103.)* Gary has a spinal cord syndrome called *Brown-Séquard's syndrome,* or hemisection of the spinal cord. The lesion is not at the cervical level because motor functions of the upper limbs were considered normal. The examiner can pinpoint the location of the lesion by using the "sensory level," or level at which the loss of pain and temperature begin, by remembering that the lesion affects fibers that have entered the spinal cord one or two levels below it, and then cross to the contralateral side. Therefore, a loss of sensory function at the T10 level indicates a lesion at the T8 or T9 level. A level at which motor deficits begin can be helpful as well, but in lesions of the thoracic spinal cord, muscles innervated by thoracic nerves are difficult to test. The examiner still expects weakness in the lower extremities, and this helps to make the diagnosis. Brown-Séquard's syndrome may occur as a result of different types of tumors or infections of the spinal cord.

5-23. The answer is a. *(Cotran, pp 1343–1346. Rubin, pp 1515–1518.)* The features listed in the question are characteristic of a high-grade astrocytoma, which is commonly called a glioblastoma multiforme. Astrocytomas, the most common primary brain tumors in adults, range from low grade to very high grade (glioblastoma multiforme). These grades of astrocytomas include grade I (the least aggressive and histologically difficult to differentiate from reactive astrocytosis), grade II (some pleomorphism microscopically), grade III (anaplastic astrocytoma, characterized histologically by increased pleomorphism and prominent mitoses), and grade IV (glioblastoma multiforme). Glioblastoma multiforme is a highly malignant tumor characterized histologically by endothelial proliferation and serpentine areas of necrosis surrounded by peripheral palisading of tumor cells. It frequently crosses the midline ("butterfly tumor").

In contrast to the highly malignant glioblastoma, schwannomas are benign tumors that generally appear as extremely cellular spindle cell neoplasms, sometimes with metaplastic elements of bone, cartilage, and skeletal muscle. Medulloblastomas, however, are malignant tumors that occur exclusively in the cerebellum and microscopically are highly cellular with uniform nuclei, scant cytoplasm, and, in about one-third of cases, rosette formation centered by neurofibrillary material. Oligodendrogliomas, which are marked by foci of calcification in 70% of cases, commonly show a pattern of uniform cellularity and are composed of round cells with small dark nuclei, clear cytoplasm, and a clearly defined cell membrane.

5-24. The answer is b. (*Moore and Dalley, p 15.*) The flexor pollicis brevis has two heads and there is a sesamoid bone associated with each of the tendons of these heads. Sesamoid bones are isolated islands of bone that may occur in tendons passing over joints. The patella is the classic example. The adductor pollicis also has two heads (transverse and oblique), but they are not associated with sesamoid bones.

5-25. The answer is e. (*Parslow, pp 376–379.*) This patient has a classic case of hereditary angioedema. This disease is characterized by a deficiency of complement control proteins such as C1 esterase inhibitor, leading to overactive complement. Uncontrolled generation of vasoactive peptides causes increased blood vessel permeability, causing hereditary angioedema. Edema, especially of the larynx, obstructs the airways. Abdominal pain may indicate that the patient has angioedema of the gut.

5-26. The answer is d. (*Rubin, pp 326–332. Cotran, pp 421–422. Braunwald, pp 159, 161–162.*) Cyanide causes cellular damage by binding to cytochrome oxidase and inhibiting cellular respiration. Cyanide is used in industry; an industrial accident in India in 1984 killed more than 2000 people. Cyanide is also a component of amygdalin, which is found in the pits of several fruits, such as apricots and peaches. It is also found in laetrile, a drug that is used outside of the United States. Cyanide poisoning produces a cherry-red color of the skin and also produces the odor of bitter almonds on the breath.

In contrast, acute arsenic toxicity causes central nervous toxicity and renal tubular necrosis. Chronic arsenic exposure causes GI disturbances, peripheral neuropathies, and skin changes (thick areas of skin with increased pigmentation called arsenical keratosis). Arsenic is also associated with cancers of the skin, respiratory tract, and liver (angiosarcomas). Arsenic accumulates in the hair and nails (forming transverse ridges called Mees' lines). Carbon monoxide is a colorless, odorless gas that is produced by natural gas heaters and is found in car exhaust. It replaces oxygen in hemoglobin, causing the formation of carboxyhemoglobin. This results in extreme cyanosis and anoxia. It produces a characteristic cherry-red color of the skin and blood. Finally, carbon tetrachloride can produce liver damage (with steatosis), while ethylene glycol, commonly used as an antifreeze, is toxic to humans (and cats and dogs) because it causes a metabolic acidosis and acute tubular necrosis in the kidney, as ethylene glycol is metabolized to calcium oxalate (polarizable crystals), which are deposited in the renal tubules.

5-27. The answer is b. (*Craig, p 237; Hardman, p 789.*) Abrupt discontinuation of clonidine has been associated with a rapidly developing and severe "rebound" phenomenon that includes excessive cardiac stimulation and a spike of blood pressure that may be sufficiently great as to cause stroke or other similar complications. Recall that clonidine is a "centrally acting α-adrenergic agonist." Through its central effects it reduces sympathetic nervous system tone. This, in turn, appears to cause supersensitivity of peripheral adrenergic receptors to direct-acting adrenergic agonists, including endogenous norepinephrine and epinephrine. Once, and soon after, the drug is stopped, endogenous catecholamines trigger hyperresponsiveness of all structures under sympathetic control.

When ACE inhibitors (or angiotensin receptor blockers), hydrochlorothiazide, or nifedipine (long-acting or otherwise) are abruptly stopped, blood pressure will begin to rise from treatment levels, but there will be no sudden "spike" of pressure nor an "overshoot" of it.

Digoxin discontinuation is not associated with the symptoms noted in the question. Besides, the half-life of digoxin (about 36 to 40 h if renal function is normal) is such that stopping the drug abruptly would not lead to any significant events occurring "within a day or two" of discontinuation.

There is no reason to predict that suddenly stopping warfarin would cause tachyarrhythmias, hypertension, or hemorrhagic stroke—and certainly not within 24 to 48 h.

5-28. The answer is b. (*Adams, pp 443–445, 453–459.*) This case is an example of a lesion of the left (usually dominant) parietal lobe, most often in the angular gyrus, with some involvement of the precentral gyrus in the posterior frontal lobe. There is contralateral UMN weakness (with a positive Babinski sign), as well as several cortical sensory defects—specifically, right-left confusion, agraphia (inability to write, independent of motor weakness), acalculia (the inability to calculate), and finger agnosia (the inability to designate the fingers). The latter four elements are sometimes referred to as the *Gerstmann syndrome* by neurologists, and all represent spatial discriminatory functions of the parietal lobe (often the dominant parietal lobe, which is usually the left). The parietal lobe also subserves other visual-spatial functions such as construction of complex drawings. There are other locations within the CNS where UMN weakness can occur; however, the combination with parietal lobe signs can occur only in this location. If the damage was slightly more extensive, it may have involved Broca's area, causing aphasia.

5-29. The answer is b. (*Boron, pp 431, 509. Guyton, pp 248–249.*) Systolic murmurs are caused by mitral or tricuspid regurgitation or by aortic or pulmonic stenosis. Aortic stenosis increases the resistance of the aortic valve, producing a large pressure drop between the ventricle and aorta. Under normal conditions, the aortic valve offers almost no resistance to flow, and, therefore, there would be virtually no pressure gradient between the left ventricle and the aorta.

5-30. The answer is b. (*Cotran, pp 1084–1089. Rubin, pp 1020–1024.*) Gestational trophoblastic diseases include benign hydatidiform mole (partial and complete), invasive mole (chorioadenoma destruens), placental site trophoblastic tumor, and choriocarcinoma. Hydatidiform moles are composed of avascular, grapelike structures that do not invade the myometrium. In complete (classic) moles, all the chorionic villi are abnormal and fetal parts are not found. They have a 46,XX diploid pattern and arise from the paternal chromosomes of a single sperm by a process called androgenesis. In partial moles, only some of the villi are abnormal and fetal parts may be seen. These moles have a triploid or a tetraploid karyotype and arise from the fertilization of a single egg by two sperm. About 2% of complete moles may develop into choriocarcinoma, but partial moles are rarely followed by malignancy. Invasive moles penetrate the myometrium and may even embolize to distant sites. A similar lesion is the placental site trophoblastic tumor, which is characterized by invasion of the myometrium by intermediate trophoblasts. Gestational choriocarcinomas, composed of malignant proliferations of both cytotrophoblasts and syncytiotrophoblasts without the formation of villi, can arise from either normal or abnormal pregnancies: 50% arise in hydatidiform moles, 25% in cases of previous abortion, 22% in normal pregnancies, and the rest in ectopic pregnancies or teratomas. Both hydatidiform moles and choriocarcinomas have high levels of human chorionic gonadotropin (hCG); the levels are extremely high in choriocarcinoma unless considerable tumor necrosis is present.

5-31. The answer is d. (*Guyton, pp 72–73. Boron, pp 235, 525–527.*) Titin is a large protein that located between the Z line at the end of the sarcomere to the M line in the middle of the sarcomere. The resistance of the muscle to stretch is determined by the elasticity of the titin molecule. The titin in cardiac muscle is much stiffer than in the skeletal muscle, so it is more difficult to stretch cardiac muscle cells than it is to stretch skeletal muscle fibers.

5-32. The answer is d. *(Kandel, pp 1151–1157. Siegel, pp 950–965.)* The primary regions shown to be affected by Alzheimer's disease include the basal nucleus of Meynert (which contains cholinergic neurons that project widely to the forebrain, including the cerebral cortex), the hippocampal formation, and the cerebral cortex. The other choices included structures that have not been significantly implicated in this disorder. The neurotransmitter that has been most implicated in this disorder is ACh. Alzheimer's brains have been shown to have reduced levels of ACh and cholinergic markers, especially after damage to cholinergic neurons of the basal nucleus of Meynert. While reductions in other neurotransmitter levels may also occur, the other choices of neurotransmitters presented have not been clearly implicated in this disorder. One of the clearest neuropathological characteristics of Alzheimer's disease is the presence of amyloid deposits and neurofibrillary tangles in the cerebral cortex. In fact, there has been a new and promising strategy that has been applied for the treatment of Alzheimer's disease. It involves the attempt to administer small molecules that retard the aggregation of amyloid-β peptides that form fibrillar amyloid plaques, which affect the normal functions of neurons.

5-33. The answer is d. *(Henry, pp 505–508.)* Abnormalities of red cells can help to identify the disease process that is present. Schistocytes, which are red cell fragments, indicate the presence of hemolysis, and they can be seen with hemolytic anemia, megaloblastic anemia, or severe burns. Other red cell shapes characteristic of hemolysis include triangular cells and helmet cells. Acanthocytes and echinocytes are considered by some to be fragmented red blood cells. Acanthocytes are irregularly spiculated red cells found in patients with abetalipoproteinemia or liver disease. Echinocytes, in contrast, have regular spicules (undulations) and may either be artifacts (crenated cells) or be found in hyperosmolar diseases such as uremia.

In contrast, drepanocytes are sickle cells, while target cells (red cells with a central dark area) are called dacrocytes. These cells are the result of excess cytoplasmic membrane material and are found in patients with liver disease, such as obstructive jaundice, or in any of the hypochromic anemias. Pappenheimer bodies are red cell inclusions composed of iron, while Heinz bodies are formed by denatured hemoglobin. The latter, which are not seen with routine stains, are found in patients with glucose-6-phosphatase dehydrogenase deficiency and the unstable hemoglobinopathies.

5-34. The answer is e. *(Craig, pp 187–188; Hardman, pp 956, 1579, 1585; Katzung, pp 232–234, 630, 633.)* Amiodarone, an iodine-rich drug, has several actions that can lead to clinical hypothyroidism (or, less often and mainly in persons with iodine-deficient diets, hyperthyroidism). It inhibits a deiodinase (an enzyme that removes iodine on both the 5 and 5′ positions) that converts thyroxine to triiodothyronine (T_3), mainly in the liver. This process is the main contributor to the production of endogenous (circulating) T_3 that is used by most target tissues in the body. Inhibit this enzyme and the peripheral tissues have less T_3 to utilize, and signs and symptoms of hypothyroidism can ensue.

The excess iodine derived from metabolism of amiodarone may also contribute to the hypothyroidism. The mechanism is analogous to the way in which administering large doses of iodide are clinically useful for suppressing thyroid function in hyperthyroid individuals: iodide limits its own transport into follicular cells, and, acutely at least, high circulating levels of iodide inhibit thyroid hormone synthesis.

5-35. The answer is h. *(Parslow, pp 128–129, 401–405, 426–430. Levinson, pp 423–428. Braunwald, pp 1922–1925.)* Loss of tolerance by the immune system to certain self-components can lead to the formation of antibodies, causing tissue and organ damage. Such diseases are referred to as *autoimmune diseases.* There are a host of autoimmune diseases characterized by the autoantibodies. The presence of a "butterfly" rash is a classic cutaneous sign of SLE and is characterized by a rash over the bridge of the nose and on the cheeks.

5-36. The answer is b. *(Murray, pp 580–597. Scriver, pp 3127–3164. Sack, pp 121–138.)* Ferrous iron (Fe^{2+}) is the form absorbed in the intestine by ferritin, transported in plasma by transferrin, and stored in the liver in combination with ferritin or as hemosiderin. There is no known excretory pathway for iron, either in the ferric or ferrous form. For this reason, excessive iron uptake over a period of many years may cause hemochromatosis (235200), the likely diagnosis for this man. This is a condition of extensive hemosiderin deposition in the liver, myocardium, pancreas, and adrenals. The resulting symptoms include liver cirrhosis, congestive heart failure, diabetes mellitus, and changes in skin pigmentation.

5-37. The answer is d. (*Cotran, pp 856–864. Chandrasoma, pp 641–643.*) Several types of viruses are implicated as being causative agents of viral hepatitis. Each of these has unique characteristics. Hepatitis A virus, an RNA picornavirus, is transmitted through the fecal-oral route (including shellfish) and is called infectious hepatitis. It is associated with small outbreaks of hepatitis in the United States, especially among young children at day care centers. Hepatitis B virus, which causes "serum hepatitis," is associated with the development of a serum sickness-like syndrome in about 10% of patients. Immune complexes of antibody and HBsAg are present in patients with vasculitis. Hepatitis C virus is characterized by episodic elevations in serum transaminases and also by fatty change in liver biopsy specimens. Hepatitis D virus is distinct in that it is a defective virus and needs HBsAg to be infective. Hepatitis E virus is characterized by waterborne transmission. It is found in underdeveloped countries and has an unusually high mortality in pregnant females. It is important to remember that the liver may be infected by other viruses, such as yellow fever virus, Epstein-Barr virus (EBV, the causative agent of infectious mononucleosis), CMV, and/or herpes virus. The latter is characterized histologically by intranuclear eosinophilic inclusions (Cowdry bodies) and nuclei that have a ground-glass appearance.

5-38. The answer is e. (*Brooks, pp 550–552. Levinson, p 310. Murray— 2002, pp 664–667. Ryan, pp 660–664.*) *C. albicans* is the most important species of *Candida* and causes thrush, vaginitis, skin and nail infections, and other infections. It is part of the normal flora of skin, mouth, GI tract, and vagina. It appears in tissues as an oval budding yeast or elongated pseudohyphae. It grows well on laboratory media and is identified by germ-tube formation. A vaccine is not available, and serologic and skin tests have little value.

5-39. The answer is b. (*Craig, p 533; Hardman, pp 1212–1213; Katzung, p 375, 1112.*) Cefoperazone (third-generation cephalosporin) or cefotetan (second-generation) inhibit aldehyde dehydrogenase and cause accumulation of acetaldehyde (as does disulfiram), and so can cause all the typical and potentially serious consequences of a disulfiram-like reaction. Cefmetazole, a second-generation cephalosporin, also causes a similar adverse interaction with alcohol. (Note that these three cephalosporins are also the ones that are associated with vitamin K-related bleeding problems, as addressed in Question 434.)

Erythromycin (whether administered as the base or one of the common salts, e.g., ethylsuccinate, estolate, or stearate) can inhibit the hepatic P450 system sufficient to cause adverse interactions with (excessive effects of) such drugs as warfarin, carbamazepine, and theophylline. However, based on current evidence there is no specific inhibition of aldehyde dehydrogenase, nor resulting accumulation of acetaldehyde, that would correctly qualify as a disulfiram-like interaction.

Amoxicillin, penicillin G, and other penicillins do not participate in disulfiram-like reactions.

Linezolid inhibits monoamine oxidase (MAO), albeit weakly, and so can trigger potentially significant adverse interactions in persons receiving such sympathomimetics as cocaine, ephedrine, or pseudoephedrine. However, the drug does not inhibit alcohol metabolism or cause the adverse responses noted in this question.

5-40. The answer is a. (*Braunwald, pp 2169–2170.*) Prolactin is the major stimulator of breast milk production. Overproduction of prolactin leads to galactorrhea. Estrogen, progesterone, thyroxine, and cortisol are all needed for proper breast development but play no role in actual milk production.

5-41. The answer is h. (*Nolte, pp 65–69, 375–390, 451–453, 513–524, 559–561, 565–582.*) This figure is a horizontal view of the brain at the level of the head of the caudate nucleus and the internal capsule. The posterior limb of the internal capsule (F) contains fibers that arise from the leg region of the cerebral cortex and project to lumbar levels of the spinal cord, thus serving as UMNs for the elicitation of voluntary movement of the contralateral leg. Fibers in the anterior limb of the internal capsule (H) project in large numbers to deep pontine nuclei and represent first-order neurons in a pathway linking the cerebral cortex with the cerebellum. These fibers comprise a part of the reciprocal feedback circuit linking the cerebellar and cerebral cortices. Disruption of a part of this circuit can result in the ability to produce smooth, coordinated, purposeful movements. Pseudobulbar palsy is characterized in part by a weakness of the muscles controlling swallowing, chewing, breathing, and speaking. It results from a lesion of the UMNs associated with the head region of the cortex, which pass through the genu of the internal capsule (G) en route to brainstem cranial nerve nuclei upon which they synapse. The descending column of the fornix (B), situated along the midline of the brain, contains fibers that arise from the hippocampal formation and project to the septal area and to the medial hypothalamus, including the mammillary bodies. This pathway plays an important role in the regulation of emotional behavior and short-term memory functions. Disruption of the hippocampal formation or its output pathway, the fornix, would affect levels of emotionality and short-term memory.

The head of the caudate nucleus (D) is part of an important element of the motor systems called the *basal ganglia*. It receives significant inputs from several regions associated with motor functions. These include the cerebral cortex and the dopamine-containing region of the substantia nigra (i.e., the pars compacta). Huntington's disease is associated with a loss of GABA levels within the neostriatum and, in particular, the caudate nucleus. The mediodorsal thalamic nucleus (E) projects large quantities of axons to extensive regions of the rostral half of the frontal lobe, including the prefrontal cortex. It also receives significant projections from the prefrontal region of the cortex.

5-42. The answer is a. (*Cotran, pp 649–650. Chandrasoma, pp 433–443.*) Lymph nodes may be enlarged (lymphadenopathy) secondary to reactive processes, which can be either acute or chronic. Acute reaction (acute nonspecific lymphadenitis) can result in focal or generalized lymphadenopathy. Focal lymph node enlargement is usually the result of bacterial infection (bacterial lymphadenitis). Sections from involved lymph nodes reveal infiltration by neutrophils. In contrast, generalized acute lymphadenopathy is usually the result of viral infections and usually produces a proliferation of reactive T lymphocytes called T immunoblasts. These reactive T cells tend to have prominent nucleoli and can be easily mistaken for malignant lymphocytes or malignant Hodgkin cells.

5-43. The answer is c. (*Cotran, p 1151. Rubin, pp 1180–1183.*) Parathyroid hyperplasia may be associated with either primary or secondary hyperparathyroidism. In contrast to primary hyperparathyroidism, secondary hyperparathyroidism results from hypocalcemia and causes secondary hypersecretion of parathyroid hormone (PTH). This results in the combination of hypocalcemia and increased PTH. This abnormality is principally found in patients with chronic renal failure, where phosphate retention is thought to cause hypocalcemia. Since the failing kidney is not able to synthesize 1,25-dihydroxycholecalciferol, the most active form of vitamin D, this deficiency leads to poor absorption of calcium from the gut and relative hypocalcemia, which stimulates excess PTH secretion. Chronic renal failure is the most important cause, but secondary hyperparathyroidism also occurs in vitamin D deficiency, malabsorption syndromes, and pseudo-hypoparathyroidism. In any of the causes of parathyroid hyperplasia, all four parathyroid glands are typically enlarged. Parathyroid hyperplasia can be differentiated from parathyroid adenomas by the fact that parathyroid hyperplasia, either primary or secondary, results in enlargement of all four glands, while a parathyroid adenoma or parathyroid carcinoma produces enlargement of only one gland. In most cases the other three glands are smaller than normal.

5-44. The answer is d. (*Murray, pp 474–480. Scriver, pp 4029–4240. Sack, pp 121–138.*) Milk intolerance may be due to milk protein allergies during infancy, but it is commonly caused by lactase deficiency in older individuals. Intestinal lactase hydrolyzes the milk sugar lactose into galactose and glucose, both reducing sugars that can be detected as reducing substances in the stool. The symptoms of lactose intolerance (lactase deficiency) and other conditions involving intestinal malabsorption include diarrhea, cramps, and flatulence due to water retention and bacterial action in the gut. In nontropical sprue, symptoms seem to result from the production of antibodies in the blood against fragments of wheat gluten. It seems likely that a defect in intestinal epithelial cells allows tryptic peptides from the digestion of gluten to be absorbed into the blood, as well as to exert a harmful effect on intestinal epithelia. Gallbladder inflammation (cholecystitis) usually presents with acute abdominal pain (colic) with radiation to the right shoulder. The normal composition of bile is about 5% cholesterol, 15% phosphatidylcholine, and 80% bile salt in a micellar liquid form. Increased cholesterol from high-fat diets or genetic conditions can upset the delicate micellar balance, leading to supersaturated cholesterol or cholesterol precipitates that cause gallstone formation. Removal of the gallbladder is a common treatment for this painful condition. Mobilization of fats with the production of ketone bodies occurs during fasting and starvation, but ketone production is well controlled. During uncontrolled diabetes mellitus, ketogenesis proceeds at a rate that exceeds the buffering capacity of the blood to produce ketoacidosis.

5-45. The answer is c. (*McPhee, p 167. Braunwald, p 2602.*) This is the classic presentation of a confusional state caused by carbon monoxide poisoning, which, in addition to confusion, includes shortness of breath, tachycardia, and reddish appearance of the mucous membranes. ABGs would show a normal Po_2; O_2 saturation by "pulse oximetry" would be essentially normal. Oxygen saturation by "CO-oximetry" would be low.

5-46. The answer is e. *(Behrman, pp 1380–1385. Cotran, pp 481–482.)* Sudden infant death syndrome (SIDS) is a heterogeneous, multifactorial disorder, but by definition it refers to sudden death of an infant under 1 year of age that is unexplained after thorough examination. Most cases of SIDS occur between 2 and 4 months of life, and the child usually dies during sleep ("crib death" or "cot death"). A risk factor for SIDS is sleeping in a prone position. Therefore healthy infants should sleep on their back or side. Maternal factors associated with SIDS include age less than 20, being unmarried, low socioeconomic group, smoking, and drug abuse. Infant factors associated with SIDS include prematurity, low birth weight, male sex, and a history of SIDS in a sibling. In contrast to SIDS, death from respiratory complications after being born 10 weeks prematurely is suggestive of hyaline membrane disease, while evidence of repeated bone fractures and bilateral retinal hemorrhages is suggestive of trauma, child abuse, or "shaken baby" syndrome.

5-47. The answer is b. *(Cotran, pp 195, 1252–1253.)* A variety of different diseases have an association with certain HLA (human leukocyte antigen) types. The exact mechanism of this association is unknown. These diseases can be grouped into three broad categories: inflammatory diseases, inherited errors of metabolism, and autoimmune diseases. The classic example of an inflammatory disease associated with a certain HLA is the association of ankylosing spondylitis with HLA-B27. Ankylosing spondylitis is one type of spondyloarthropathy that lacks the rheumatoid factor found in rheumatoid arthritis. Other seronegative spondyloarthropathies include Reiter's syndrome, psoriatic arthritis, and enteropathic arthritis. All of these are associated with an increased incidence of HLA-B27. Ankylosing spondylitis, also known as rheumatoid spondylitis or Marie-Strümpell disease, is a chronic inflammatory disease that primarily affects the sacroiliac joints of adult males. Calcification of the vertebral and paravertebral ligaments produce low back pain and stiffness and are seen radiographically as a "bamboo spine."

HLA types are also associated with inherited errors of metabolism and autoimmune diseases. An example of an inherited error of metabolism being associated with a certain HLA type is the association of hemochromatosis with HLA-A3, while autoimmune diseases can be associated with the DR locus. Two examples of this are the associations of rheumatoid arthritis with DR4 and of insulin-dependent diabetes with DR3/DR4.

5-48. The answer is d. (*Scriver, pp 3–45. Sack, pp 57–84.*) The case described represents one of the more common chromosomal causes of reproductive failure, Turner mosaicism. Turner's syndrome represents a pattern of anomalies including short stature, heart defects, and infertility. Turner's syndrome is often associated with a 45,X karyotype (monosomy X) in females, but mosaicism (i.e., two or more cell lines with different karyotypes in the same individual) is common. However, chimerism (i.e., two cell lines in an individual arising from different zygotes, such as fraternal twins who do not separate) is extremely rare. Trisomy refers to three copies of one chromosome, euploidy to a normal chromosome number, and monoploidy to one set of chromosomes (haploidy in humans).

5-49. The answer is c. (*Braunwald, pp 312–313, 1102, 1107.*) The rash is impetigo, which is caused by group A streptococci, occasionally by other streptococci, and also by *Staphylococcus aureus*. It occurs in children who have poor hygiene, and the streptococci, which colonize the skin, gain entrance through a break in the skin, such as a scratch or an insect bite. The rash is painless, unlike herpes simplex or shingles, which is due to herpesvirus varicellae. Herpes simplex occurs on the face and mouth and genitals; shingles follows the distribution of a nerve, mainly the temporal nerve and the intracostal nerves. Scarlet fever, also due to streptococci, characteristically covers the trunk and extremities with a fine papular rash, sparing the palms and soles. Erysipelas is a streptococcal cellulitis.

5-50. The answer is a. (*Boron, pp 656–659. Guyton, pp 266, 390–391.*) Polycythemia vera is a disease in which an abnormally large number of red blood cells are produced. The large number of red blood cells causes an increase in blood viscosity by two or three times normal. Patients with polycythemia vera often have high blood pressure (because of increased blood volume) and cyanosis (because of increased oxygen extraction from blood flowing slowly through capillaries).

BLOCK 6

Answers

6-1. The answer is a. *(Cotran, pp 84–87.)* An abscess is a localized collection of neutrophils and necrotic debris. It is basically a localized form of suppurative (purulent) inflammation, which is associated with pyogenic bacteria and is characterized by edema fluid admixed with neutrophils and necrotic cells (liquefactive necrosis or pus). *S. aureus* classically produces abscesses, because it is coagulase-positive and coagulase helps to produce fibrinous material that localizes the infection. In contrast to an abscess, an ulcer is a defect of an epithelium in which the full-thickness of the epithelial lining is sloughed and is replaced by inflammatory necrotic material. Partial sloughing of the epithelium is called an erosion.

Other morphologic patterns of inflammation include serous inflammation, fibrinous inflammation, and pseudomembranous inflammation. Serous inflammation produces a thin fluid, such as is present in skin blisters or body cavities. There is not enough fibrinogen present in serous inflammation to form fibrin. In contrast, fibrinous inflammation is associated with the deposition of fibrin in body cavities, which subsequently stimulates coagulation. Histologically, fibrin is seen as amorphic eosinophilic material. Fibrinous inflammation within the pericardial cavity (fibrinous pericarditis) produces a characteristic "bread-and-butter" appearance grossly.

6-2. The answer is c. *(Guyton, pp 52–55. Boron, pp 814–817.)* Orange juice contains a significant amount of K^+. Consuming a large amount of K^+ when the extracellular volume is low (dehydration) can cause a significant rise in extracellular K^+. An increase in extracellular K^+ makes the membrane potential more positive. Depolarizing the membrane opens K^+ channels causing an increase in membrane conductance. Prolonged depolarization, whether caused by an increase in extracellular K^+ or by an action potential causes Na^+ channels to inactivate. Inactivation, which decreases the excitability of the nerve membrane, is observed in hyperkalemia and during the absolute and relative refractory periods following a normal action potential. The activity of the Na-K pump can be reduced by a reduction, not an increase, in extracellular K^+ concentration.

6-3. The answer is d. (*Craig, pp 101–102, 112t; Hardman, p 228; Katzung, pp 136–137, 212–213.*) Dobutamine behaves, for all practical purposes, as a selective β_1 agonist. Norepinephrine is a β_1 agonist that also activates α-adrenergic receptors effectively. However, when it is administered with phentolamine (prototype α blocker) its spectrum of activity is, qualitatively, identical to that of dobutamine.

High doses of dopamine cause positive inotropic and chronotropic effects, but also release neuronal norepinephrine and probably activate α-adrenergic receptors directly (causing unwanted vasoconstriction). These vasoconstrictor effects would negate vasodilator effects due to stimulation of dopamine D_1 receptors found in some arterioles, and of D_2 receptors found on some ganglia, and in the cardiovascular control center of the CNS.

Ephedrine weakly activates all adrenergic receptors and also leads to norepinephrine release. Overall, its effects are quite similar to those produced by norepinephrine itself. Regardless, if one administers ephedrine with propranolol, the prototypic nonselective (β_1 and β_2) beta blocker, ephedrine's remaining actions amount to selective α-adrenergic activation (i.e., phenylephrine-like)—not at all like dobutamine.

Phenylephrine (α agonist) plus atropine (muscarinic antagonist) causes effects that in no way resemble those of dobutamine or the norepinephrine-phentolamine combination.

6-4. The answer is d. (*Scriver, pp 3–45. Sack, pp 97–158.*) The figure shows the correctly drawn pedigree with generations indicated by Roman numerals and individuals by Arabic numbers. As the McKusick numbers indicate, achondroplasia is autosomal dominant, cystic fibrosis autosomal recessive. Since neither parent is affected with achondroplasia, the risk for their next child to be affected is virtually zero (rare chances for germ-line mosaicism or incomplete penetrance are ignored). The person who prompted genetic concern is the proband (III-1). George has a brother with cystic fibrosis, making his parents (I-3, I-4) obligate carriers. He has a ¼ chance of being normal, a ¾ chance of being a carrier, and a ¼ chance of being affected with cystic fibrosis. Since George's possibility of being affected is eliminated by circumstance (he is normal), his odds of being a carrier are ⅔. George's wife is definitely a carrier, giving their next child a ⅙ chance to have cystic fibrosis (⅔ chance George is a carrier × ¼ chance the child is affected if both are carriers). Although the DF_{508} (three–base pair deletion of phenylalanine codon at position 508 in the cystic fibrosis transmembrane regulator gene) accounts for 70% of cystic fibrosis mutations in whites, George's family may have a different mutation than was detected by DNA analysis in his wife. Their child may therefore have a risk of being a compound heterozygote (two different abnormal cystic fibrosis alleles) but will still be affected.

6-5. The answer is b. (*Parslow, pp 575–576, 699–700, 703–706.*) There are three forms of immunity: active, passive, and adoptive. Active immunity involves an individual making his or her own antibodies either naturally, by infection, or artificially, by immunizations. Passive immunity refers to the transfer of preformed antibodies from one individual to another either naturally (transplacental or enteromammary antibodies from mother to fetus) or artificially through gamma globulin injections such as antitoxins, anti-Rh, and antivenoms (black widow spider bites, etc.). Finally, adoptive immunity refers to the transfer of lymphoid cells from an actively immunized donor and does not involve antibody transfer.

6-6. The answer is d. (*Carlson, pp 259–267.*) Most of the human research on sleep has found that after a few days of sleep deprivation people report perceptual distortions or, in a few cases, even hallucinations. These studies have documented statements such as "the floor seems wavy" or "steam seems to be rising from the floor," indicating that sleep deprivation affects cerebral functioning. Another research finding is that being sleepy is distinctly different from being tired, as after exercise. Sleepiness can occur even without any activity and sleep deprivation does not appear to interfere with the ability to perform physical exercise. Likewise, there is no evidence of a physiologic stress response to sleep deprivation, indicated by little change in blood levels of cortisol and epinephrine. Sleep does appear to be necessary for the brain to function normally. After a period of sleep deprivation a rebound phenomenon does occur. The individual will sleep longer and spend a much greater time in REM sleep, but will not regain the number of sleepless hours lost.

6-7. The answer is d. (*Murray, pp 358–373. Scriver, pp 3–45. Sack, pp 1–40.*) The gene that produces the deadly toxin of *Corynebacterium diphtheriae* comes from a lysogenic phage that grows in the bacteria. Prior to immunization, diphtheria was the primary cause of death in children. The protein toxin produced by this bacterium inhibits protein synthesis by inactivating elongation factor 2 (EF-2, or translocase). Diphtheria toxin is a single protein composed of two portions (A and B). The B portion enables the A portion to translocate across a cell membrane into the cytoplasm. The A portion catalyzes the transfer of the adenosine diphosphate ribose unit of NAD_1 to a nitrogen atom of the diphthamide ring of EF-2, thereby blocking translocation. Diphthamide is an unusual amino acid residue of EF-2.

6-8. The answer is d. *(Levinson, pp 398–399. Braunwald, pp 739–742.)* Graft-versus-host disease (GVHD) can develop in immunosuppressed persons who receive allogeneic bone marrow transplants that contain allogeneic T cells transferred with the donor's stem cells or develop from it. The donor cells respond to histocompatibility antigens present on the recipient's cells, which are not present on the donor cells. Bone marrow contains immunocompetent T cells; liver, kidney, and skin do not have a sufficient number of immunocompetent T cells to elicit GVH reactions. MHC I proteins identical in donor and recipient do not play a role in GVHD, but GVHD can ensue from a mismatch of MHC I and II proteins between donor and recipient. Antibody and nitric oxide are not involved in GVHD.

6-9. The answer is c. *(Craig, pp 197, 739–740; Katzung, p 189.)* Sildenafil (and the related drugs, tadalafil and vardenafil), a wildly popular and widely prescribed drug for erectile dysfunction (ED), prolongs and enhances erection by a nitric oxide–dependent mechanism. Of course, its effects are systemic—not limited to the penile vasculature. Nitroglycerin causes its vaso- (veno-)dilator effects via a NO/G protein–dependent mechanism also. The ED drug can profoundly intensify nitrate-induced vasodilation and cause life-threatening hypotension and myocardial and cerebral ischemia.

Note the important mechanistic links between vasodilation/hypotension, sexual intercourse, and potentially fatal cardiac responses. Sexual arousal—and, especially orgasm—causes a massive activation of the sympathetic nervous system. One consequence of that, α-mediated vasoconstriction that tends to keep blood pressure up, is too feeble to overcome the hypotensive effects of the sildenafil-nitroglycerin combination. Along with a fall of blood pressure is a fall of coronary perfusion pressure (diastolic blood pressure), i.e., reduced myocardial blood flow/oxygen supply. Yet the sympathetic activation concomitantly causes significant increases of cardiac rate and contractility, i.e., increased myocardial oxygen demand. Oxygen demand rises, supply falls, and the stage is set for acute myocardial ischemia.

6-10. The answer is c. (*Moore and Dalley, p 159.*) The patient has a left pneumothorax. The lucidity of the left pleural cavity with the lack of pulmonary vessels indicates that the left lung has collapsed into a small, dense mass adjacent to the mediastinum. Such a nontraumatic pneumothorax may result from the rupture of a pulmonary bleb, especially in a young person. The right lung is normal. There is no pleural fluid level indicative of hemothorax, and the near symmetry of the domes of the two hemidiaphragms on inspiration indicates normal function of the phrenic nerves. The pleural cavities normally extend superior to the first rib into the base of the neck. The heart, measuring less than one-half of the chest diameter, is of normal size, but is shifted to the right. Both the pulmonary trunk and the left ventricle would be inferior to the arrow on the left heart border.

6-11. The answer is E. (*Afifi, pp 187–213. Nolte, pp 266–277.*) The inferior colliculus (E) is situated in the caudal aspect of the tectum and is an important relay nucleus for the transmission of auditory information to the cortex from lower levels of the brainstem. Damage to the inferior colliculus would likely result in some loss of auditory discrimination, acuity, and ability to localize sound in space. The decussation of the superior cerebellar peduncle (B) is also present at caudal levels of the midbrain and is usually seen together with the inferior colliculus. These crossing fibers arise from the dentate and interposed nuclei and terminate in the contralateral red nucleus and ventrolateral nucleus of the thalamus. Damage to the cerebellum would likely result in degeneration of the fibers contained within the superior cerebellar peduncle. The crus cerebri (C) contains fibers that arise from all regions of the cortex and project to all the levels of the brainstem and the spinal cord. As noted previously, damage to the corticospinal tract at any level would result in a UMN paralysis. The trochlear nucleus (cranial nerve IV) (A), which is situated just below the periaqueductal gray at the level of the inferior colliculus, receives direct inputs from ascending fibers of the medial longitudinal fasciculus that arise from vestibular nuclei. The trochlear nucleus governs the downward movements of the eyes, in particular, when they are in a medial position. A fourth nerve paralysis is particularly seen when the patient is attempting to walk down a flight of stairs and cannot move his eyes downward. The midbrain periaqueductal gray (D) contains dense quantities of enkephalin-positive cells and nerve terminals. The transmitter (or neuromodulator) enkephalin plays an important role in the regulation of pain, cardiovascular functions, and emotional behavior.

6-12. The answer is c. *(Levinson, pp 114, 121.)* Among children 1 month of age and younger, the gram-negative bacilli, mainly *E. coli* and other enteric bacilli, are the most common cause of meningitis. Group B streptococci and *Listeria monocytogenes* also cause meningitis in this age group of children, but not as often as do the gram-negative bacilli. Group B streptococci septic infections that occur very early do so as a result of spread of the organism to the newborn from the maternal genital tract. *N. meningitidis* is a common cause of meningitis in children older than 1 month of age, and among older children, adolescents, and adults, *N. meningitidis* and *S. pneumoniae* are the two most common pathogens of meningitis. *H. influenzae* is a common cause of meningitis among older children and adolescents.

6-13. The answer is c. *(Kaplan, pp 737–741.)* Sleep is divided into two distinct states: D sleep (desynchronized EEG pattern sleep) and S sleep (synchronized EEG pattern sleep). D sleep is also known as REM (rapid-eye-movement) or dreaming sleep; S sleep as NREM (non-rapid-eye-movement), orthodox, or quiet sleep. S sleep (NREM) is divided into stages 1, 2, 3, and 4; stage 1 is the lightest and stage 4 the deepest. NREM sleep lasts from 60 to 100 min, followed by 10 to 40 min of REM sleep, and the cycle is continued throughout the night. Typically, about 80% of an adult's sleep time is spent in NREM sleep and 20% in REM sleep. REM sleep tends to increase during the second half of the night. The amount of REM sleep appears to determine the amount of rest. When REM sleep is interrupted, tiredness tends to develop. A newborn spends about 50% of sleep time in REM sleep. Deep sleep begins to be replaced by longer periods of lighter sleep after the age of 30.

6-14. The answer is b. *(McPhee, pp 630–634. Cotran, pp 1056, 1079.)* Secondary amenorrhea refers to absent menses for 3 months in a woman who had previously had menses. Causes of secondary amenorrhea include pregnancy (the most common cause), hypothalamic/pituitary abnormalities, ovarian disorders, and end organ (uterine) disease. Pregnancy can be diagnosed by obtaining a clinical history along with a pregnancy test that determines serum or urine β-human chorionic gonadotropin (β-hCG) levels. Placental human chorionic gonadotropin (hCG), secreted by syncytiotrophoblasts, functions early in pregnancy to stimulate the corpus luteum to continue secreting progesterone until the mature placenta, working together with the mother and the fetus, can produce progesterone. Levels of hCG reach a peak at approximately 8 to 10 weeks of development and then rapidly decline.

The remainder of the disorders causing secondary amenorrhea can be differentiated by examining gonadotropin (FSH and LH) levels along with the results of a progesterone challenge test. Withdrawal bleeding following progesterone administration indicates that the endometrial mucosa had been primed with estrogen, which in turn indicates that the hypothalamus/pituitary axis and ovaries are normal. Hypothalamic/pituitary disorders, which are characterized by decreased FSH and LH levels, include functional gonadotropin deficiencies, such as can be seen in patients with a weight loss syndrome. In these patients, markedly decreased body weight (>15% below ideal weight) causes decreased secretion of GnRH from the hypothalamus. Decreased gonadotropin levels decrease estrogen levels, which results in amenorrhea and an increased risk for osteoporosis. Because of the decreased estrogen levels, a progesterone challenge does not result in withdrawal bleeding. Ovarian conditions, such as surgical removal of the ovaries, would most likely produce elevated gonadotropin levels due to the lack of negative feedback from estrogen and progesterone. Because of the decreased estrogen levels, a progesterone challenge would not result in withdrawal bleeding. Uterine (end organ) disorders are characterized by normal FSH and LH levels. An example is Asherman's syndrome, in which numerous and overly aggressive dilatation and curettage of the endometrium for menorrhagia removes the stratum basalis and no glandular epithelium remains. A patient with Asherman's syndrome would have no response to progesterone.

6-15. The answer is c. (*Murray, pp 556–579. Scriver, pp 2863–2914. Sack, pp 205–222.*) Nitroglycerin causes release of nitric oxide (NO), which activates guanyl cyclase, produces cyclic GMP, and causes vasodilation. NO is formed from one of the guanidino nitrogens of the arginine side chain by the enzyme nitric oxide synthase. NO has a short half-life, reacting with oxygen to form nitrite and then nitrates that are excreted in urine. Coronary vasodilation caused by nitroglycerin is thus short-lived, making other measures necessary for long-term relief of coronary occlusion. The neurotransmitter formed by condensation of acetyl CoA and choline is acetylcholine, which does not play a role in dilation of coronary arteries.

6-16. The answer is e. (*Adams, pp 799, 1383. Afifi, pp 125–127, 141–143.*) Emma had a stroke resulting from occlusion of medial branches of the left vertebral artery, presumably secondary to atherosclerosis (i.e., cholesterol deposits within the artery, which eventually occlude it). The resulting syndrome is called the *medial medullary syndrome,* because the affected structures are located in the medial portion of the medulla. These structures include the pyramids, the medial lemniscus, the medial longitudinal fasciculus, and the nucleus of the hypoglossal nerve and its outflow tract. Emma's symptoms resulted from damage to the aforementioned structures and may have been caused by the same process (atherosclerosis) that resulted in her heart disease. The weakness of her right side was caused by damage to the medullary pyramid on the left side. Her face was spared because fibers supplying the face exited above the level of infarct. However, a lesion in the corticospinal tract of the cervical spinal cord above C5 could cause arm and leg weakness and spare the face, because facial fibers exit in the rostral medulla. A lesion in the inferior portion of the precentral gyrus of the left frontal lobe would cause right-sided weakness, but would include the face, because this area is represented more inferiorly than are the extremities. Her unsteady gait was a result of the weakness of her right side, but may also have been the result of the loss of position and vibration sense on that side from damage to the medial lemniscus (as demonstrated by the inability to identify the position of her toe with her eyes closed, and the inability to feel the vibrations of a tuning fork). Without position sense, walking becomes unsteady because it is necessary to feel the position of one's feet on the floor during normal gait. Damage to both the medial lemniscus and pyramids at this level causes problems on the contralateral side because this lesion is located rostral to the level where both of these fiber bundles cross to the opposite side of the brain. Damage to the descending component of the medial longitudinal fasciculus could only affect head and neck reflexes, but not gait. Gait is also unaffected by pain inputs. Deviation of the tongue occurs because fibers from the hypoglossal nucleus innervate the genioglossus muscle on the ipsilateral side of the tongue. This muscle normally protrudes the tongue toward the contralateral side. Therefore, if one side is weak, the tongue will deviate toward the side ipsilateral to the lesion when protruded. A lesion in the precentral gyrus causes protrusion of the tongue toward the side that is contralateral to the lesion because it is rostral to the crossing of fibers into the hypoglossal nucleus. Emma's speech was dysarthric (slurred) because her tongue was weak on the left side. The physician saw this during the exam when her tongue deviated to the left when protruded. Since the weakness of the tongue is purely a motor problem, rather than an effect that is manifested by a lesion to higher centers in the cortex (which mediate the structure and function of speech), the grammar, content, and meaning of Emma's speech remained intact, as would be expected with an aphasia or agnosia.

6-17. The answer is e. (*Guyton, pp 239–241, 449.*) Orthopnea or dyspnea associated with lying down is caused by redistribution of blood from the periphery to the chest, leading to an increase in pulmonary capillary pressure. Pulmonary capillary pressure is elevated in patients with heart failure. When the patient lies down, the pulmonary capillary pressure is increased, causing the orthopnea. A third heart sound is often heard in heart failure and when associated with a high heart rate produces a gallop rhythm. The third heart sound can also be heard in patients with cor pulmonale (an enlargement of the right heart) and constrictive pericarditis. Neither, however, produces orthopnea. Mitral regurgitation can produce dyspnea but is not associated with a third heart sound.

6-18. The answer is b. (*Cotran, pp 43–45. Henry, pp 195–196.*) Calcification within tissue can be classified as being dystrophic or metastatic. Dystrophic calcification is characterized by calcification in abnormal (dystrophic) tissue, while metastatic calcification is characterized by calcification in normal tissue. Examples of dystrophic calcification include calcification within severe atherosclerosis, calcification of damaged or abnormal heart valves, and calcification within tumors. Small (microscopic) laminated calcifications within tumors are called psammoma bodies and are due to single-cell necrosis. Psammoma bodies are characteristically found in papillary tumors, such as papillary carcinomas of the thyroid and papillary tumors of the ovary (especially papillary serous cystadenocarcinomas), but they can also be found in meningiomas or mesotheliomas. Dystrophic calcification within tumors of the central nervous system (CNS), which can be seen with x-rays, is useful in the differential diagnosis of these CNS tumors. For example, calcification of a tumor of the cortex in an adult is suggestive of an oligodendroglioma, while calcification of a hypothalamus tumor is suggestive of a craniopharyngioma. Additional periventricular calcification in children is most commonly caused by infection with cytomegalovirus (CMV) or toxoplasmosis. With dystrophic calcification the serum calcium levels are normal, while with metastatic calcification the serum calcium levels are elevated (hypercalcemia). Causes of hypercalcemia include certain paraneoplastic syndromes, such as secretion of parathyroid hormone–related peptide, hyperparathyroidism, iatrogenic causes (drugs), immobilization, multiple myeloma, increased milk consumption (milk-alkali syndrome), and sarcoidosis.

6-19. The answer is c. (*Brooks, pp 594–595. Levinson, p 335. Murray— 2002, pp 757–758. Ryan, pp 797–798.*) Consumption of raw fish causes endemic diphyllobothriasis in Scandinavia and the Baltic countries. While most people do not become ill, a small percentage (2%) develop vitamin B_{12} deficiency anemia. The adult fish tapeworm has an affinity for vitamin B_{12} and may induce a serious megaloblastic anemia. Parvovirus B19 causes acute hemolytic anemia primarily in immunosuppressed patients. *Yersinia* infection is common in Scandinavia but is not fish-borne and does not cause anemia. The larval stage of *T. solium* is called *cysticercus*. Humans usually acquire cysticercosis by ingestion of food and water contaminated by infected human feces.

6-20. The answer is d. (*Braunwald, pp 1382–1383.*) The goal of LDL-lowering should be less than 100 mg/dL. Risk factor modification for atherosclerotic coronary artery disease is a crucial part of management of any patient who has suffered a myocardial infarction. This patient's risk factor modification would be classified as secondary, because he already has known disease, given the fact that he has suffered an infarction. Primary prevention refers to preventing the first event. Modifiable risk factors for atherosclerosis include discontinuation of smoking, alteration of obesity, treatment of lipid disorders, treatment of hypertension, and aggressive treatment of diabetes mellitus. Unmodifiable risk factors include age, genetics (family history), and gender. Cholesterol goals for secondary prevention are straightforward. The LDL goal of any patient who has known atherosclerotic coronary disease is to lower the LDL to less than 100 mg/dL.

The total cholesterol goal is currently to lower the total cholesterol to less than 200 mg/dL. The benefit of a lower LDL has been clearly shown in multiple large outcome trials. In addition to addressing lipid levels (several therapeutic choices exist, the most effective is the statin drugs), the physician also must aggressively address smoking postmyocardial infarction, hypertension, and diabetes mellitus. Control of all these factors can substantially decrease this patient's incidence of a second myocardial infarction. Several medications have been associated with decreased risk of a second myocardial infarction; the most important two are simple aspirin therapy and beta-blockade therapy. These drugs must be included in any discussion with the patient of decreasing his risk for a second myocardial infarction.

6-21. The answer is b. (*Cotran, pp 636–637, 985–986. Rubin, pp 1104–1105.*) A fulminating septic state should always be considered whenever the constellation of fever, deteriorating mental status, skin hemorrhages, and shock develops. Such conditions can be seen in gram-negative rod septicemia caused by any of the coliforms (gram-negative endotoxic shock) or fulminant meningococcemia (Waterhouse-Friderichsen syndrome). However, a form of nonbacterial vasculitis termed thrombotic thrombocytopenic purpura (TTP) is notorious for producing a clinical syndrome very similar to fulminating infective states. TTP is characterized by arteriole and capillary occlusions by fibrin and platelet microthrombi and is usually unassociated with any of the predisposing states seen in disseminated intravascular coagulopathy (DIC), such as malignancy, infection, retained fetus, and amniotic fluid embolism. Macrocytic hemolytic anemia, variable jaundice, renal failure, skin hemorrhages, and central nervous system dysfunction are all seen in TTP and are related to the fibrin thrombi, which can be demonstrated with biopsies of skin, bone marrow, and lymph node. There is less coagulopathy in TTP than is found in DIC, and hemolytic anemia is generally not found in idiopathic or autoimmune thrombocytopenic purpura. The condition of patients with TTP may be improved by plasmapheresis, with 80% survival.

6-22. The answer is e. (*Craig, pp 444–445; Hardman, p 723; Katzung, pp 597–598.*) It has been said that the initial phase of uricosuric therapy is the most worrisome period. Probenecid is a uricosuric drug, but that effect depends on having high (therapeutic) blood levels that are sufficient to inhibit active *tubular reabsorption* of urate. At subtherapeutic blood levels the main effect is inhibition of *tubular secretion* of urate, which reduces net urate excretion and raises serum urate levels (sometimes to the point of causing clinical gout). It is only once drug levels are therapeutic that the desired effects to inhibit tubular reabsorption of urate predominate. Thus, and intuitively, once a patient starts probenecid therapy drug levels must pass through that stage in which urate excretion will actually go down.

Some texts suggest using a short course of colchicine or another (nonaspirin) NSAID that is indicated for gout when probenecid therapy is started. That is for prophylaxis of acute gout that might occur. Although that may be acceptable, other rules are perhaps more important: (1) do not administer a uricosuric during a gout attack; (2) if the patient has had a gout attack recently, suppress the inflammation for 2 to 3 months with a suitable anti-inflammatory and consider starting a uricosuric only after that 2- to 3-month symptom-free interval; and (3) do not use uricosurics for patients with "severe hyperuricemia" and/or poor renal function. Doing otherwise is associated with a great risk of potentially severe renal tubular damage as the uricosuric shifts large amounts of uric acid from the blood (with its large volume, that keeps urate relatively "dilute") into a small volume of acidic urine, which concentrates urate and lowers its solubility via pH-dependent mechanisms.

(The patient who skips doses of probenecid also becomes very vulnerable to the "paradoxical" extra risk, because doing this may allow drug levels to fall into that subtherapeutic range in which more urate is retained than eliminated.)

6-23. The answer is e. (*Moore and Dalley, pp 278–279.*) Because of an enlarged liver and the history of alcohol consumption, you suspect cirrhosis of the liver, which had resulted in portal hypertension. Because the blood is bright red, suggesting that it has not been exposed to duodenal or gastric secretions, the most likely source would be esophageal varices, as blood is trying to return from portal system to the systemic circulatory system.

6-24. The answer is c. (*Cotran, pp 788–789, 805.*) Several congenital abnormalities of the gastrointestinal tract present with specific symptoms. Infants with congenital hypertrophic pyloric stenosis present in the second or third week of life with symptoms of regurgitation and persistent severe vomiting. Physical examination reveals a firm mass in the region of the pylorus. Surgical splitting of the muscle in the stenotic region is curative. Diaphragmatic hernias, if large enough, may allow abdominal contents—including portions of the stomach, intestines, or liver—to herniate into the thoracic cavity and cause respiratory compromise. Congenital aganglionic megacolon (Hirschsprung's disease) is caused by failure of the neural crest cells to migrate all the way to the anus, resulting in a portion of distal colon that lacks ganglion cells and both Meissner's submucosal and Auerbach's myenteric plexuses. This results in a functional obstruction and dilation proximal to the affected portion of colon. Symptoms of Hirschsprung's disease include failure to pass meconium soon after birth followed by constipation and possible abdominal distention.

6-25. The answer is d. *(Brooks, pp 292–293. Levinson, pp 157–158. Murray—2002, pp 391–393. Ryan, pp 430–431.)* Leptospirosis is a zoonosis of worldwide distribution. Human infection results from ingestion of water or food contaminated with leptospirae. Rats, mice, wild rodents, dogs, swine, and cattle excrete the organisms in urine and feces during active illness and during an asymptomatic carrier state. Drinking, swimming, bathing, or food consumption may lead to human infection. Children acquire the disease from dogs more often than do adults. Treatment can include doxycycline, ampicillin, or amoxicillin. Symptoms in humans range from fever and rash to jaundice through aseptic meningitis.

6-26. The answer is e. *(Craig, pp 415–416, 780; Hardman, pp 430–431, 434–435, 1755–1756; Katzung, pp 368–372.)* Thiamine, administered parenterally with glucose, is the specific intervention for Wernicke's encephalopathy. It dramatically ameliorates the signs and symptoms as well as the underlying causes. Thiamine deficiency is also responsible for Korsakoff's psychosis, another accompaniment of severe, long-term alcohol consumption (especially without adequately nutritional diets). Unfortunately, the signs and symptoms of Korsakoff's (short-term memory problems, a tendency to fabricate, polyneuropathies) are not reversible.

6-27. The answer is a. *(Afifi, p 489. Nolte, p 323.)* Uncinate fits (hallucinations) are characterized by seizure activity involving portions of the anterior aspect of the temporal lobe. The structures most often implicated include the uncus, parahippocampal gyrus, the region of the amygdala and adjoining tissue, and the pyriform cortex. During the occurrence of uncinate fits, a person experiences olfactory hallucinations of a highly unpleasant nature.

6-28. The answer is b. (*Craig, pp 643–644; Hardman, pp 1399–1404, 1512; Katzung, pp 907–908.*) This essential technique to reduce host cell toxicity in response to MTX therapy is known as leucovorin rescue. Methotrexate, a folic acid analog/antimetabolite, can be curative for women with choriocarcinoma and is also useful for non-Hodgkin's lymphomas and acute lymphocytic leukemias in children. The drug kills responsive cancer cells by inhibiting dihyrofolate, an enzyme necessary for forming tetrahydrofolic acid (FH_4). The FH_4, in turn, is critical for eventual synthesis of DNA, RNA, and proteins. Inhibition of thymidylate synthesis is probably the single most important consequence in the overall reaction scheme.

Some cancer cells are resistant to MTX because they lack adequate mechanisms for transporting the drug intracellularly. These include some head and neck cancers and osteogenic sarcomas. In such cases we need to give very large doses of MTX to establish a high concentration gradient that essentially "drives" it into the cells. Unfortunately, normal host cells depend on folate metabolism, they take up MTX well, and they will be affected.

To protect normal cells we administer leucovorin (also called citrovorum factor or folinic acid) right after giving the MTX. It is taken up by the normal cells, bypasses the block induced by the MTX, and so spares normal cell metabolism. The leucovorin does not spare cancer cells: just as they cannot take up MTX well, they cannot take up the rescue agent and save themselves from cytotoxicity.

Leucovorin rescue is not done "automatically" in every case when MTX is given. When low MTX doses are used leucovorin may be withheld until and unless blood counts show evidence of MTX-induced bone marrow suppression. However, it is quite usually given along with MTX when MTX doses are very high (as in severe or MTX-resistant cases), and host toxicity is very probable.

The main adverse responses to MTX, regardless of the purpose for which it is given, include bone marrow suppression, pulmonary damage (infiltrates, fibrosis), stomatitis, and lesions elsewhere in the GI tract. High doses can be nephrotoxic (risk reduced by maintaining adequate hydration and alkalinizing the urine). MTX is also teratogenic.

Recall that deferoxamine is used to treat iron poisoning (it is an iron chelator). N-acetylcysteine is mainly used either as a mucolytic (mucus-thinning) drug for certain pulmonary disorders or as an antidote for acetaminophen poisoning. Penicillamine is mainly a copper chelator, used for copper poisoning or Wilson's disease. Vitamin K is used for deficiency states, for combating excessive effects of warfarin, or for managing bleeding disorders in newborns of mothers who have been taking certain drugs (e.g., anticonvulsants such as phenytoin) during pregnancy.

6-29. The answer is a. (*Cotran, pp 685, 1129. Rubin, pp 1161, 1364–1365.*) Diabetes insipidus (DI) results from a deficiency of antidiuretic hormone (ADH) and is characterized by polyuria and polydipsia, but not the polyphagia or hyperglycemia of diabetes mellitus. The hallmark of DI is a dilute urine (low urine osmolarity) with an increased serum sodium (hypernatremia). Many cases of diabetes insipidus are of unknown cause (idiopathic), but DI may be the result of hypothalamic tumors, inflammations, surgery, or radiation therapy. Multifocal Langerhans cell histiocytosis (Hand-Schüller-Christian disease) is one of the Langerhans cell histiocytoses (histiocytosis X). The disorder, which usually begins between the second and sixth years of life, is associated with the characteristic triad of bone lesions (particularly in the calvarium and the base of the skull), diabetes insipidus, and exophthalmos.

6-30. The answer is c. (*Damjanov, pp 1429–1431. Cotran, pp 520–521.*) Classic polyarteritis nodosa (PAN) is a systemic disease characterized by necrotizing inflammation of small or medium-sized muscular arteries, typically involving the visceral vessels but sparing the small blood vessels of the lungs and kidneys. Histologically, there is intense localized acute inflammation and necrosis of vessel walls with fibrinoid necrosis and often thrombosis of the vessel with ischemic infarcts of the affected organ. Healed lesions display fibrosis in the walls of affected blood vessels with focal aneurysmal dilations. Clinically, PAN is a protracted, recurring disease that affects young adults. It is a multisystem disease affecting many organs of the body, and this makes it difficult to diagnose unless the vasculitis is recognized by biopsy. Symptoms include fever, weight loss, malaise, abdominal pain, headache, and myalgia. Skin involvement results in palpable purpura. The etiology is not known, but 30% of patients with classic PAN have circulating hepatitis B antigen in their serum.

6-31. The answer is b. *(Moore and Dalley, pp 546, 561.)* Perforating branches of the deep femoral artery are the principal blood supply to the posterior thigh. The other arteries supply anterior, medial, and gluteal regions of the thigh.

6-32. The answer is b. *(Kandel, p 988.)* In this syndrome, produced experimentally in monkeys and also seen in cats, there is an extreme change in the personality of the animal. Its responses to emotion-laden stimuli are much reduced. It appears very tame. Aggressive tendencies are not evident. It also manifests oral tendencies and displays hypersexuality. This syndrome is the result of lesions of the temporal lobe in which parts of the amygdala are involved. Lesions of other regions such as the hypothalamus, cingulate cortex, or septal area do not produce the Klüver-Bucy syndrome.

6-33. The answer is c. *(Boron, p 948.)* Gluten-sensitivity enteropathy is characterized by an autoimmune-induced decrease in the absorptive surface area of the small intestine. In addition to a decrease in the area available for absorption of nutrients, minerals, electrolytes and water, the membrane transporters of the remaining villous tip cells are impaired or absent.

6-34. The answer is b. *(Craig, p 401; Hardman, p 420; Katzung, p 469.)* We are describing some of the symptoms and signs of Tourette's syndrome. It is effectively treated with haloperidol, a high-potency antipsychotic. If patients are unresponsive or do not tolerate haloperidol, they might be switched to pimozide.

6-35. The answer is b. *(Henry, pp 264–266. Cotran, pp 848–851.)* Jaundice is caused by increased blood levels of bilirubin, which result from abnormalities in bilirubin metabolism. Bilirubin, the end product of heme breakdown, is taken up by the liver, where it is conjugated with glucuronic acid by the enzyme bilirubin UDP-glucuronosyl transferase (UGT) and then secreted into the bile. Unconjugated bilirubin is not soluble in an aqueous solution, is complexed to albumin, and cannot be excreted in the urine. Unconjugated hyperbilirubinemia may result from excessive production of bilirubin, which occurs in hemolytic anemias. It can also result from reduced hepatic uptake of bilirubin, as occurs in Gilbert's syndrome, a mild disease associated with a subclinical hyperbilirubinemia. Unconjugated hyperbilirubinemia may result from impaired conjugation of bilirubin. Examples of diseases resulting from impaired conjugation include physiologic jaundice of the newborn and Crigler-Najjar syndrome, which result from either decreased UGT activity (type II) or absent UGT activity (type I). Individuals with type II Crigler-Najjar syndrome may not need any therapy, or their condition may be managed with phenobarbital, which is metabolized in the smooth endoplasmic reticulum in hepatocytes. Therapy with this drug causes hyperplasia of the smooth endoplasmic reticulum in hepatocytes and indirectly increases the levels of bilirubin-UDP-glucuronyl transferase.

In contrast to unconjugated bilirubin, conjugated bilirubin is water-soluble, nontoxic, and readily excreted in the urine. Conjugated hyperbilirubinemia may result from either decreased hepatic excretion of conjugates of bilirubin, such as in Dubin-Johnson syndrome, or impaired extrahepatic bile excretion, as occurs with extrahepatic biliary obstruction. Finally aspartate aminotransferase and gamma-glutamyl transpeptidase are both liver enzymes; galactosylceramide beta-galactosidase is deficient with Krabbe disease, while *L*-iduronosulfate sulfatase is deficient with Hunter's syndrome.

6-36. The answer is c. (*Afifi, pp 481–484. Nolte, pp 326–342.*) Since the auditory relay system is a highly complex pathway in which auditory signals are bilaterally represented at all levels beyond the receptor level, lesions at these levels would not produce a solely unilateral deafness. Such a loss could only result when the lesion involves either the receptor or the first-order neurons of the nerve (i.e., cranial nerve VIII itself). The medial lemniscus is not related to the auditory system.

6-37. The answer is c. (*Braunwald, p 1388.*) This 72-year-old female experienced significant chest pain of approximately 8 hours' duration and her EKG shows an acute antero-septal myocardial injury. The myoglobin level will definitely be elevated after 8 h of significant chest pain and all the cardiac enzymes, including the MB isoenzyme and troponin, will be elevated at 8 h as well. Cardiac isoenzymes assist in making the diagnosis of an acute myocardial infarction. The creatine phosphokinase level usually rises within 4 to 8 h and the troponin level usually rises slightly earlier. The earliest enzyme to rise is the myoglobin level, although several other causes of elevated myoglobin exist. The patient's EKG may or may not show development of Q waves, providing she is aggressively treated with reestablishment of perfusion. The MB isoenzyme of creatine phosphokinase is significantly more specific to cardiac muscle and elevates at approximately the same time as the creatine phosphokinase.

6-38. The answer is a. (*Boron, pp 50–53, 80–81. Guyton, pp 272–273.*) When water is ingested from the intestine, it enters the plasma and rapidly achieves osmotic equilibrium with the interstitial and intracellular compartments. A sodium concentration of 125 mM is equivalent to an osmolarity of 250 milliosmoles/L. Assuming that her normal osmolarity of 285 millimoles/L was reduced to 250 milliosmoles by the ingestion of water, she drank approximately 5 L. The amount of water ingested by the patient was not likely this high because she probably lost significant amount of salt as sweat while under the influence of ecstasy. Her signs and symptoms are due to the brain swelling caused by hypotonicity.

$$\text{Osmolarity} = \frac{\text{Milliosmoles}}{\text{Volume}}$$

$$250 \text{ milliosmoles/L} = \frac{60 \text{ kg} \times 60\% \times 284}{\text{Volume}}$$

$$\text{Total Volume} = \frac{10{,}224 \text{ milliosmoles}}{250 \text{ milliosmoles/L}} \approx 41 \text{ L}$$

$$\text{Volume Consumed} = \text{Total Volume} - \text{Original volume}$$

$$\text{Volume Consumed} = 41 \text{ L} - 36 \text{ L} = 5 \text{ L}$$

6-39. The answer is b. (*Brooks, pp 192–193. Levinson, p 114. Murray—2002, pp 245–247. Ryan, pp 302–305.*) Except during a meningococcal epidemic, *H. influenzae* is the most common cause of bacterial meningitis in children. The organism is occasionally found to be associated with respiratory tract infections or otitis media. *H. influenzae, N. meningitidis, S. pneumoniae,* and *Listeria* account for 80 to 90% of all cases of bacterial meningitis. A purified polysaccharide vaccine conjugated to protein for

H. *influenzae* type B is available. A tetravalent vaccine is available for N. *meningitidis* and a 23-serotype vaccine for *S. pneumoniae*. No vaccine is available for *Listeria*.

6-40. The answer is c. (*Cotran, pp 284–286.*) There are several mechanisms through which proto-oncogenes (p-oncs) can become oncogenic (c-oncs). Normal cellular genes (proto-oncogenes) may become oncogenic by being incorporated into the viral genome (forming v-oncs), or they may be activated by other processes to form cellular oncogenes (c-oncs). These other processes include gene mutations, chromosomal translocations, and gene amplifications. Gene mutations, such as point mutations, are associated with the formation of cancers by mutant c-*ras* oncogenes. Chromosomal translocations are associated with the development of many types of cancers, one example of which is Burkitt's lymphoma. The most common translocation associated with Burkitt's lymphoma is t(8;14), in which the c-*myc* oncogene on chromosome 8 is brought in contact with the immunoglobulin heavy-chain gene on chromosome 14. Two other examples of chromosomal translocations are the association of chronic myelocytic leukemia (CML) with t(9;22), which is the Philadelphia chromosome, and the association of follicular lymphoma with the translocation t(18;14). The former involves the proto-oncogene c-*abl*, which is rearranged in proximity to a break point cluster region (bcr) on chromosome 22. The resultant chimeric c-*abl/bcr* gene encodes a protein with tyrosine kinase activity. The t(18;14) translocation involves the *bcl-2* oncogene on chromosome 18. Expression of the oncogene *bcl-2* is associated with the prevention of apoptosis in germinal centers. Examples of associations that involve gene amplification include N-*myc* and neuroblastoma, c-*neu* and breast cancer, and *erb*-B and breast and ovarian cancer. Gene amplifications can be demonstrated by finding doublet minutes or homogenous staining regions.

6-41. The answer is c. (*Craig, p 768; Hardman, pp 1691–1692; Katzung, p 703.*) Serum glucose reacts nonenzymatically with hemoglobin to form glycated hemoglobin products (e.g., Hb A_{1C}). The rate of Hb A_{1C} formation is related to ambient glucose levels, and the amount of Hb A_{1C} measured in any given blood sample reflects the average blood glucose levels over the last 2 to 3 months. Thus, although the patient's serum glucose levels may be acceptable after a couple of days' fast, Hb A_{1C} measurements give the big picture about how good glycemic control was on a more long-term (and more important) timeline. Note that although measuring HbA_{1C} gives important information about the long-term, it does not provide any information about day-to-day fluctuations in glucose levels or what's happening "right now", and such information is important to optimal control of diabetes and its symptoms. Nonetheless, regular, periodic checks of Hb A_{1C} should be part of the monitoring for every patient with diabetes (type 1 or 2), not so much as a way to assess for noncompliance as to make sure that the current treatment plan with which the patient is complying is working. It is a common and relatively inexpensive assay.

Having the clinical lab measure glucose in a venous blood sample won't give any additional or meaningful information: hand-held glucometers, used properly, are remarkably accurate. Glucose tolerance tests, even those done with oral glucose, will provide little historic information, and they are expensive. Few clinical labs are set up to measure serum concentrations of most oral antidiabetic drugs, and the cost for these nonstandard tests would be quite expensive. Measuring urine ketone levels are of no benefit for our purposes. All that they might prove is that our patient has fasted for several days. Urine glucose monitoring is not very enlightening either. Recall that glucose appears in the urine only when serum concentrations exceed a renal threshold for reabsorption (around 180 mg/dL or so). A glucose-free urine sample, then, would only indicate that serum glucose levels are below the threshold: they still could be unacceptably high, or normal, or low, and you would never know just by urine testing.

6-42. The answer is b. (*Braunwald, pp 2171–2175. Sadler, pp 13–14, 353. Moore and Persaud, Developing, p 165.*) Cells from a patient with the most common form of Klinefelter's syndrome (47,XXY genotype) will have one inactive X chromosome and, therefore, one Barr body. The formula is the number of Barr bodies equals the number of X chromosomes minus one. Klinefelter's syndrome occurs at a ratio of about 1:500 males and is due to meiotic nondisjunction of the chromosomes. The nondisjunction is more frequent in oogenesis than in spermatogenesis, and increased occurrence is directly proportional to increasing maternal age. Klinefelter's may occur as 47,XXY, 48,XXYY, 48,XXXY, and 49,XXXXY. A combination of abnormal and normal genotype occurs in mosaic individuals who generally have less severe symptoms. Females have two X chromosomes, one of maternal and the other of paternal origin. Only one of the X chromosomes is active in the somatic, diploid cells of the female; the other X chromosome remains inactive and is visible in appropriately stained interphase cells as a mass of heterochromatin. Detection of the Barr body (sex chromatin) has been an efficient method for the determination of chromosomal sex and abnormalities of X-chromosome number; however, it is not definitive proof of maleness or femaleness. The genotypic sex of Klinefelter's syndrome and XXX individuals would be male and female as determined by the presence or absence of the testis-determining Y chromosome. In Turner's syndrome (XO), no Barr bodies would be present. In comparison, "superfemales" (XXX) would possess two inactive X chromosomes (2 Barr bodies) and one active X chromosome. Buccal scrapings for Barr body analysis are being used less—chromosomal analysis is becoming the standard test now.

6-43. The answer is e. (*Cotran, pp 1333–1334. Rubin, pp 1502–1504.*) The degenerative diseases of the CNS are diseases that affect the gray matter and are characterized by the progressive loss of neurons in specific areas of the brain. In Parkinson's disease, characterized by a masklike facial expression, coarse tremors, slowness of voluntary movements, and muscular rigidity, there is degeneration and loss of pigmented cells in the substantia nigra, resulting in a decrease in dopamine synthesis. Lewy bodies (eosinophilic intracytoplasmic inclusions) are found in the remaining neurons of the substantia nigra. The decreased synthesis of dopamine by neurons originating in the substantia nigra leads to decreased amounts and functioning of dopamine in the striatum. This results in decreased dopamine inhibition and a relative increase in acetylcholine function, which is excitatory in the striatum. The effect of this excitation, however, is to increase the functioning of GABA neurons, which are inhibitory. The result, therefore, is increased inhibition or decreased movement. The severity of the motor syndrome correlates with the degree of dopamine deficiency. Therapy may be with dopamine agonists or anticholinergics.

6-44. The answer is a. (*Scriver, pp 3–45. Sack, pp 57–76.*) A missing band suggests an interstitial (internal) deletion rather than removal of the distal short or long arm (known as a terminal deletion). The shorthand notation 15q− implies a terminal deletion of the long arm of chromosome 15. Pericentric (surrounding the centromere) or paracentric (not including the centromere) inversions result from crossover of a chromosome with itself and then breakage and reunion to produce an internal inverted segment. Interstitial deletion 15q11q13 is seen in approximately 50% of patients with Prader-Willi and Angelman's syndromes. Other patients with these syndromes inherit both chromosomes 15 from their mother (Prader-Willi) or both from their father (Angelman's), a situation known as uniparental disomy. Genomic imprinting of the 15q11q13 region is different on the chromosome inherited from the mother than on the chromosome inherited from the father. The normal balance of maternal and paternal imprints is thus disrupted by deletion or uniparental disomy, leading to reciprocal differences in gene expression that present as Angelman's or Prader-Willi syndromes.

6-45. The answer is e. *(Craig, p 517; Hardman, pp 1161, 1176; Katzung, p 775.)* Sulfonamides cross the placenta and enter the fetus in concentrations sufficient to produce toxic effects. They compete with and displace bilirubin from plasma protein binding sites, raising free bilirubin levels and causing the jaundice and other manifestations of kernicterus. For the same reason, sulfonamides should also not be given to neonates, especially premature infants. This woman should not have been given the sulfonamide, whether alone or in combination with trimethoprim.

6-46. The answer is b. *(Braunwald, pp 2452–2457. Cotran, 1326–1327. Kierszenbaum, pp 210–212. Junqueira, p 171.)* The patient is suffering from multiple sclerosis (MS), a demyelinating disease in which both CD4+ and CD8+ T cells as well as autoantibodies are targeted to oligodendrocytes. MS is twice as prevalent in women as in men and demyelination is most commonly found in the anterior corpus callosum. Alterations in the CSF shows pleocytosis (increase in the number of mononuclear cells above normal levels), increase in protein, and elevated gamma globulin (antibodies to oligodendrocytes as represented by oligoclonal bands on gel electrophoresis). Microglia (answer a) are the phagocytes of the CNS, astrocytes (answer c) induce and maintain the blood-brain barrier and form the glial scar following injury, and Schwann cells (answer d) are responsible for myelination in the PNS. On autopsy, plaques are found that contain lymphocytes and monocytes in infiltrates around small veins in what is known as *perivascular cuffing*. Axons (answer e) are generally preserved. The main identifying feature on histopathological examination is the paucity of oligodendrocytes. Astrocytic proliferation and gliosis may increase with the duration of MS.

6-47. The answer is b. (*Cotran, pp 567–568. McPhee, pp 281–283.*) Aortic stenosis (AS) is usually the result of a bicuspid aortic valve (AV), degenerative calcification of a bicuspid valve, or rheumatic heart disease. Patients with aortic stenosis may present with angina (chest pain), syncopal episodes with exertion, and heart failure. Angina results from the mismatch between increased oxygen demand of the hypertrophied left ventricle (LV) and decreased blood flow, while syncope results from the inability to increase stroke volume as necessary with a stenotic AV. AS is the most common valvular disease that is associated with angina and syncope. The characteristic heart murmur of AS is a crescendo-decrescendo midsystolic ejection murmur that has a paradoxically split S_2. In order to pump the blood into the aorta across a stenotic AV, the pressure in the LV must be much greater than the resultant pressure in the aorta. In order to produce this increased pressure, the LV undergoes concentric hypertrophy, which increases contractility. This concentric hypertrophy also makes the wall of the LV stiffer (decreased compliance). This stiff LV is unable to dilate until the time the LV starts to fail.

6-48. The answer is d. (*Braunwald, p 1627.*) Chronic obstructive uropathy commonly results in polyuria and nocturia due to impaired urinary concentrating ability. A distal renal tubular acidosis may result with accompanying hyperkalemia (Type IV RTA). Because the process develops gradually, frequency and urgency and a sense of incomplete emptying are the main complaints, but pain is uncommon. With an elevated serum creatinine, some degree of hydronephrosis would be found on ultrasound.

6-49. The answer is d. (*Boron, pp 79–81. Guyton, pp 269–273.*) Drinking water after losing a significant volume of water as sweat decreases the osmolarity of the extracellular fluid. The decrease occurs because the salt lost from the extracellular fluid in sweat is not replaced by the ingested water. When the extracellular osmolarity is decreased, water flows from the extracellular to the intracellular body compartment, causing intracellular volume to increase. The patient's symptoms are caused by swelling of the brain.

6-50. The answer is b. (*Parslow, pp 76–77. Levinson, pp 360–361.*) Haptens (incomplete antigens) are not themselves antigenic, but when coupled to a cell or carrier protein become antigenic and induce antibodies that can bind the hapten alone (in the absence of the carrier protein). They are small molecules that are generally less than 1000 Da. While haptens react with antibodies, they are not immunogenic because they do not activate T cells and cannot bind the major histocompatibility complex (MHC). Haptens are significant in disease; penicillin is a hapten and can cause severe life-threatening allergic reaction by destruction of erythrocytes. Catechols in the oils of poison ivy plants are haptens and cause a significant skin inflammatory response. Chloramphenicol is a hapten that can lead to the destruction of leukocytes and cause agranulocytosis. Sedormid is a hapten that can cause thrombocytopenia and purpura (bleeding) through the destruction of platelets.

BLOCK 7

Answers

7-1. The answer is d. (*Braunwald, p 1591.*) All of these diseases are common in older persons. Amyloidosis and light-chain deposition disease are related to paraprotein deposition in the kidney and typically present with nephrotic syndrome. The subacute presentation and erythrocyte casts in the urine along with the rapid decline in renal function are most consistent with vasculitis. A positive antineutrophil cytoplasmic antibody (ANCA) would be supportive. Erythrocyte casts are not seen in the other diseases.

7-2. The answer is b. (*Boron, p 733. Guyton, pp 689–691.*) In a normal sleep cycle, a person passes through the four stages of slow-wave sleep before entering REM sleep. In narcolepsy, a person may pass directly from the waking state to REM sleep. REM sleep is characterized by irregular heart beats and respiration and by periods of atonia (loss of muscle tone). Hypoventilation is characteristic of both REM and non-REM sleep because sleep depresses the central chemoreceptors. Brain activity during REM sleep is higher than during wakefulness so there is an increase in brain metabolism. It is also the state of sleep in which dreaming occurs.

7-3. The answer is a. (*Murray, pp 163–170, 613–619. Scriver, pp 4517–4554. Sack, pp 121–138.*) One of the world's most common enzyme deficiencies is glucose-6-phosphate-dehydrogenase deficiency (305900). This deficiency in erythrocytes is particularly prevalent among African and Mediterranean males. A deficiency in glucose-6-phosphate dehydrogenase blocks the pentose phosphate pathway and NADPH production. Without NADPH to maintain glutathione in its reduced form, erythrocytes have no protection from oxidizing agents. This X-linked recessive deficiency is often diagnosed when patients develop hemolytic anemia after receiving oxidizing drugs such as pamaquine or after eating oxidizing substances such as fava beans.

7-4. The answer is b. (*Craig, pp 342, 344; Hardman, pp 188, 312–316; Katzung, pp 410–411.*) Although a rare occurrence, halothane and other inhaled volatile liquid anesthetics may cause malignant hyperthermia, the signs and symptoms of which we have described in the question. Apparently, this occurs mainly in genetically susceptible individuals (whether a personal or familial history, as the predisposition seems to be heritable). The prevalence of the reaction is increased by concomitant use of succinylcholine.

7-5. The answer is d. (*Adams, pp 802–805. Afifi, pp 163–168, 180–182.*) This is an example of the *locked-in syndrome*, or pseudocoma, caused by an infarction of the basilar pons. Because the tracts mediating movement of the limbs and face run through this region, the patient is unable to move the face, as well as both arms and legs. Consciousness and eye movements are preserved. The pontine basilar pons is supplied mainly by the basilar artery. Complete occlusion of this artery causes deficits on both sides, since this artery supplies both sides of the pons. Basilar artery occlusion causes damage to the basilar pons, where the corticospinal and corticobulbar tracts run. These tracts contain motor fibers mediating movement of the limb and face, respectively. This results in complete paralysis to both sides of the body and the face. None of the tracts in the other choices mediate conscious movement. Sensory loss, including loss of proprioception (feeling the movement of a limb), also occurs as a result of damage to the medial lemniscus bilaterally. This tract contains fibers from the dorsal columns and also runs through the pontine tegmentum. Patients with the locked-in syndrome are often mistaken for comatose patients due to their inability to move or speak. If the lesion spares the reticular formation, an area mediating consciousness in the pons, the patient will remain alert.

7-6. The answer is e. (*Cotran, pp 919–920. Henry, pp 215–218.*) Major factors involved in the pathogenesis of type 2 diabetes mellitus include beta cell dysfunction, peripheral insulin resistance, and excessive hepatic glucose production. Beta cell dysfunction, which causes impaired insulin secretion, may result from glucotoxicity (prolonged increased serum glucose inhibits beta cells) and lipotoxicity (prolonged increased serum free fatty acids also inhibit beta cells). Peripheral insulin resistance is associated with obesity and abnormalities of the peroxisome proliferator-activator receptor (PPAR). More than 80% of type 2 DM individuals are overweight, which can produce peripheral insulin resistance as obesity is associated with downregulation of insulin receptors. Gamma-PPAR, which is found in adipose tissue, is important for adipocyte differentiation. One theory about a possible cause of insulin resistance is the "thrifty" gene hypothesis, which involves abnormal functioning of gamma-PPAR. This hypothesis is somewhat based on humans ability to gain weight quickly ("thrifty") when food is abundant between times of famine. With too much food available, however, fat gets deposited in wrong places, such as the liver, muscle, and islet cells of the pancreas, which in turn can modulate gamma-PPAR and lead to insulin resistance. Finally recall that antibodies to beta cells of the pancreas are seen with type 1 DM, antibodies to insulin may develop in these same individuals, while excess production of cortisol is seen with Cushing's syndrome, which is a cause of secondary DM.

7-7. The answer is e. (*Braunwald, p 1760.*) Hematemesis or vomiting of bright red blood represents an upper gastrointestinal (GI) source of blood loss, in this case from esophageal varices, a common complication of chronic alcoholism. Bleeding from the colon will be manifested either by no change in the color of the stools or by black, tarry-like stools (melena). Pulmonary embolism can cause bleeding from the lungs with blood in the sputum (hemoptysis). Hematemesis is not found in the other three diseases.

7-8. The answer is d. (*Levinson, pp 61, 91, 94, 107–108, 140–141. Ryan, pp 198, 220–221, 269–270, 305–307, 484–488.*) The patient is infected with *Yersinia pestis* and has bubonic plague. Ceftriaxone or cefotaxime are preferred in the treatment of childhood meningitis because they have the highest activity against the three major causes, namely *Haemophilus influenzae*, *N. meningitidis*, and *S. pneumoniae*.

7-9. The answer is a. (*Cotran, pp 651–655, 659–661. Rubin, pp 1131–1132. Hoffman, pp 1218–1225, 1293–1294.*) In general, the non-Hodgkin's lymphomas (NHLs) can be divided histologically into nodular forms and diffuse forms. All nodular NHLs, one of which is seen in the picture associated with this question, are the result of neoplastic proliferations of B lymphocytes. Histologically these nodules somewhat resemble the germinal centers of lymphoid follicles, but instead they are characterized by increased numbers (crowding) of nodules, their location in both the cortex and the medulla, their uniform size, and their composition (a monotonous proliferation of cells).

In contrast to the nodular NHLs, the diffuse NHLs may be derived from either B or T lymphocytes. Two types of NHL that are always diffuse in appearance are small lymphocytic NHL (SLL) and lymphoblastic lymphomas. Finally, one type of Hodgkin's disease (HD) is characterized histologically by the formation of nodules, and that is nodular sclerosis HD (not lymphocyte predominate HD, which has a diffuse pattern). In contrast to nodular NHL, however, the malignant cell in HD is the Reed-Sternberg cell.

7-10. The answer is a. (*Murray, pp 374–395. Scriver, pp 3–45. Sack, pp 245–257.*) Imbalance of globin chain synthesis occurs in the thalassemias. Deficiency of α-globin chains (α-thalassemia) is common in Asian populations and may be associated with abnormal hemoglobins composed of four β-globin chains (hemoglobin H) or (in fetuses and newborns) of four γ-globin chains (hemoglobin Bart's). Mutation in a transcription factor necessary for expression of α-globin could ablate α-globin expression, since the same factor could act in *trans* on all four copies of the α-globin genes (two α-globin loci). Mutation of a regulatory sequence element that acts in *cis* would inactivate only one α-globin gene, leaving others to produce α-globin in reduced amounts (mild α thalassemia). Deletions of one α-globin would produce a similar mild phenotype, and deficiencies of transcription factors regulating α- and β-globin genes would not produce chain imbalance.

7-11. The answer is c. (*Kandel, pp 758–765.*) A CT scan of Helen's head was done in the emergency room, which showed a new infarct or stroke in the genu and anterior portion of the posterior limb of the left internal capsule. This is the region of the internal capsule through which most of the fibers of the corticospinal and corticobulbar tracts pass in a somatotopically organized fashion before entering the brainstem. Because most of these fibers pass through a very small region, a small infarct can cause deficits in a wide distribution of areas. In this case, Helen had weakness in her face and tongue, causing her slurred speech, in addition to weakness of her arm and leg. In addition, since somatosensory fibers destined for the postcentral gyrus occupy a position in the internal capsule caudal to the corticospinal tract fibers, these fibers were spared and Helen had no sensory deficits. The only other area in the CNS that can cause a pure motor hemiparesis is the basilar pons, an area through which corticospinal and corticobulbar fibers also run. The vascular supply of this region consists of perforators from the basilar artery, which are small and subject to atherosclerotic disease.

7-12. The answer is b. (*Cotran, p 1350–1351. Rubin, pp 1519–1520.*) A tumor that is attached to the dura is most likely to be a meningioma. This type of tumor arises from the arachnoid villi of the brain or spinal cord. Although they usually occur during middle or later life, a small number occur in persons 20 to 40 years of age. They commonly arise along the venous sinuses (parasagittal, sphenoid wings, and olfactory groove). Although meningiomas are benign and usually slow-growing, some have progesterone receptors and rapid growth in pregnancy occurs occasionally. The rare malignant meningioma may invade or even metastasize. The typical case, however, does not invade the brain, but displaces it, causing headaches and seizures. Histologically, many different patterns can be seen, but psammoma bodies and a whorled pattern of tumor cells are somewhat characteristic. In contrast to this histologic appearance, Antoni A areas with Verocay bodies are seen in schwannomas, endothelial proliferation and serpentine areas of necrosis are seen in glioblastoma multiformes, a "fried-egg" appearance of tumor cells is characteristic of oligodendrogliomas, and true rosettes and pseudorosettes can be seen in medulloblastomas.

7-13. The answer is b. (*Brooks, pp 375–376. Levinson, pp 221–224. Murray—2002, pp 479–481. Ryan pp 559–561.*) Human papillomaviruses (HPV) are the causative agents of cutaneous warts as well as proliferative squamous lesions of mucosal surfaces. Although most infections by human papillomavirus are benign, some undergo malignant transformation into in situ and invasive squamous cell carcinoma. Both HPV and polyomavirus have icosahedral capsids and DNA genomes. JC virus, a polyomavirus, was first isolated from the diseased brain of a patient with Hodgkin's lymphoma who was dying of progressive multifocal leukoencephalopathy (PML). This demyelinating disease occurs usually in immunosuppressed persons and is the result of oligodendrocyte infection by JC virus. JC virus has also been isolated from the urine of patients suffering from demyelinating disease. Cryotherapy and laser treatment are the most popular therapies for warts, although surgery may be indicated in some cases. At the present time, there is no effective antiviral therapy for treatment of infection with polyomavirus or HPV. West Nile virus (WNV) is an arbovirus. Although prevalent in Europe, Africa, and the Middle East, it was not seen in the United States until the summer of 1999. It is transmitted by mosquitoes and birds, especially crows; these animals are a reservoir. WNV causes a rather mild encephalitis in humans, the exception being older patients or those who may be immunocompromised.

Primary HSV-1 infections are usually asymptomatic. Symptomatic disease occurs most frequently in small children (one to five years old). Buccal and gingival mucosa are most often involved, and lesions, if untreated, may last two to three weeks. Acyclovir treatment is effective therapy and should be started immediately. The classic location of latent HSV-1 infection is the trigeminal ganglia. Reactivation results in sporadic vesicular lesions and may also be treated with acyclovir. B cell activation would be unusual, and there appears to be no greater risk for cancer development than that seen in the general population.

7-14. The answer is d. *(Baum, pp 219–220.)* Uncontrollable bouts of pain are most apt to be the patient's major source of stress. She probably feels that she could cope with her slowly developing disability and loss of self-esteem if she could have relief from or control over the bouts of pain. She may know that about 60% of patients with rheumatoid arthritis become progressively disabled and that there is no cure for the disease. Pain is more severe among patients who are anxious or depressed. She must somehow learn to cope with the pain, swelling, and fatigue.

Staying busy tends to be an effective way of distracting attention from the pain. Concern for her future could also be very much on her mind as she sees and feels the chronic, progressive, and debilitating aspect of her disease and becomes increasingly concerned for her future welfare, care, and loss of independence. Some behavioral and cognitive behavioral approaches could be effective in reducing the patient's pain and distress, along with stress management and coping skill instruction.

7-15. The answer is e. *(Sadler, 90, 187, 378, 463. Moore and Persaud, Developing, pp 171, 172, 178, 439.)* Vitamin A is a member of the retinoic acid family. Retinoic acid directs the polarity of development in the central nervous system, the axial skeleton (vertebral column), and probably the appendicular skeleton as well. Retinoic acid turns on various combinations of homeobox genes, depending on the tissue type and location (distance and direction from the source of retinoic acid). Exogenous sources of retinoic acid may induce the wrong sequence or combination of homeobox genes, leading to structural abnormalities in the nervous and skeletal systems. The other organ systems listed are not as susceptible to vitamin A (answers a, b, c, and d).

7-16. The answer is b. (*Craig, pp 292t, 297; Hardman, pp 326–327; Katzung, pp 411–412, 415–416.*) The scenario describes most of the classic responses to ketamine, a "dissociative anesthetic": analgesia; an ostensibly light sleep-like state; a trance-like and cataplectic state (including increased muscle tone); and activation of most cardiovascular parameters (in patients with normal cardiovascular status to begin with). The various psychosis-like emergence reactions are the main disadvantages to using a drug that, otherwise, causes many of the desired elements of complete anesthesia, usually without the need for complicated and expensive anesthesia administration devices or personnel. Ketamine undergoes significant metabolism in humans, with about 20% of the absorbed dose recovered as metabolites. Halothane can cause postoperative jaundice and hepatic necrosis with repeated administration in rare instances.

7-17. The answer is d. (*Craig, pp 235–236; Hardman, pp 787–788; Katzung, p 166.*) A Coombs-positive finding is, among all the antihypertensives, uniquely associated with methyldopa. It occurs in up to about 20% of patients taking this drug long term. Although rare, it may progress to hemolytic anemia. The cause is formation of a hapten on erythrocyte membranes, which induces an immune reaction (IgG antibodies) directed against and potentially lysing the red cell membrane. Many drugs can cause an immunohemolytic anemia. Other drugs with similar actions, and the potential to cause an immunohemolytic anemia, are penicillins, quinidine, procainamide, and sulfonamides.

7-18. The answer is b. (*Moore and Dalley, p 366.*) Bulges in the anterior wall of the vagina are most likely due to the bladder falling posteriorly into the anterior vaginal wall. A bulge on the posterior wall of the vagina would most likely be a rectocele. Cervical cancer generally would not present as described. A didelphic uterus is a duplication of the uterus as result of failure of the right and left paramesonephric duct to fuse in the midline. An indirect inguinal hernia would generally present as a mass within the labia major.

7-19. The answer is d. (*Cotran, pp 1173–1177. Rubin, pp 1277–1280.*) Melanocytic hyperplasia, which causes hyperpigmentation of the skin, can be classified into several types of lesions. A lentigo consists of melanocytic hyperplasia in the basal layers of the epidermis along with elongation and thinning of the rete ridges. Two types of lentigines are lentigo simplex and lentigo senilis ("liver spots"). Increased numbers of melanocytes may form clusters located at the tips of the rete ridges in the epidermis (junctional nevus), within the dermis (intradermal nevus), or both at the tips of the rete ridges and within the dermis (compound nevus). A blue nevus is composed of highly dendritic melanocytes that penetrate more deeply into the dermis. This deep location gives the lesion its characteristic blue color. The Spitz tumor (epithelioid cell nevus) is a benign lesion composed of groups of epithelioid and spindle melanocytes and is found in children and young adults. It may be mistaken histologically for a malignant melanoma. A freckle (ephelis) is a pigmented lesion caused by increased melanin pigmentation within keratinocytes of the basal layer of the epidermis. There is no increase in the number of melanocytes. These lesions fade with lack of sun exposure.

7-20. The answer is b. (*Cotran, pp 180–181. Rubin, pp 227, 234.*) Several genetic diseases are characterized by a deletion of part of an autosomal chromosome. The 5p⁻ syndrome is also called the cri-du-chat syndrome, as affected infants characteristically have a high-pitched cry similar to that of a kitten. Additional findings in this disorder include severe mental retardation, microcephaly, and congenital heart disease. 4p⁻, also called Wolf-Hirschhorn syndrome, is characterized by pre- and postnatal growth retardation and severe hypotonia. Affected infants have many defects including micrognathia and a prominent forehead. The 11p⁻ syndrome is characterized by the congenital absence of the iris (aniridia) and is often accompanied by Wilms' tumor of the kidney. The 13q⁻ syndrome is associated with the loss of the Rb suppressor gene and the development of retinoblastoma. Deletions involving chromosome 15 (15q⁻) may result in either Prader-Willi syndrome or Angelman's syndrome depending on whether the defect involves the paternal or the maternal chromosome (genetic imprinting). 17p⁻, also known as Smith-Margens syndrome, is associated with self-destructive behavior.

7-21. The answer is c. *(Boron, pp 410–411, 641.)* Reducing alveolar ventilation will decrease the pH toward a normal value. However, in this circumstance, it is an inappropriate therapy because the high pH is keeping most of the aspirin in an ionized form in which it cannot easily cross the blood-brain barrier. When the patient was placed on a ventilator, to prevent muscle fatigue, the hyperventilation was not sustained, the aspirin crossed the blood brain barrier, and the situation became far worse.

7-22. The answer is d. *(Moore and Dalley, pp 100–103, 162–163.)* The lobe indicated by the asterisk is the left upper (or superior) lobe. The general orientation when viewing CTs is that the observer is looking up from the patient's feet. Therefore, the patient's left is on your right. In addition, on the left, the inferior (lower) lobe begins relatively high in the thoracic cavity and is posterior to the upper lobe.

7-23. The answer is e. *(Craig, pp 155–156; Katzung, pp 209–211.)* Vasodilator therapy for CHF has gained prominence in the past 10 years. The ACE inhibitors, such as enalapril, are among the best agents for this purpose, although Ca channel inhibitors and nitroglycerin can also be used. The ACE inhibitors dilate arterioles and veins (reducing preload), as well as inhibit aldosterone production (reducing blood volume), factors considered beneficial in CHF therapy. Both β-adrenergic antagonists and ACE inhibitors have been shown to increase survival in CHF.

7-24. The answer is d. *(Ryan, pp 561–562. Brooks, pp 376–377. Murray—2002, pp 482–483.)* HSV meningitis or encephalitis is difficult to diagnose by laboratory tests, as there is a low titer of virus present in the cerebrospinal fluid. Neonatal HSV infects the child during the birth process. While culture, Tzanck smear, and even antibody tests may be useful in adults, particularly those with HSV-rich lesions, they are not useful for CSF testing. Only PCR is sensitive enough to detect HSV DNA in the CSF. Once diagnosed rapidly, HSV encephalitis or meningitis can be treated with acyclovir.

7-25. The answer is b. *(Sierles, pp 76–80. Wedding, pp 274–275.)* Contingency management is the technical term often used for positive reinforcement or stepping. It involves the process of changing the frequency of a behavior by controlling the consequences of that behavior with positive reinforcement to encourage or discourage a particular behavior. The procedure is used daily in our family and professional lives, such as rewarding (or punishing) children for their behavior and receiving (or being denied) a raise at work. Thus, a particular behavior becomes associated with a certain positive or negative consequence and the individual eventually accepts the desired behavior as being preferable. Behavior therapists have developed a wide range of applications for this learning procedure. A successful example is the token economy program (receiving tokens redeemable for snacks, movies, special privileges, and the like) which rewards destructive individuals for exhibiting appropriate behavior such as participating in rehabilitation activities. Contingency management has been effective with chronically hospitalized schizophrenic patients, such as the patient in the question who was disrupting the ward by shouting in the hall. Often, well-timed praise or friendliness will serve as an appropriate reinforcer to foster patient compliance, as will a lollipop for a child, or a follow-up phone call to a patient who has recovered or stopped smoking to reinforce your interest in their wellness, as well as their illness.

In stimulus control, the attempt is to eliminate the stimulus or cue that triggers undesired behavior. Modeling exposes the individual to desirable behavior or stimuli (e.g., posters or advertisements showing high status persons resisting smoking or explaining how to resist peer pressure).

7-26. The answer is d. *(Craig, p 481; Hardman, pp 694, 709, 1011–1012, 1018; Katzung, pp 299, 309, 1043.)* Misoprostol is a long-acting synthetic analog of PGE_1, and its only use (outside of reproductive medicine) is prophylaxis of NSAID-induced gastric ulcers. Its main effects are suppression of gastric acid secretion and enhanced gastric mucus production (a so-called mucotropic or cytoprotective effect). The need for the drug arises, of course, because such drugs as indomethacin (and most other COX-nonselective inhibitors) inhibit PGE_1 synthesis (as well as that of other prostaglandins, prostacyclin, and thromboxane A_2).

Although cimetidine might help reduce gastric acid secretion (via H_2 blockade) and diphenhydramine may too (via antimuscarinic effects), their antisecretory effects are weak and nonspecific in this situation, and they don't increase formation of the stomach's protective mucus.

Celecoxib (and other coxibs) are associated with a lower risk or incidence of peptic ulcers than more traditional NSAIDs, mainly because the former are relatively selective COX-2 inhibitors: it is the COX-1 pathway that, when inhibited, mainly allows gastric HCl secretion to rise and mucus production to fall. However, we asked about which drug would be an add-on to indomethacin therapy, and adding a COX-2 inhibitor would be of little benefit. Sumatriptan, a serotonin receptor agonist, also would be of little benefit in this situation and would not be prescribed for this purpose.

7-27. The answer is e. (*Hardman, pp 1055–1056; Katzung, p 1058.*) Pancrelipase is an alcoholic extract of hog pancreas that contains lipase, trypsin, and amylase. (The related drug, pancreatin, is similar.) The goal here is not so much to control the diarrhea, but do so by attacking the cause, which is endogenous pancreatic enzyme deficiency (lipases, amylase, chymotrypsin, and trypsin) that leads to impaired fat digestion and absorption. None of the other drugs mentioned have actions that would be as effective or specific as pancrelipase. "Traditional" antidiarrheals, for example, would only treat the symptoms, not the underlying cause.

Note: You may find pancrelipase administered with antacids, or an acid secretion inhibitor (H_2 blocker or proton pump inhibitor). The purpose of combined therapy is not related to preventing adverse effects of acid on the gastric mucosa, but rather to raise gastric pH and prevent the pancrelipase from being hydrolyzed and inactivated by acid.

7-28. The answer is e. (*Guyton, pp 742–744, 768–769.*) Analysis of serum electrolytes reveals low potassium (hypokalemia), low chloride (hypochloremia), and metabolic alkalosis. These abnormalities arise from two sources. First, gastric juice contains potassium and chloride in concentrations higher than found in the plasma. Loss of gastric juice through vomiting or drainage leads to depletion of these electrolytes from the plasma. Second, the metabolic abnormalities are exacerbated by the student's dehydration. Contraction of the vascular volume leads to orthostatic hypotension and the activation of renal mechanisms important for conserving volume. As a result, water, sodium, and bicarbonate are reabsorbed at the expense of increased potassium and hydrogen excretion.

7-29. The answer is c. (*Murray, pp 30–39. Scriver, pp 3–45. Sack, pp 1–3.*) Glycosaminoglycans (mucopolysaccharides) are polysaccharide chains that may be bound to proteins as proteoglycans. Each proteoglycan is a complex molecule with a core protein that is covalently bound to glycosaminoglycans—repeating units of disaccharides. The amino sugars forming the disaccharides contain negatively charged sulfate or carboxylate groups. The primary glycosaminoglycans found in mammals are hyaluronic acid, heparin, heparan sulfate, chondroitin sulfate, and keratan sulfate. Inborn errors of glycosaminoglycan degradation cause neurodegeneration and physical stigmata described by the outmoded term "gargoylism." Glycogen is a polysaccharide of glucose used for energy storage and has no sulfate groups. Collagen and fibrillin are important proteins in connective tissue. γ-aminobutyric acid is a γ-amino acid involved in neurotransmission.

7-30. The answer is c. (*Gilroy, pp 6–9. Rowland, pp 7–10.*) The language problem is an example of Broca's aphasia, a deficit seen with lesions of Broca's area and manifested by defects in the motor aspect of speech, leaving the patient's speech halting and nonfluent. People with Broca's aphasia tend to repeat certain phrases, as well as leave out pronouns. Since the language centers are usually located on the dominant side of the brain (the left side for a right-handed person), this lesion must be on the left side of Joe's brain. Wernicke's aphasia is a problem with the sensory aspect of speech, where the patient can speak fluently, but the speech sounds like gibberish. The area of disruption in this type of aphasia is usually in Wernicke's area, a region of the posterior superior temporal lobe. Dysarthria is slurred speech, but makes grammatical sense. Alexia is the inability to read. Pure-word deafness is a type of sensory aphasia whereby language, reading, and writing are only mildly disturbed, but auditory comprehension of words is very abnormal. This arises from lesions of the posterior temporal lobe.

7-31. The answer is a. (*Craig, pp 649–650, 707, 709–710; Hardman, pp 1440–1441, 1613–1614; Katzung, pp 679–680, 916–917.*) Tamoxifen is often referred to as a selective estrogen receptor modifier (SERM). It blocks estrogen receptors in some tissues and stimulates them in some others. The drug can be used to prevent or treat estrogen-dependent breast cancers, and it works as an estrogen receptor antagonist there. A receptor-agonist action also accounts for one of the drug's more distressing and common side effects, hot flashes. In contrast, the drug activates estrogen receptors in the uterus, increasing the risk of endometrial cancers. Other estrogen-activating (estrogen-like) consequences include a reduced risk of osteoporosis, desirable changes in serum cholesterol profiles (reduced LDL and total cholesterols; increased HDL), and an increased risk of thromboembolic events. The related drug, raloxifene, is largely tamoxifen-like with one main exception: it does not activate uterine estrogen receptors, and so does not increase the risk of endometrial cancers.

7-32. The answer is c. (*Moore and Dalley, p 1092.*) Information from the nasal retinal field crosses the midline at the optic chiasm; thus images from the right visual fields strike the left retinal fields of both eyes and from the right eye cross at the optic chiasm (see figure on page 380). The images that strike the left temporal retina (from the right visual field) of the left eye stay on the left and join the nasal retinal field of the right eye in the left optic tract. An aneurysm in the left middle cerebral artery, if large enough, would likely impinge on the left optic tract. A pituitary tumor would likely compress the optic chiasm leading to a loss of the temporal visual fields in both eyes, or tunnel vision (or bitemporal hemianopsia). A tumor in the right orbit that compresses the right optic nerve would just lead to loss of vision in the right eye. Compromise of the right optic tract would lead to loss of left visual fields in both eyes. A tumor in the occipital visual cortex would be very unlikely to produce the symptoms described.

7-33. The answer is b. (*Craig, pp 597–598; Hardman, pp 1298–1299; Katzung, pp 792–794.*) Amphotericin B, given intravenously, often alters kidney function. The most common and most easily detected manifestation of this is decreased creatinine clearance. If this occurs, the dose must be reduced. Amphotericin B also commonly increases potassium (K^+) loss, leading to hypokalemia; and can cause anemia and neurologic symptoms. A liposomal preparation of amphotericin B may reduce the incidence of renal and neurologic toxicity. Vancomycin may cause renal damage, but the overall incidence is lower, the severity less.

7-34. The answer is c. (*McKenzie, p 21. Junqueira, p 40.*) Tay-Sachs disease is one of the lysosomal storage diseases. Lysosomes contain an array of specific hydrolases. In Tay-Sachs disease, hexosaminidase A is deficient, resulting in the buildup of GM2 ganglioside and leading to mental retardation, blindness, and mortality. A pharmacological approach would target reducing GM2 ganglioside levels by increasing hexosaminidase A activity (answer c). Increase in GM2 levels (answers a and b) or increased transport (answer d) to a lysosome deficient in hexosaminidase would worsen the disease. The table on page 104 summarizes the enzyme deficiencies and resulting effects in some of the more prominent lysosomal disorders. Mannose-6-phosphate and its receptor are involved in the trafficking of proteins to the lysosomal compartment. Removal of mannose 6-phosphate (answer e), as occurs in inclusion-cell (I-cell) disease, would result in default of lysosomal enzymes to the secretory pathway, and the hexosaminidase deficiency would worsen.

7-35. The answer is b. *(Braunwald, pp 1644–1645.)* Patients with esophageal spasm usually have more severe pain than patients with hypertensive (hypercontracting) LES (and the other disorders). The symptoms of esophageal spasm often are confused with the pain of cardiac origin. Patients with esophageal spasm and hypertensive (hypercontracting) LES usually present at an earlier age than patients with achalasia.

7-36. The answer is a. *(Cotran, pp 620–621. Rubin, pp 1085–1086.)* Cold-antibody autoimmune hemolytic anemia (cold AIHA) is subdivided into two clinical categories based on the type of antibodies involved. These two types of cold antibodies are cold agglutinins and cold hemolysins. Cold agglutinins are monoclonal IgM antibodies that react at 4 to 6°C. They are called agglutinins because the IgM can agglutinate red cells due to its large size (pentamer). Additionally, IgM can activate complement, which may result in IV hemolysis. Mycoplasma pneumonitis and infectious mononucleosis are classically associated with cold-agglutinin formation. Vascular obstruction by the red cell agglutination can produce Raynaud's phenomenon, which is characterized by ischemia in the fingers when exposed to the cold.

In contrast to cold agglutinins, cold hemolysins are seen in patients with paroxysmal cold hemoglobinuria (PCH). These cold hemolysins are unique because they are biphasic antierythrocyte autoantibodies. These antibodies are IgG that is directed against the P blood group antigen. They are called biphasic because they attach to red cells and bind complement at low temperatures, but the activation of complement does not occur until the temperature is increased. This antibody, called the Donath-Landsteiner antibody, was previously associated with syphilis, but may follow various infections, such as mycoplasmal pneumonia.

7-37. The correct answer is c. (*Craig, pp 49–50; Hardman, pp 20–21; Katzung, pp 34–47.*) Regardless of which administration route has been used, if we plot the log of blood concentration of a drug vs. time (and assuming first-order kinetics, which applies to the elimination of most drugs), we get a straight line. It is described by the equation

$$\ln C = \ln C_0 - Kt$$

The slope of this line, κ, is the *elimination rate constant*.

An arguably more useful (and familiar) measure of the rate at which a drug is eliminated is the half-life ($t_{1/2}$). It is equal to $0.693/\kappa$, and is defined as the time it takes for the concentration of a drug in the blood to fall to precisely one half of what it is now (or at any specified time).

The *area under the curve* (AUC) is the integration of a time vs. concentration plot for a drug. It is a linear—not a logarithmic or semilog—plot. One use for plots of AUC is to estimate one's "total exposure" to a drug, usually from "time zero" (instantaneously upon administration) until blood concentrations of drug are no longer reliably detectable or further measurements are impractical. The AUC can be used to estimate total body clearance of a drug, without the need to know the drug's volume of distribution or its half-life, since

$$\text{Clearance} = \frac{\text{Dose}}{\text{AUC}}$$

Determining AUC also enables us to calculate a drug's *bioavailabity.* Bioavailability (*F*) is a measure of the fraction of an administered dose that is absorbed systemically and is detectable in the plasma. Note that when a drug is given intravenously, bioavailability is, by definition, 1.0 (100%), since there are no barriers that might prevent the absorption of drug from the administration site. So by administering a drug intravenously, and also giving it by another route, we can calculate bioavailability. For example, assume the other route we use is oral (PO).

$$\text{Bioavailability} = \left(\frac{\text{Dose}_{IV}}{\text{Dose}_{PO}} \right) \times \left(\frac{\text{AUC}_{PO}}{\text{AUC}_{IV}} \right)$$

If we do our bioavailability determinations by giving the same dose of the drug, the dosage units in the above equation cancel out, and so

$$\text{Bioavailability} = \frac{AUC_{PO}}{AUC_{IV}}$$

The *extraction ratio* (E) is a measure of a drug's removal from the blood as it passes through an organ (e.g., the liver) that can metabolize (or otherwise extract) it, e.g., from the artierial to the venous side of that organ.

The rate of drug entry to an organ is the product of blood flow (Q) and the arterial concentration of the drug (C_A). The rate at which the drug leaves is flow × the venous concentration (C_V). If flow into and out of an organ are identical (as it often is), then the extraction ratio can be expressed as

$$E = \frac{(C_A - C_V)}{C_A}$$

We can also use the extraction ratio to calculate the organ clearance of a drug—i.e., the volume per unit time from which an organ removes a drug

Organ clearance = Blood flow × Extraction ratio

The *volume of distribution* (V_d) relates the amount of drug in the body to its concentration in the blood (or plasma). It is typically calculated as the administered dose divided by the concentration of drug in the blood

$$V_d = \frac{D}{C}$$

To simplify things, we typically give the drug intravenously (so we know how much drug enters the system) and measure the concentration immediately thereafter (or use a plot of the log of drug concentration vs. time) to extrapolate drug concentration at "time zero" (the y-axis intercept).

7-38. The answer is c. (*Brooks, pp 476–478. Levinson, pp 243–244. Murray—2002, pp 529–530. Ryan, pp 506–507.*) Parainfluenza viruses are important causes of respiratory diseases in infants and young children. The spectrum of disease caused by these viruses ranges from a mild febrile cold to croup, bronchiolitis, and pneumonia. Parainfluenza viruses contain RNA in a nucleocapsid encased within an envelope derived from the host cell membrane. Infected mammalian cell culture will hemabsorb red blood cells owing to viral hemagglutinin on the surface of the cell.

7-39. The answer is f. (*Craig, p 66; Hardman, pp 1892–1893; Katzung, p 992.*) Cyanide reacts with Fe(III) in mitochondrial cytochrome oxidase, inhibiting oxidative phosphorylation. The shift in metabolism from aerobic to glycolytic soon leads to not only ATP depletion, but also severe lactic acidosis.

Cyanide normally reacts with endogenous sulfur-containing compounds, mainly thiosulfate, and under catalysis by rhodanese forms relatively less toxic thiocyanate that is formed and excreted in the urine. In cyanide poisoning, endogenous sulfur-containing substrate stores are quickly depleted. We manage this, then, by IV infusion of an aqueous sodium thiosulfate solution. (This is the same approach we use for "therapeutic cyanide poisoning," as can arise when nitroprusside doses are too great.)

Ammonium chloride would be ineffective and may actually make matters worse by exacerbating metabolic acidosis. Deferoxamine, an iron chelator, would be of no benefit in terms of signs, symptoms, or their causes or consequences. Dimercaprol is a heavy metal (mainly lead) chelator that would be of no benefit. Mannitol, an osmotic diuretic that is sometimes used to hasten the renal excretion of some toxins (via "forced diuresis"), would not alleviate or shorten signs and symptoms. Pralidoxime is a cholinesterase reactivator that is effective only for poisoning with organophosphate insecticides, nerve gases (sarin, soman), or other drugs that cause profound and largely permanent inactivation of acetylcholinesterase.

7-40. The answer is D. (*Afifi, pp 59–83. Nolte, pp 220–235.*) Sensory fibers that terminate in the medulla are located in the dorsal columns. Fibers mediating conscious proprioception from the upper limb are contained in the fasciculus cuneatus (A). The lateral spinothalamic tract (D) transmits pain and temperature information directly to the thalamus. The lateral corticospinal tract (B) originates in the contralateral cortex and crosses over at the level of the lower medulla. This important pathway mediates control over volitional movements. When these fibers are cut, there is a clear loss of ability to produce volitional movements. The rubrospinal tract (C), situated adjacent to the lateral corticospinal tract, originates from the red nucleus of the midbrain and facilitates the actions of flexor motor neurons. The lateral vestibulospinal tract (E) powerfully facilitates alpha motor neurons of extensor muscles. This tract is located in the ventral funiculus adjacent to the gray matter. The axons of the cells situated in this part of the gray matter (i.e., ventral horn) innervate extensor motor neurons. The posterior (or dorsal) spinocerebellar tract (H) transmits information from muscle spindles to the cerebellum via the inferior cerebellar peduncle. This tract is located on the lateral aspect of the lateral funiculus of the cord, just above the anterior (or ventral) spinocerebellar tract. Pain and temperature fibers from the periphery terminate directly in the region of the dorsal horn, called the *substantia gelatinosa* (I). A smaller component of the corticospinal tract, the anterior corticospinal tract (F), originates from the cerebral cortex and passes ipsilaterally to the spinal cord. In its ventromedial position, the fibers are ipsilateral to their cortical origin. Just prior to their termination, many of the fibers are distributed to the contralateral side of the cord. The anterior (or ventral) spinocerebellar tract (G) arises from wide regions of the gray matter of the cord. These fibers pass contralaterally to the lateral aspect of the lateral funiculus to reach a position just below the dorsal spinocerebellar tract. These fibers then ascend to the cerebellum via the superior cerebellar peduncle, conveying information from Golgi tendon organs located in the lower limbs.

7-41. The answer is a. (*Cotran, pp 1130–1131. Henry, pp 310–313.*) Tests used to determine thyroid function include serum thyroxine (T_4), resin T_3 uptake (RTU), thyroxine uptake (TU), free thyroxine index (FTI), and thyroid-stimulating hormone (TSH) levels. Serum T_4 measures the total T_4, which includes T_4 bound to thyroid-binding globulin (TBG) and free T_4. Therefore, increased total serum T_4 levels can be from increased free T_4 (such as Graves' disease) or from increased TBG. The resin T_3 uptake (RTU) essentially measures the TBG concentration by measuring the binding of radioactive T_3 to TBG; note that this is not the serum T_3 concentration. The same thing is essentially determined using the thyroxine uptake (TU). These values then can be used to artificially determine the free thyroxine index (FTI), which is an estimate of the free thyroxine. The FTI (T_7) can be determined using either T_4 times TU or T_4 times T_3U.

To illustrate, consider the following. If a person is euthyroid, then their free T_4 will be within normal limits. If the TBG in this person is normal, then the serum T_4 will also be normal, but if their TBG is increased, which can be the result of increased estrogen from birth control pills or pregnancy, then the total serum T_4 will be increased. Because the TBG is increased, however, the resin triiodothyronine uptake will be decreased. Because they are euthyroid and their free T_4 is normal, then their TSH will also be normal. Note that the measurement of serum TSH levels is the best test to determine if thyroid function is normal or abnormal. A normal TSH level indicates that free T_3 and free T_4 levels in the serum are normal. Increased serum TSH indicates low free T_3 and T_4 levels (primary hypothyroidism), while decreased serum TSH levels indicate either decreased production by the pituitary (hypopituitarism) or increased thyroid production by the thyroid gland (hyperthyroidism).

7-42. The answer is c. (*Braunwald, pp 2034–2035.*) This is the common CT finding and clinical presentation for craniopharyngioma. Empty sella does not usually cause marked enlargement of the sella, and there is no cystic structure with calcification. Pituitary macroadenomas can expand the sella but are not commonly cystic and calcified. Optic glioma and hypothalamic hamartoma are rarely cystic.

7-43. The answer is a. (*Murray, pp 40–48. Scriver, pp 4571–4636. Sack, pp 3–17.*) The woman would exhibit respiratory acidosis due to shortness of breath and decreased efficiency of gas exchange in the lungs. Emphysema involves dilated and dysfunctional alveoli from alveolar tissue damage, usually secondary to cigarette smoking. The hypoxia leads to tissue deoxygenation and acidosis, exacerbated by the hypercarbia (CO_2 accumulation) that distinguishes respiratory acidosis (higher bicarbonate than expected) from metabolic acidosis (very low bicarbonate, usually with low P_{CO_2} due to compensatory hyperventilation). Choice a shows the only set of values indicating acidosis (pH lower than 7.4), hypoxia (P_{O_2} lower than 95), and hypercarbia (P_{CO_2} greater than 44).

The tetrameric structure of hemoglobin allows cooperative binding of oxygen in that binding of oxygen to the heme molecule of the first subunit facilitates binding to the other three. This enhanced binding is due to allosteric changes of the hemoglobin molecule, accounting for its S-shaped oxygen saturation curve as compared with that of myoglobin (see the figure in question 143). At the lower oxygen saturations in peripheral tissues (P_{O_2} 30 to 40), hemoglobin releases much more oxygen (up to 50% desaturated) than myoglobin with its single polypeptide structure. The amount of oxygen released (and CO_2 absorbed as carboxyhemoglobin) is further increased by the Bohr effect—increasing hydrogen ion (H^+) concentration (lowering pH) and increasing CO_2 partial pressure (P_{CO_2}) shift the sigmoidal-shaped oxygen binding curve for hemoglobin further to the right.

7-44. The answer is e. (*Cotran, pp 812–815. Rubin, pp 711–717.*) The causes of malabsorption are vast, but in a few cases biopsy specimens of the small intestine may provide clues to a specific diagnosis. Whipple's disease is a systemic disease associated with malabsorption, fever, skin pigmentation, lymphadenopathy, and arthritis. Biopsy of the small intestine typically reveals the lamina propria to be infiltrated by numerous PAS-positive macrophages that contain glycoprotein and rod-shaped bacteria. The organism, *Tropheryma whippelii*, is a gram-positive actinomycete. The disease responds promptly to broad-spectrum antibiotic therapy. Abetalipo-proteinemia is a genetic defect in the synthesis of apolipoprotein B that leads to an inability to synthesize prebetalipoproteins (VLDLs), beta-lipoproteins (LDLs), and chylomicrons. These individuals have no chylomicrons, VLDLs, or LDLs in their blood. A biopsy of the small intestine reveals the mucosal absorptive cells to be vacuolated by lipid (triglyceride) inclusions, and peripheral smear reveals numerous acanthocytes, which are red blood cells that have numerous irregular spikes on their cell surface. The symptoms of malabsorption may be partially reversed by ingestion of medium-chain triglycerides rather than long-chain triglycerides, because these medium-chain triglycerides are absorbed directly into the portal system and are not incorporated into lipoproteins. Tropical and nontropical (celiac) sprue are both characterized by shortened to absent villi in the small intestines (atrophy). Celiac sprue is a disease of malabsorption related to a sensitivity to gluten, which is found in wheat, oats, barley, and rye. This disease is related to HLA-B8 and to previous infection with type 12 adenovirus. These patients respond to removal of gluten from their diet. Tropical sprue is an acquired disease found in tropical areas, such as the Caribbean, the Far East, and India. It is the result of a chronic bacterial infection. Granulomas in mucosa and submucosa of an intestinal biopsy, if infectious causes have been excluded, are highly suggestive of Crohn's disease. Fibrosis of the lamina propria and submucosa may be seen in patients with systemic sclerosis. Bacterial overgrowth, a result of numerous causes such as the blind loop syndrome, strictures, achlorhydria, or immune deficiencies, may also cause malabsorption. Treatment is with appropriate antibiotics.

7-45. The answer is b. (*Cotran, pp 5–11.*) With prolonged ischemia, certain cellular events occur that are not reversible, even with restoration of oxygen supply. These cellular changes are referred to as irreversible cellular injury. This type of injury is characterized by severe damage to mitochondria (vacuole formation), extensive damage to plasma membranes and nuclei, and rupture of lysosomes. Severe damage to mitochondria is characterized by the influx of calcium ions into the mitochondria and the subsequent formation of large, flocculent densities within the mitochondria. These flocculent densities are characteristically seen in irreversibly injured myocardial cells that undergo reperfusion soon after injury. Less severe changes in mitochondria, such as mitochondrial swelling, are seen with reversible injury. Cytochrome c released from damaged mitochondria can induce apoptosis, a process through which irreversibly injured cells can shrink and increase the eosinophilia of their cytoplasm. These shrunken apoptotic cells (apoptotic bodies) may be engulfed by adjacent cells or macrophages. Myelin figures are derived from plasma membranes and organelle membranes and can be seen with either reversible or irreversible injury. Psammoma bodies are small, laminated calcifications, while Russell bodies are round, eosinophilic aggregates of immunoglobulin.

7-46. The answer is d. (*Boron, pp 960–964, 969–971.*) Removal of the terminal ileum can lead to diarrhea and steatorrea. The terminal ileum contains specialized cells responsible for the absorption of primary and secondary bile salts by active transport. Bile salts are necessary for adequate digestion and absorption of fat. In the absence of the terminal ileum there will be an increase in the amounts of bile acids and fatty acids delivered to the colon. Fats and bile salts in the colon increase the water content of the feces by promoting the influx (secretion) of water into the lumen of the colon.

7-47. The answer is b. (*Afifi, pp 130–134. Gilroy, pp 590–591. Greenberg, pp 92–93.*) The cranial nerve that was directly affected was the glossopharyngeal nerve (cranial nerve IX). This is a mixed and complex nerve containing (1) special visceral efferents from the nucleus ambiguus that supply the stylopharyngeus muscle (for elevation of pharynx in speech); (2) special visceral afferent fibers that transmit taste impulses from the posterior third of the tongue and general visceral afferent fibers associated with the inferior ganglion whose receptors lie in the carotid sinus that regulates cardiovascular functions; (3) general somatic afferents whose cell bodies lie in the superior ganglion of cranial nerve IX and which mediate somatosensory information, including pain from the pharynx; and (4) general visceral efferent fibers that originate in the inferior salivatory nucleus, which are preganglionic and synapse in the otic ganglion. The postganglionic fiber from the otic ganglion innervates the parotid gland and mediates, in part, salivation. Thus, when this nerve is affected by an infectious agent, it results in the constellation of symptoms presented earlier in this case. Since the cell bodies of motor (or visceral motor) fibers (mediating motor and visceral effects) as well as the terminals of sensory afferents (mediating pain from the pharynx) lie in different regions of the medulla, it is very unlikely that such an effect could be the result of damage centrally. A much more likely occurrence is that the infectious agent produced disruption of the glossopharyngeal nerve peripherally, such as at the base of the skull or jugular foramen, where all the components run together and can be more easily affected.

7-48. The answer is c. (*Brooks, p 485. Levinson, p 245. Murray—2002, p 567. Ryan, pp 519–520.*) The highest risk of fetal infection with rubella occurs during the first trimester. In seronegative patients, the risk of infection exceeds 90%. However, before other measures (such as termination of pregnancy) are considered, a rubella immune status must be performed. A rubella titer of 1:10 is protective.

7-49. The answer is b. (*Boron, pp 425–426. Guyton, pp 420–421.*) Plasminogen is the inactive precursor of plasmin, the proteolytic enzyme involved in clot dissolution. An infusion of tissue plasminogen activator (tPA) soon after a heart attack (and possibly a thrombolytic stroke) can lessen the chances of permanent damage. Thrombin, the enzyme ultimately responsible for the formation of fibrin monomers, is generated from prothrombin by activated factor X. Activation of factor X occurs via both extrinsic and intrinsic pathways. Kininogens are enzymes responsible for the production of peptides (kinins) associated with inflammation. Heparin is an anticlotting agent found on endothelial cell surfaces.

7-50. The answer is a. (*Cotran, pp 751–753. Rubin, p 666.*) Malignant mesothelioma and adenocarcinoma are two neoplasms that may involve the pleural surfaces, as seen in the gross photograph. Malignant mesothelioma arises from the pleural surfaces and develops with significant and chronic exposure to asbestos (usually occupationally incurred). As the malignant mesothelioma spreads, it lines the pleural surfaces, including the fissures through the lobes of the lungs, and results in a tight and constricting encasement. This restricts the excursions of the lungs during ventilation. Adenocarcinoma of the lung also may invade the pleural surfaces and spread in an advancing manner throughout the pleural lining. The differential diagnosis histologically between an epithelial type of malignant mesothelioma and an adenocarcinoma may be difficult and sometimes impossible without special techniques. A characteristic feature seen by electron microscopy is numerous long microvilli on the surface of cells from mesotheliomas. Other histologic characteristics that favor the diagnosis of malignant mesothelioma over adenocarcinoma include positive acid mucopolysaccharide staining that is inhibited by hyaluronidase, perinuclear keratin staining (not peripheral), and negative staining with CEA and Leu-M$_1$.

BLOCK 8

Answers

8-1. The answer is e. (*Boron, pp 686–693.*) The F_{ACO_2} (the fraction of CO_2 in the alveolar gas) equals the ratio of partial pressure of CO_2 to the total dry atmospheric pressure ($P_{atm} - P_{water\ vapor} = (760 - 47)$ mmHg at sea level and body temperature.

$$F_{ACO_2} = P_{ACO_2}/(P_{atm} - P_{water\ vapor}) = 44\ \text{mmHg}/(760 - 47)\ \text{mmHg}$$

$$F_{ACO_2} = 44\ \text{mmHg}/(760 - 47)\ \text{mmHg}$$

$$F_{ACO_2} = 0.06$$

8-2. The answer is e. (*Cotran, pp 1297–1298.*) Increased intracranial pressure can result from mass lesions in the brain, cerebral edema, or hydrocephalus. Increased intracranial pressure can cause swelling of the optic nerve (papilledema), headaches, vomiting, or herniation of part of the brain into the foramen magnum or under a free part of the dura.

Brain herniations are classified according to the area of the brain that is herniated. Subfalcine herniations are caused by herniation of the medial aspect of the cerebral hemisphere (cingulate gyrus) under the falx, which may compress the anterior cerebral artery. Transtentorial herniation, which occurs when the medial part of the temporal lobe (uncus) herniates over the free edge of the tentorium, may result in compression of the oculomotor nerve, which results in pupillary dilation and ophthalmoplegia (the affected eye points "down and out"). Tentorial herniation may also compress the cerebral peduncles, within which are the pyramidal tracts. Ipsilateral compression produces contralateral motor paralysis (hemiparesis), while compression of the contralateral cerebral peduncle against Kernohan's notch causes ipsilateral hemiparesis. Further caudal displacement of the entire brainstem may cause tearing of the penetrating arteries of the midbrain (Duret hemorrhages). This caudal displacement may also stretch the trochlear nerve (cranial nerve VI), causing paralysis of the lateral rectus muscle (the abnormal eye turns inward). Masses in the cerebellum may cause tonsillar herniation, in which the cerebellar tonsils are herniated into the foramen magnum. This may compress the medulla and respiratory centers, causing death. Tonsillar herniation may also occur if a lumbar puncture (LP) is performed in a patient with increased intracranial pressure. Therefore, before performing an LP, check the patient for the presence of papilledema.

8-3. The answer is c. (*Brooks, pp 270–272. Levinson, pp 136, 137. Murray—2002, pp 325–327. Ryan, pp 415–419.*) The symptoms of Legionnaires' disease are similar to those of mycoplasmal pneumonia and influenza. Affected persons are moderately febrile, complain of pleuritic chest pain, and have a dry cough. Unlike *Klebsiella* and *Staphylococcus, L. pneumophila* exhibits fastidious growth requirements. Charcoal yeast extract agar either with or without antibiotics is the preferred isolation medium. While sputum may not be the specimen of choice for *Legionella,* the discovery of small, gram-negative rods by direct fluorescent antibody (FA) technique should certainly heighten suspicion of the disease. *L. pneumophila* is a facultative intracellular pathogen and enters macrophages without activating their oxidizing capabilities. The organisms bind to macrophage C receptors, which promote engulfment.

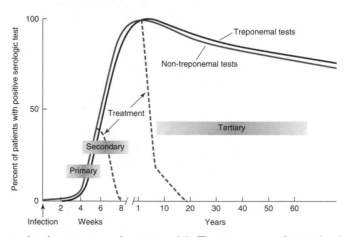

Treponemal and nontreponemal tests in syphilis. The time course of treated and untreated syphilis in relation to serologic tests is shown. The nontreponemal tests (VDRL, RPR) rise during primary syphilis and reach their peak in secondary syphilis. They slowly decline with advancing age. With treatment they revert to normal over a few weeks. The treponemal tests (FTA-Abs, MHTP) follow the same course but remain elevated even following successful treatment. (*Reprinted, with permission, from Ryan KJ et al. Sherris Medical Microbiology, 4e. New York: McGraw-Hill, 2001, 429.*)

8-4. The answer is c. (*Cotran, pp 956–958. Rubin, pp 874–875.*) Focal seg-mental glomerulosclerosis (FSGS) is a glomerular disorder that accounts for about 10% of the cases of nephrotic syndrome. FSGS, which affects children and adults, begins as a focal process, affecting only some glomeruli. In the earliest stage, only some of the juxtamedullary glomeruli show changes. Eventually, some glomeruli in other parts of the cortex are affected. In the late stages of the disease, the process may become diffuse, affecting most or all glomeruli. Initially, the process is also segmental, involving some but not all of the lobules within an individual glomerular tuft. The involved area shows sclerosis and may show hyalinosis lesions. Eventually some glomeruli show sclerosis of the entire tuft (global sclerosis). Electron microscopy shows increased mesangial matrix and dense granular mesan-gial deposits. Immunofluorescence typically shows granular mesangial fluo-rescence for IgM and C3. Because of the focal nature of FSGS, early cases can be difficult to distinguish from minimal change disease (MCD). Clini-cally, the nephrotic syndrome of FSGS is more severe than that of MCD and is nonselective. The process is much less responsive to steroids and is much more prone to progress to chronic renal failure. It tends to recur in trans-planted kidneys. FSGS can be seen in the setting of AIDS nephropathy and heroin nephropathy. [Note: FSGS, with no cellular proliferation, is different from focal segmental glomerulonephritis (FSGN), which involves cellular proliferation. The main cause of FSGN is IgA (Berger's) nephropathy, while FSGS is most notably seen in patients with AIDS.]

8-5. The answer is c. (*Craig, p 138; Hardman, pp 167–168; Katzung, pp 116–117.*) These are among the classic signs and symptoms of atropine (antimuscarinic) poisoning. Although you may have not learned this this way, put a Lewis Carroll/Alice in Wonderland spin on what the main find-ings are. Maybe that will help your memory. The antimuscarinic drug-poisoning syndrome has the patient

red as a beet (characteristic facial flushing; a so-called "atropine flush");
dry as a bone (no exocrine gland secretions, no fecal or urinary output because bowel and bladder motility are inhibited);
hot as a furnace (profound fever; a CNS "problem" compounded by a lack of body heat loss normally afforded by sweating);
blind as a bat (paralysis of accommodation and dilated pupils do not respond to even very bright light);
mad as a hatter (CNS problems, including delirium).

You may never see true atropine poisoning. As you know, that proto-type antimuscarinic is not used clinically that much, except in some partic-ular specialties. However, you should realize that many common groups of drugs (see Question 80), some of which are available over-the-counter, exert strong antimuscarinic effects; the signs and symptoms of "atropine poison-ing" are an important component of their overdose syndromes.

8-6. The answer is d. *(Baron, pp 352–357. Guyton, pp 561–563.)* Free nerve endings contain receptors for temperature, pain, and crude touch. However, fine touch, pressure, and vibration are detected by nerve endings contained within specialized capsules that transmit the stimulus to the sen-sory receptors. Muscle length is encoded by the primary nerve endings of Ia fibers, which are located on intrafusal fibers within the muscle spindle.

8-7. The answer is c. *(Braunwald, pp 686–687.)* The direct Coombs' test detects IgG or C3 on the surface of erythrocytes in persons with autoim-mune hemolytic anemia, as in this case. This test utilizes an anti-IgG or an anti-C3 to agglutinate erythrocytes when IgG or C3 are present. About one-fourth of persons who develop autoimmune hemolytic anemia suffer an underlying disease such as systemic lupus erythematosus or lymphoid neo-plasms. Factor VIII assay assists in replacement therapy in hemophiliacs; von Willebrand's factor is assayed in the diagnosis of von Willebrand's dis-ease; vitamin B_{12} absorption test is used in the diagnosis of pernicious ane-mia; and, prothrombin time guides anticoagulant therapy and it is increased in liver disease and vitamin K deficiency.

8-8. The answer is c. *(Taylor, pp 570–572.)* The behavioral conditioning process is very active in cancer patients who are receiving chemotherapy. The conditioned response of anticipatory nausea occurs because certain personal, environmental, or situational stimuli may elicit nausea before the administration of the chemotherapy that can cause nausea in its own right. About one-third of cancer patients on chemotherapy develop anticipatory nausea. It also occurs more frequently in patients who are less hopeful and more pessimistic, isolated, and inhibited, and those who have more chronic anxiety. The anticipatory nausea also appears to be related to the severity of the dose of chemotherapy. The major stimuli involved can be the hospital, the clinic, the nurse, or the smells encountered before admin-istration of the chemotherapy.

8-9. The answer is a. (*Afifi, pp 171–177. Nolte, pp 294–301.*) The spinal trigeminal nucleus receives its sensory inputs from first-order neurons contained in the ipsilateral descending tract of cranial nerve V. A central property of the spinal trigeminal nucleus is that it is uniquely associated with pain inputs (to the exclusion of the main sensory nucleus and mesencephalic nucleus). Fibers from this nucleus mainly project contralaterally to the ventral posteromedial nucleus of the thalamus. Surgical interruption of these descending first-order pain fibers is a practical approach and one that has been carried out by neurosurgeons. Destruction of the ventral posterolateral nucleus would not necessarily destroy the major pain inputs to the cerebral cortex and would additionally be a more difficult structure to destroy surgically. The main sensory nucleus of the trigeminal nerve is not known to convey pain inputs to thalamus and cortex. The substantia gelatinosa conveys pain and temperature sensation from the body and not the head. The midbrain periaqueductal gray constitutes part of a pain-inhibitory system, not one that transmits pain sensations to the cerebral cortex.

8-10. The answer is d. (*Cotran, pp 1281–1283. Rubin, 1420–1423.*) Duchenne's muscular dystrophy (DMD) is a noninflammatory inherited myopathy that causes progressive, severe weakness and degeneration of muscles, particularly the proximal muscles, such as the pelvic and shoulder girdles. The defective gene is located on the X chromosome and codes for dystrophin, a protein found on the inner surface of the sarcolemma. Histologically, muscle fibers in patients with DMD show variations in size and shape, degenerative and regenerative changes in adjacent myocytes, necrotic fibers invaded by histiocytes, and progressive fibrosis. There are rounded, atrophic muscle fibers mixed with hypertrophied fibers. These muscle changes cause creatine kinase levels in the serum to be elevated. The weak muscles are replaced by fibrofatty tissue, which results in pseudohypertrophy. In Duchenne's muscular dystrophy, symptoms begin before the age of 4, are progressive and lead to difficulty in walking, and are eventually followed by involvement of respiratory muscles, which causes death from respiratory failure before the age of 20. The classification of the muscular dystrophies is based on the mode of inheritance and clinical features. X-linked inheritance characterizes Duchenne's muscular dystrophy, autosomal dominant inheritance characterizes both myotonic dystrophy and the fascioscapulohumeral type, and limb-girdle dystrophy is autosomal recessive. Sustained muscle contractions and rigidity (myotonia) are seen in myotonic dystrophy, the most common form of adult muscular dystrophy.

In contrast, dermatomyositis is an autoimmune disease that is one of a group of idiopathic inflammatory myopathies. The inflammatory myopathies are characterized by immune-mediated inflammation and injury of skeletal muscle and include polymyositis, dermatomyositis, and inclusion-body myositis. These diseases are associated with numerous types of autoantibodies, one of which is the anti-Jo-1 antibody. The capillaries are the principle target in patients with dermatomyositis. Damage is by complement-mediated cytotoxic antibodies against the microvasculature of skeletal muscle. In addition to proximal muscle weakness, patients typically develop a lilac discoloration around the eyelids with edema. Patients may also develop erythema over their knuckles (Gorton's sign). Histologically, examination of muscles from patients with dermatomyositis reveals perivascular inflammation within the tissue around muscle fascicles. This is in contrast to the other types of inflammatory myopathies, where the inflammation is within the muscle fascicles (endomysial inflammation). In particular, inclusion-body myositis is characterized by basophilic granular inclusions around vacuoles ("rimmed" vacuoles). Werdnig-Hoffmann disease is a severe lower motor neuron disease that presents in the neonatal period with marked proximal muscle weakness ("floppy infant").

8-11. The answer is b. (*Murray, pp 5–13. Scriver, pp 1471–1488. Sack, pp 217–218.*) The man is acidotic as defined by the pH lower than the normal 7.4. His hyperventilation with Kussmaul respirations can be interpreted as compensation by the lungs to blow off CO_2, lower P_{CO_2}, increase $[HCO_3^-]/[CO_2]$ ratio, and raise pH. The correct answer therefore includes a low P_{CO_2}, eliminating choices c through e. Using the Henderson-Hasselbalch equation indicates that the pH minus the pK for carbonic acid ($7.3 - 6.1 = 1.2$) equals $\log [15]/[0.03 \times 30 \text{ mmHg}]$ or $\log [15/0.9]$. These values correspond to those in choice b. The man has compensated his metabolic acidosis (caused by the accumulation of ketone bodies such as acetoacetic acid) by increasing his respiratory rate and volume.

8-12. The answer is d. (*Braunwald, pp 719–720.*) These findings describe chronic lymphocytic leukemia (CLL). It is a monoclonal B cell disease and the lymphocytes show CD5 antigen. About one-fourth of persons with CLL show trisomy 12 and in some cases chromosome 13 also shows abnormalities. The B cells in the other diseases do not express CD5 antigen nor are "smudge" cells seen on the peripheral smear.

8-13. The answer is d. (*Cotran, pp 371–373. Rubin, pp 370–372, 1094.*) Infectious mononucleosis is a benign lymphoproliferative disorder caused by infection with the Epstein-Barr virus (EBV). It typically occurs in young adults and presents with systemic symptoms, lymphadenopathy, and pharyngitis. Hepatosplenomegaly may be present. Peripheral blood shows an absolute lymphocytosis, and many lymphocytes are atypical with irregular nuclei and abundant basophilic vacuolated cytoplasm. These represent CD8+ T killer cells induced by EBV-transformed B lymphocytes. These atypical lymphocytes are usually adequate for diagnosis, along with a positive heterophil or monospot test (increased sheep red cell agglutinin). Administration of ampicillin for a mistaken diagnosis of streptococcal pharyngitis results in a rash in many patients.

8-14. The answer is e. (*Boron, p 663.*) Carbon monoxide poisoning reduces the amount of oxygen that can combine with hemoglobin but does not reduce the arterial oxygen tension. Because the peripheral chemoreceptors do not increase ventilation until the arterial P_{O_2} is less than 60 mmHg, severe hypoxemia can occur without any respiratory or cardiovascular symptoms being apparent to the victim of CO poisoning. This is the reason that it is so important to install carbon monoxide detectors in homes and businesses.

8-15. The answer is d. (*Brooks, pp 239–244. Levinson, pp 127–128. Murray—2002, pp 288–289. Ryan, pp 379–380.*) Until recently, both erythromycin and ciprofloxacin were the drugs of choice for *C. jejuni* enterocolitis. Recently, resistance to the quinolones (ciprofloxacin) has been observed. Ampicillin is ineffective against this gram-negative, curved rod. While Pepto-Bismol may be adequate for a related ulcer-causing bacterium, *Helicobacter*, it is not used for *C. jejuni*. While the pathogenesis of *C. jejuni* suggests an enterotoxin, an antitoxin is not available.

8-16. The answer is d. (*Moore and Dalley, p 396.*) The blood is limited to the superficial perineal space which is bound by the superficial membranous fascia (superficially; including Scarpa's fascia on the anterior abdominal wall and Colles' fascia on the urogenital triangle) and the deep perineal mem-

brane (deep). The superficial membranous fascia is attached to deep structures at the following locations: superiorly the superficial membranous fascia
attaches to the deep fascia of the anterior abdominal muscles about half way
between the pubis symphysis and the umbilicus; attaches to the inguinal ligament, laterally; and attaches to the fascia lata, laterally; and attaches to the
posterior edge of the perineal membrane just anterior to the anus.

8-17. The answer is d. *(Cotran, pp 798–802. Rubin, pp 696–699.)* "Signet
ring cell" carcinoma is a morphologic variant of adenocarcinoma most
often seen in the stomach. In these tumors, intracellular mucin vacuoles
coalesce and distend the cytoplasm of tumor cells, which compresses the
nucleus toward the edge of the cell and creates a signet ring appearance.
Tumors of this type are usually deeply invasive and fall into the category of
advanced gastric carcinoma. There is often a striking desmoplasia with
thickening and rigidity of the gastric wall, which may result in the so-called
linitis plastica ("leather bottle") appearance. Advanced gastric carcinoma is
usually located in the pyloroantrum, and the prognosis is poor, with 5-year
survival of only 5 to 15%.

In contrast, cystosarcoma phyllodes is a type of breast tumor (phyllodes refers to its leaflike appearance), and peau d'orange refers to breast
tumors that cause the overlying skin to have the appearance of an orange.
Rodent ulcer refers to the clinical appearance of some basal cell carcinomas
of the skin, while sarcoma botryoides is a malignant vaginal tumor that has
a grapelike gross appearance.

8-18. The answer is d. *(Braunwald, p 275.)* This patient has two possible
causes of hyponatremia, cirrhosis, or SIADH due to small-cell lung cancer.
In both cases the serum osmolarity will be low because true hyponatremia
is present. There is inappropriate excretion of vasopressin in both cases and
therefore urine osmolarity will be inappropriately high because of water
retention. However, in cirrhosis the effective circulating volume is
decreased due to venodilatation, and therefore renal sodium retention will
occur. In SIADH, the patient would be euvolemic and no increase in
sodium avidity is present.

8-19. The answer is d. *(Craig, p 342; Hardman, pp 203, 205; Katzung, p 433.)*
While this may seem like a trick question, the point is that even with
markedly deficient cholinesterase activity, the succinylcholine eventually

will be metabolized and its effects will disappear. All that needs to be done is to maintain adequate mechanical ventilatory support.

Succinylcholine exerts its effects by activating nicotinic receptors on skeletal muscle (powerfully but normally briefly, owing to prompt metabolism) and depolarizing the myocytes. Atropine will not work. It blocks only muscarinic receptors. Bethanechol is a muscarinic agonist. Although it may have some nicotinic activating actions at extraordinarily high doses, that effect would add to, not resolve, the effects of the succinylcholine.

Some texts note that under some conditions succinylcholine can cause what is termed Phase II block: a type of neuromuscular blockade that is curare-like (i.e., nondepolarizing). Because nondepolarizing blockade can be (and is, clinically) reversed with acetylcholinesterase inhibitors (mainly neostigmine; physostigmine would work but is not used because of its CNS effects), the implication is that we could administer a cholinesterase inhibitor here and reverse the paralysis. However, this so-called Phase II block is a manifestation of excessive (toxic) doses of succinylcholine and is not likely to apply here. Regardless, the approach is to give nothing and to ventilate the patient as long as needed, as noted above.

8-20. The answer is d. (*Boron, pp 918–924, 963–965.*) The process of fat digestion begins in the stomach and is completed in the proximal small intestine, predominately by enzymes synthesized and secreted by the pancreatic acinar cells. The major lipolytic pancreatic enzyme is the carboxylic esterase, known as lipase. Full activity requires the protein cofactor colipase, as well as an alkaline pH, bile salts, and fatty acids.

8-21. The answer is b. (*Afifi, pp 168–169, 194–196, 209–222, 227–232.*) The third cranial nerve (oculomotor) controls four of the six extraocular muscles that move the eye. When this nerve fails to function, the eye remains deviated laterally due to the unopposed action of the other two extraocular muscles. When the eyes no longer move together, patients have double vision because the visual cortex now receives two different images. In addition, fibers originating in the third nerve nucleus innervate the levator palpebrae superioris, a muscle that helps to lift the eyelid. Damage to the optic nerve causes loss of vision, blurred vision, and a central scotoma (blind spot in the center of the visual field). Damage to the cervical sympathetic fibers causes Horner's syndrome, consisting of ptosis (drooping of the eyelid), miosis (constriction of the pupil), and anhydrosis (loss of sweating), not eye movement abnormalities. The actions of the superior oblique, the muscle innervated by the trochlear nerve, include intorsion, depression, and abduction. The abducens nerve mediates the lateral rectus muscle, which abducts the eye. The eye is depressed and abducted due to the unopposed actions of the superior oblique and lateral rectus muscles, which together move the eye downward and abduct it (see earlier discussion for the actions of these muscles). The other four muscles are innervated by the oculomotor nerve, which presumably has been damaged. This is an example of Weber's syndrome, or a lesion involving the third cranial nerve outflow tract and the corticospinal and corticobulbar tracts in the cerebral peduncles of the midbrain. Weber's syndrome may occur as a result of an occlusion of the interpeduncular branches of the posterior cerebral artery (which supply this portion of the midbrain), a tumor pressing on this area, an aneurysm (circumscribed dilation of an artery) of the posterior communicating artery, or a plaque (lesion) related to multiple sclerosis. Fibers from the Edinger-Westphal nucleus are affected by lesions of the midbrain as well, and because they are instrumental in constricting the pupil, this lesion causes the patient to have a dilated pupil. If there is a mass that is external to the midbrain but pressing on the oculomotor nerve, then the preganglionic parasympathetic fibers traveling to the ciliary ganglion, which, in turn, innervate the pupillary constrictor muscles, can be damaged, also causing a dilated pupil. Cervical sympathetic fibers cause pupillary dilatation, so damage to these fibers causes pupillary constriction (see Horner's syndrome, earlier). Involvement of the cerebral peduncle causes damage to the corticospinal and corticobulbar tracts, resulting in weakness of the contralateral face, arm, and leg. The motor deficit is contralateral because the corticospinal tracts cross in the medullary pyramids, below the level of the lesion. The upper portion of Mike's face was spared in this case (as well as in any other UMN lesion) because the face is innervated bilaterally until the level of the caudal pons, so a unilateral lesion results in sparing of this portion of the face. The combination of a third-nerve palsy and contralateral hemiparesis can occur only in the midbrain. The observed effects relating to cranial nerve III could not be accounted for by cortical damage. Likewise, damage to the cervical cord would not affect the third nerve.

8-22. The answer is e. (*Cotran, pp 904–907. Goldman, pp 752–757.*) Inflammation of the pancreas (pancreatitis) may be either acute or chronic.

Patients with acute pancreatitis typically present with abdominal pain that is associated with increased serum levels of pancreatic enzymes (amylase and lipase). Most cases of acute pancreatitis are associated with either alcohol ingestion or biliary tract disease (gallstones). Alcohol ingestion is the most common cause, and pancreatitis usually follows an episode of heavy drinking. Other, less frequent causes include hypercalcemia, hyperlipidemias, shock, infections (CMV and mumps), trauma, and drugs. Acute pancreatitis usually presents as a medical emergency. Symptoms of acute pancreatitis include abdominal pain that is localized to the epigastrium and radiates to the back, vomiting, and shock, the latter being the result of hemorrhage and kinins released into the blood. In severe pancreatitis there may be hemorrhage in the subcutaneous tissue around the umbilicus (Cullen's sign) and in the flanks (Turner's sign). Activation of the plasma coagulation cascade may lead to disseminated intravascular coagulopathy (DIC). Laboratory confirmation of pancreatic disease involves the finding of elevated serum amylase levels in the first 24 h and rising lipase levels over the next several days. Other pancreatic enzymes, such as trypsin, chymotrypsin, and carboxypeptidases, have not been as useful for diagnosis as have amylase and lipase. Complications seen in patients who survive the acute attack include pancreatic abscess formation, pseudocyst formation, or duodenal obstruction. Diabetes mellitus almost never occurs after a single attack of pancreatitis.

8-23. The answer is e. (*Craig, pp 325–326; Hardman, pp 546–548; Katzung, pp 505–507, 509.*) Adding pentazocine to an analgesic regimen involving morphine will counteract key effects of morphine. In this case, the patient's pain will grow worse, not become less. Pentazocine is classified as a partial agonist (or mixed agonist-antagonist). Recall that morphine causes the following effects by acting as a "pure" agonist on μ receptors: analgesia, respiratory depression, euphoria, sedation, physical dependence, and decreased gut motility. Pentazocine, given alone, causes analgesia, sedation, and decreased gut motility by acting as an agonist on κ receptors. However, it is a weak agonist. But it antagonizes the actions of morphine on μ receptors in a concentration-dependent fashion, and so pain returns in this patient.

8-24. The answer is b. (*Greenberg, pp 138–145.*) Calcification of the internal carotid artery could serve to disrupt nerve fibers proximal to it.

One such group of fibers includes parts of the optic nerve. In this case, the component of the right optic nerve affected includes the lateral aspect, or those fibers that mediate vision associated with the nasal visual field of the right eye. If the damage were more extensive and if it involved the entire nerve, then total blindness of the right eye would have occurred.

8-25. The answer is a. (*Braunwald, pp 268–271.*) Detrusor instability, decreased contractility, and failure are all part of a continuum. Decreased contractility is implied by the decreased force of the stream. Instability alone has only frequency and urgency. Failure implies an inability to urinate due to muscle failure. With acute obstruction, the patient cannot void, and there is significant pain. With chronic urinary obstruction, starting the stream is also a problem.

8-26. The answer is c. (*Murray, p 546. Scriver, pp 3421–3452. Sack, pp 121–138.*) The two major groups of lysosomal storage disease are sphingolipidoses and mucopolysaccharidoses. An absence of α-L-iduronidase, as in Hurler's syndrome (252800) and Scheie's syndrome (252800), leads to accumulations of dermatan sulfate and heparan sulfate. Scheie's syndrome is less severe, with corneal clouding, joint degeneration, and increased heart disease. Hurler's syndrome has the same symptoms plus mental and physical retardation leading to early death. The later onset in this child is compatible with a diagnosis of Scheie's syndrome. Note that Hurler's and Scheie's syndromes result from mutations at the same locus—hence their identical McKusick numbers. The reasons for the differences in disease severity are unknown. All of the other enzyme deficiencies listed lead to the lack of proper breakdown of sphingolipids and their accumulation as gangliosides, glucocerebrosides, and sphingomyelins. Symptoms of lipidoses may include organ enlargement, mental retardation, and early death.

8-27. The answer is c. (*McKenzie, p 163. Alberts, p 1103. Braunwald, pp 1430–1431, 2298–2299.*) The patient in the scenario suffers from Marfan's syndrome, an autosomal dominant disease in which persons develop abnormal elastic tissue. Pneumothorax in Marfan's patients occurs seemingly without explanation. Decreased elasticity of lung tissue causes an increased tendency toward spontaneous pneumothorax, also known as a collapsed lung. The aorta is the most affected organ because of the extensive elastin in the wall, and dissecting aortic aneurysms are common in these patients. Marfan malformations include cardiovascular (valve problems as well as aortic aneurysm), skeletal (abnormal height and severe chest deformities), and ocular systems. The molecular basis of the disease is a mutation in the fibrillin gene. The lens is also often affected in patients with Marfan's syndrome. The result is the dislocation of the lens because of loss of elasticity in the suspensory ligament.

8-28. The answer is b. (*Craig, p 259; Hardman, pp 1343–1345; Katzung, pp 545–547.*) Heparin binds to antithrombin III (a plasma protease inhibitor), thereby enhancing its activation. The heparin-antithrombin III complex interacts with thrombin. This inactivates thrombin and other coagulation factors such as VIIa, IXa, Xa, and IIa. Heparin accelerates the rate of thrombin-antithrombin binding, resulting in the inhibition of thrombin. The latter effect is not typically seen with low-molecular-weight heparins that are not of sufficient length to catalyze the inhibition of thrombin.

8-29. The answer is a. (*Brooks, pp 242–244. Levinson, pp 133–134. Murray—2002, p 319. Ryan, pp 397–401.*) Meningitis caused by *H. influenzae* cannot be distinguished on clinical grounds from that caused by pneumococci or meningococci. The symptoms described are typical for all three organisms. *H. influenzae* is a small, gram-negative rod with a polysaccharide capsule. It is able to grow on laboratory media if two factors are added. Heme (factor X) and NAD (factor V) provide for energy production. Use of the conjugate vaccine (type b polysaccharide) reduces the disease incidence more than 90%. Pneumococci are gram-positive diplococci, and meningococci are gram-negative diplococci, which grow on blood agar and chocolate agar with no X and V factors needed, respectively.

8-30. The answer is d. (*Craig, pp 66t, 261, 781–782; Hardman, pp 1349–1350, 1584–1585; Katzung, pp 552, 556.*) Phytonadione (vitamin K_1) is the antidote. It overcomes (reverses, antagonizes) warfarin's hepatic anticoagulant effects, which involve inhibited synthesis of clotting factors (VII, IX, X, and prothrombin).

Aminocaproic acid is a backup (to whole blood, packed red cells, or fresh-frozen plasma) for managing bleeding in response to excessive effects of thrombolytic drugs [e.g., alteplase (tPA), streptokinase, tenecteplase]. It is not indicated for warfarin-related bleeding. Epoetin alfa is a hematopoietic growth factor that stimulated erythrocyte production in peritubular cells in the proximal tubules of the kidney. Its uses include management of anemias associated with chronic renal failure, chemotherapy (of nonmeleloid malignancies), or zidovudine therapy in patients with acquired immunodeficiency syndrome. It is inappropriate for this patient. Ferrous sulfate (or fumarate or gluconate) is indicated for prevention or treatment of iron-deficiency anemias. It will do nothing to lower the patient's INR or alleviate related symptoms. Protamine sulfate is the antidote for heparin overdoses. It acts electrostatically with heparin, in the blood, to form a complex that lacks anticoagulant activity. It does nothing to the hepatic vitamin K–related problems that are at the root of excessive warfarin effects.

8-31. The answer is e. (*Cotran, pp 712–716. Braunwald, pp 1456–1460. Junqueira, p 358.*) The teenage patient is suffering from an asthmatic attack, probably allergen-induced. Mast cells are a key player in this airway disease. Mast cells in the bronchioles are stimulated to release histamine and heparin that induce the contraction of smooth bronchiolar muscle and edema in the wall. If the bronchoconstriction is chronic, the long-term result is thickening of the bronchiolar musculature. Other cells involved in asthma include eosinophils, neutrophils, macrophages, and lymphocytes, which signal to each other through a complex cytokine network. Mediators released include bradykinin, leukotrienes, and prostaglandins, which enhance bronchoconstriction, vascular congestion, and edema. The airway epithelium also is involved in response to and release of mediators. These muscle changes are usually accompanied by goblet cell hypersecretion of a viscous mucus, which can obstruct the airway. Eosinophils release proteins that destroy the airway epithelium (releasing Creola bodies). T lymphocytes are also present in more severe "attacks" and, along with B lymphocytes, may play a role in the initiation of allergic asthma. T lymphocytes also release cytokines that activate cell-mediated immunity pathways. Mucociliary transport is active in the trachea and bronchi; alveolar macrophages do not play a role in that process.

8-32. The answer is a. (*Cotran, pp 578–584. Rubin, pp 577–579.*) The cardiomyopathies (CMPs) may be classified into primary and secondary forms. The primary forms are mainly idiopathic (unknown cause). Most of the secondary cardiomyopathies result in a dilated cardiomyopathy that is characterized by congestion and four-chamber dilation with hypertrophy. The walls are either of normal thickness or they may be thinner than normal. This results in a flabby, globular, banana-shaped heart that is hypocontracting. The microscopic appearance is not distinctive. The ventricles may contain mural thrombi. The causes of secondary dilated CMP are many and include alcoholism (the most common cause in the United States), metabolic disorders, and toxins. Examples of the latter include cobalt, which has been used in beer as a foam stabilizer; anthracyclines; cocaine; and iron, the deposition of which is seen in patients with hemochromatosis. The anthracycline Adriamycin, which is used in chemotherapy, causes lipid peroxidation of myofiber membranes. One final form of DCM develops in the last trimester of pregnancy or the first 6 months after delivery. About half of these patients recover full cardiac function.

Other forms of cardiomyopathies include a hypertrophic form, a restrictive form, and an obliterative form. In hypertrophic CMP the major gross abnormality is within the interventricular septum, which is usually thicker than the left ventricle. Constrictive (restrictive) CMP is associated with amyloidosis, sarcoidosis, endomyocardial disease, or storage diseases. These abnormalities produce a stiff, hypocontracting heart.

8-33. The answer is f. (*Craig, pp 465–466; Hardman, p 644; Katzung, pp 330–331.*) Montelukast (and a related drug, zafirlukast) block receptors for leukotrienes (LTs). (When you see "leuk" or "luk" as part of these drugs' generic names, think leukotrienes or leukotriene modifiers.)

Recall that the LTs, which are pro-inflammatory and bronchoconstrictor mediators, are formed as part of normal arachidonic acid metabolism via the 5′-lipoxygenase pathway. (Recall that the other main part of arachidonic acid metabolism, involving cyclooxygenases, forms various prostaglandins and thromboxane A_2.) A somewhat related drug, zileuton, inhibits 5′-lipoxygenase directly, thereby mainly blocking LT synthesis rather than mainly blocking LT receptors.

These are oral agents, indicated for prophylaxis only. They will do virtually no good in a short enough time if they were administered to suppress ongoing bronchoconstriction, mainly because they are too slow-acting. And, although this class of drugs is the newest one to be approved for asthma in many years, they are not panaceas for all asthma patients, and for some patients their efficacy is not all that great.

Note: One probable advantage of montelukast or zafirlukast over zileuton is that they don't appear to participate in well-documented, clinically significant drug-drug interactions.

In contrast, zileuton inhibits theophylline's metabolism to a degree that is likely to be clinically significant for some patients (e.g., envisage a scenario in which these two asthma drugs are prescribed for the same patient) and also inhibits hepatic clearance of warfarin. It can also cause liver damage (as evidenced by increased transaminase levels in the blood). It is contraindicated for patients with acute liver disease and probably also should be avoided in chronic liver disease.

8-34. The answer is a. (*Cotran, pp 1040–1042. Rubin, pp 970–972.*) Several pathologic conditions are associated with the formation of white plaques on the vulva, which are clinically referred to as leukoplakia. Lichen sclerosis is seen histologically as atrophy of the epidermis with underlying dermal fibrosis. This abnormality is seen in postmenopausal women, who develop pruritic white plaques of the vulva. It is not thought to be premalignant. Loss of pigment in the epidermis (vitiligo) can also produce leukoplakia. Inflammatory skin diseases, such as chronic dermal inflammation, squamous hyperplasia (characterized by epithelial hyperplasia and hyperkeratosis), and vulvar intraepithelial neoplasia (characterized by epithelial atypia or dysplasia), can also present with leukoplakia. A term related to leukoplakia is vulvar dystrophy, but this refers specifically to either lichen sclerosis or squamous hyperplasia. Because the latter is sometimes associated with epithelial dysplasia, it is also referred to as hyperplastic dystrophy. It is most commonly seen in postmenopausal women. The male counterpart of lichen sclerosis, called balanitis xerotica obliterans, is found on the penis. Paget's disease is a malignant tumor that can be found in the breast or the vulva. The latter is seen clinically as pruritic, red, crusted, sharply demarcated maplike areas. Histologically, these malignant lesions reveal single anaplastic tumor cells surrounded by clear spaces ("halos") infiltrating the epidermis. These malignant cells stain positively with PAS and mucicarmine stains.

8-35. The answer is d. (*Boron, p 1226. Guyton, pp 428–429.*) Warfarin is often prescribed for patients at risk for thromboembolic episodes. Vitamin K is necessary for the conversion of prothrombin to thrombin. Thrombin is an important intermediate in the coagulation cascade. It converts fibrinogen to fibrin and is a powerful activator of platelets. Warfarin interferes with the activity of vitamin K and therefore reduces the likelihood of clot formation. Administering vitamin K can restore coagulation if warfarin therapy leads to excessive bleeding. Heparin prevents clotting by inhibiting thrombin. Aspirin blocks the formation of thromboxane A_2, which is necessary for platelet aggregation. Tissue plasminogen activator (tPA) is a thrombolytic agent.

8-36. The answer is d. (*Murray, pp 481–497. Scriver, pp 3897–3964. Sack, pp 121–138.*) People with bowed legs and other bone malformations were quite common in the northeastern United States following the industrial revolution. This was caused by childhood diets lacking foods with vitamin D and by minimal exposure to sunlight due to the dawn-to-dusk working conditions of the textile mills. Vitamin D is essential for the metabolism of calcium and phosphorus. Soft and malformed bones result from its absence. Liver, fish oil, and egg yolks contain vitamin D, and milk is supplemented with vitamin D by law. In adults, lack of sunlight and a diet poor in vitamin D lead to osteomalacia (soft bones). Dark-skinned peoples are more susceptible to vitamin D deficiency.

Biotin deficiency can be caused by diets with excess egg white, leading to dehydration and acidosis from accumulation of carboxylic and lactic acids. Retinoic acid is a vitamin A derivative that can be helpful in treating acne but not vitamin D deficiency. Leafy vegetables are a source of B vitamins such as niacin and cobalamin.

8-37. The answer is a. (*Moore and Dalley, pp 47–49, 287.*) The adrenal medulla is innervated from thoracic levels of the spinal cord mediated by preganglionic sympathetic nerve fibers traveling in the lesser and least splanchnic nerves, with some contribution from the greater splanchnic and lumbar splanchnic nerves. Because both the adrenal medulla and postganglionic sympathetic neurons are adrenergic and derived from neural crest tissue, the homology of the chromaffin cells and postganglionic sympathetic neurons is apparent. There appears to be no parasympathetic innervation to the adrenal medulla or cortex.

8-38. The answer is c. (*Cotran, pp 448–450. Chandrasoma, pp 160–162. Rubin, pp 349–350.*) Deficiencies of niacin (vitamin B$_3$) produce pellagra, a disease that is characterized by the triad of dementia, dermatitis ("glove" or "necklace" distribution), and diarrhea. Decreased levels of niacin may result from diets that are deficient in niacin, such as diets that depend on maize (corn) as the main staple, because niacin in maize is bound in a form that is not available. Part of the body's need for niacin is supplied by the conversion of the essential amino acid tryptophan to NAD, and therefore a deficiency of tryptophan can also produce symptoms of pellagra. Deficiencies of tryptophan can be seen in individuals with Hartnup disease, which is caused by the abnormal membrane transport of neutral amino acids and tryptophan in the small intestines and kidneys. Deficiencies of tryptophan can also be found in individuals whose diets are high in leucine (an amino acid that inhibits one of the enzymes necessary to convert tryptophan to NAD), in patients with carcinoid tumors (tumors that can convert trypto- phan into serotonin), or in patients with tuberculosis who receive isoniazid therapy (because isoniazid is a pyridoxine antagonist and pyridoxine is also necessary for the conversion of tryptophan to NAD).

In contrast to pellagra, beriberi is due to a deficiency of thiamine (vi- tamin B_1), which has three important functions. It participates in oxidative decarboxylation of α-keto acids, participates as a cofactor for transketolase in the pentose phosphate path, and participates in maintaining neural membranes. Thiamine deficiency mainly affects two organ systems, the heart and the nervous system. If the heart is affected in a patient with beriberi, it may become dilated and flabby. Patients may also develop peripheral vasodilation that leads to a high-output cardiac failure and marked peripheral edema. This combination of vascular abnormalities is called wet beriberi. The peripheral nerves in beriberi may be damaged by focal areas of myelin degeneration, which leads to footdrop, wristdrop, and sensory changes (numbness and tingling) in the feet and lower legs. These symptoms are referred to as dry beriberi. The causes of thiamine deficiency include poor diet, deficient absorption and storage, and accelerated destruction of thiamine diphosphate. This deficiency may be seen in alco- holics and prisoners of war because of poor nutrition, or it may be seen in individuals who eat large amounts of polished rice. (Polishing rice removes the outer, thiamine-containing portion of the grain.) Finally, marasmus is due to a deficiency of calories, rickets is due to a deficiency of vitamin D in children, and scurvy is due to a deficiency of vitamin C.

8-39. The answer is a. (*McPhee, pp 394–397. Braunwald, pp 591, 1770.*) The symptoms and signs and laboratory findings of increased direct biliru- bin, normal indirect bilirubin, and markedly elevated alkaline phosphatase combined with bilirubin in the urine point to extrahepatic obstructive jaundice, most likely from a carcinoma of the head of the pancreas as about 80% of these cases show jaundice due to biliary obstruction. In Gilbert's syndrome and hemolytic anemia, indirect bilirubin is elevated, but direct bilirubin and alkaline phosphatase are normal. In intrahepatic cholestasis, the indirect bilirubin and alkaline phosphatase are normal. Jaundice is usually absent in amyloidosis.

8-40. The answer is a. (*Cotran, pp 1187–1188. Rubin, pp 1294–1296.*) Two tumors that arise from fibroblasts in the dermis of the skin are the benign fibrous histiocytoma and the malignant dermatofibrosarcoma protuberans (DFSP). Benign fibrous histiocytomas are composed of a mixture of fibroblasts, histiocytes (some of which are lipid-laden), mesenchymal cells, and capillaries. Depending on which element predominates, these lesions have also been called dermatofibromas (mainly fibroblasts), fibroxanthomas (mainly histiocytes), and sclerosing hemangiomas (mainly blood vessels). Hyperplasia of the epidermis overlying a dermatofibroma is quite characteristic. In contrast, the lesions of dermatofibrosarcoma protuberans are cellular lesions composed of fibroblasts that form a characteristic pinwheel (storiform) pattern. They have irregular, infiltrative margins and are locally aggressive. They frequently extend into the underlying fat and complete excision is difficult. The overlying epidermis is characteristically thinned.

8-41. The answer is d. (*Hardman, p 479; Katzung, pp 271, 493–494, 991.*) The serotonin receptor agonist actions of the "triptans," including the prototype, sumatriptan, can trigger intense vasoconstriction in various vascular beds. The cerebral vasoconstrictor effects of these drugs contribute importantly to the relief they afford in migraine headaches. However, coronary vasospasm can occur also, and these drugs are therefore contraindicated for patients with coronary artery disease.

None of the other drugs listed have any coronary (or other) vasoconstrictor effects. Indeed, some such as phenytoin and zolpidem (a benzodiazepine-like hypnotic) actually cause slight cardiovascular changes that would actually reduce the risk of myocardial ischemia and angina.

8-42. The answer is a. (*Braunwald, pp 2028, 2175.*) Karyotype is the preferred screening test for Turner's syndrome, which is characterized by a chromosome complement of 45,X. Levels of testosterone, estradiol, FSH, or LH are not very specific. Gonadal dysgenesis accounts for one-third of patients with primary amenorrhea.

8-43. The answer is e. (*Katzung, p 762.*) There are several pieces of information you should link together to help arrive at the answer, for which a relatively new drug is the correct answer. (1) Although linezolid has several uses, it is best reserved for vancomycin-resistant enterococci (VRE) and methicillin-resistant *S. aureus* (MRSA) infections. (It's seldom a first-line antibiotic because of the risk of resistance.) (2) Linezolid is occasionally linked to bone marrow suppression that is usually reversible upon discontinuation of the drug. (Granted, such other antibiotics as chloramphenicol pose greater risks of bone marrow suppression, but this property is nonetheless associated with linezolid.) (3) The third piece of evidence is the rise of blood pressure in response to ephedrine, a mixed-acting sympathomimetic that works, in part, by releasing neuronal norepinephrine. Linezolid has monoamine oxidase inhibitory activity (albeit relatively weak compared with traditional MAO inhibitors). Piece these three lines of evidence together and the only reasonable choice is linezolid.

8-44. The answer is b. (*Hoffman, pp 431–437.*) The porphyrias are inherited or acquired disorders of heme biosynthesis with varied patterns of overproduction, accumulation, and excretion of heme synthesis intermediates. Major characteristics of the porphyrias include intermittent neurologic dysfunction and skin sensitivity to sunlight, but these changes do not occur in all of the different types of porphyria. Neurologic changes, such as hallucinations and manic-depressive episodes, can be seen with acute intermittent porphyria (AIP), hereditary coproporphyria (HCP), and variegate porphyria (VP), while skin changes, such as a bullous photosensitivity, can be seen with porphyria cutanea tarda (PCT), which is the most common type of porphyria, congenital erythropoietic porphyria (CEP), HCP, and VP. That is, AIP produces no skin photosensitivity. Abdominal pain (colic) can be seen with AIP, HCP, and VP. Therefore, the combination of neurologic changes with skin changes and abdominal pain is suggestive of either HCP or VP. These two disorders are clinically similar with increased urinary delta-aminolevulinic acid (ALA) and porphobilinogen (PBG), but VP is quite prevalent in South Africa.

8-45. The answer is a. (*Scriver, pp 3–45. Sack, pp 57–84.*) A chromosome study or karyotype delineates the number and kinds of chromosomes in one cell karyon (nucleus). Blood is conveniently sampled, so most chromosomal studies or karyotypes are performed on peripheral leukocytes in blood. A number of leukocytes are karyotyped under the microscope (10 to 25, depending on the laboratory), and a representative photograph is taken. The chromosome images are then arranged (cut out by hand or moved by computer) in order of size from the #1 pair to the #22 pair, and this ordered array is also called a karyotype. Except in cases of mosaicism (different karyotypes in different tissues), the peripheral blood karyotype is indicative of the germ-line karyotype that is characteristic for an individual. In most cases of Turner's syndrome there is a lack of one X chromosome, as in panel A, which shows one X (arrow) and no Y chromosome. Other cases involve mosaicism (45,X/46,XX or 45,X/46,XY) or isochromosomes (e.g., 46,X,isoXq). Correlation of karyotypes and phenotypic features of girls with Turner's syndrome has demonstrated that haploinsufficiency (partial monosomy) of the short arm (Xp) is what generates the characteristic manifestations (web neck, shield chest, puffy feet, coarctation). Women with Turner's syndrome also have short stature and infertility due to maldevelopment of the ovaries (streak gonads).

8-46. The answer is d. (*Carlson, pp 91–94.*) The limbic system includes regions of the limbic cortex, as well as a group of interconnected structures that surround the core of the forebrain. The limbic system forms a circuit whose primary function was formerly regarded as modulating motivation and emotional responses. Studies have discovered that the hippocampal formation and the limbic cortex that surround it are involved in learning and memory, rather than emotional behavior. However, the remaining sections of the limbic system are responsible for emotions, feelings, moods, and motivation. Thus, the 65-year-old man's limbic system is the site primarily responsible for his learning difficulty, lack of motivation, and his recent loss of emotional feelings for his grandchildren.

8-47. The answer is d. (*Moore and Dalley, p 1059.*) The palatine tonsil sits in the lateral wall of the oropharynx in the palatine arch posterior to the palatoglossus muscle and anterior to the palatopharyngeus muscle. In the bed of the palatine tonsil runs the glossopharyngeal CN (IX) that carries afferent information back to the brain regarding both general sensation and the special sense of taste from the posterior one-third of the tongue. The glossopharyngeal nerve is at risk for being cut during tonsillectomy. (Answer a) The ability to taste in the anterior two-thirds of the tongue is not at risk because that information is carried by the lingual nerve, below the tongue.

(Answer b) The ability to protrude your tongue is provided by innervation from the hypoglossal nerve, which innervates all the intrinsic tongue muscles and lies below the tongue and is not a risk. Neither the ability to open your jaw wide nor to move your jaw from side to side is controlled by the mandibular division of the trigeminal CN (V) (answers d and e, respectively), which does not course near the palatine arch and would not be at risk.

8-48. The answer is c. (*Craig, pp 443–444; Hardman, p 720; Katzung, pp 596–597.*) The main reason why many physicians are shunning oral colchicine for acute gout is that many patients develop horrible GI discomfort, vomiting, diarrhea, and the like. For some, the "cure" is almost as bad as the disorder for which the drug is given. This GI distress can be alleviated somewhat by giving colchicine IV, but more serious systemic responses can develop if the IV dose is too great or too many IV doses are given in a short period of time. Indomethacin seems to have become one of the preferred alternatives for anti-inflammatory therapy of acute gout or prophylaxis of recurrences. (And clearly indomethacin is not without side effects or toxicities; the risks are simply more acceptable, for some patients, with it.)

But when colchicine does work in acute gout, relief may be dramatic and occur literally "overnight" with just a dose or two. The likely mechanism of action involves impaired microtubular assembly or function in leukocytes, which limits their migration to the area of crystal deposition and so limits their ability to amplify the inflammatory reaction.

Bone marrow suppression can occur, but that is mainly with long-term, high-dose oral or parenteral colchicine administration (the latter of which must be avoided). The same applies to frank gastric damage (with the possibility of gastric bleeding or hemorrhage) and to blood dyscrasias (bone marrow toxicity).

8-49. The answer is d. (*Craig, pp 359–408, 411–412; Hardman, pp 412–419, 628–630; Katzung, pp 520–521.*) A long-acting benzodiazepine, such as diazepam, is effective in alleviating barbiturate withdrawal symptoms. The anxiolytic effects of buspirone take several days to develop, obviating its use for acute, severe anxiety.

8-50. The answer is c. (*Cotran, pp 658–659. Rubin, pp 1122–1126.*) Chronic lymphocytic leukemia (CLL) is the most common leukemia and is similar in many aspects to small lymphocytic lymphoma (SLL). It is typically found in patients older than 60 years of age. Histological examination of the peripheral smear reveals a marked increase in the number of mature-appearing lymphocytes. These neoplastic lymphocytes are fragile and easily damaged. This fragility produces the characteristic finding of numerous smudge cells in the peripheral smears of patients with CLL. About 95% of the cases of CLL are of B cell origin (B-CLL) and are characterized by having pan–B cell markers, such as CD19. These malignant cells characteristically also have the T cell marker CD5. The remaining 5% of cases of CLL are mainly of T cell origin. Patients with CLL tend to have an indolent course and the disease is associated with long survival in many cases. The few symptoms that may develop are related to anemia and the absolute lymphocytosis of small, mature cells. Splenomegaly may be noted. In a minority of patients, however, the disease may transform into prolymphocytic leukemia or a large cell immunoblastic lymphoma (Richter's syndrome). Prolymphocytic leukemia is characterized by massive splenomegaly and a markedly increased leukocyte count consisting of enlarged lymphocytes having nuclei with mature chromatin and nucleoli.

Bibliography

Adams RD, Victor M, Ropper AH: *Principles of Neurology,* 6/e. New York, McGraw-Hill, 1997.

Afifi AK, Bergman RA: *Functional Neuroanatomy.* New York, McGraw-Hill, 1998.

Alberts B, Johnson A, Lewis J et al: *Molecular Biology of the Cell,* 4/e. New York, Garland, 2002.

Baum A, Gatchel RJ, Krantz DS: *An Introduction to Health Psychology,* 3/e. New York, McGraw-Hill, 1997.

Behrman RE, Kliegman RM, Jenson HB: *Nelson's Textbook of Pediatrics,* 17/e. Philadelphia, Saunders, 2004.

Berman JJ, O'Leary TJ: *Gastrointestinal stromal tumor workshop.* Hum Pathol 32:578–582, 2001.

Boron WF, Boulpaep EL: *Medical Physiology.* Philadelphia, WB Saunders, 2003.

Braunwald E, Fauci AS, Kasper DL, et al (eds): *Harrison's Principles of Internal Medicine,* 15/e. New York, McGraw-Hill, 2001.

Brooks GF, et al (ed): *Jawetz's Medical Microbiology,* 22/e, New York, McGraw-Hill, 2001.

Carlson NR: *Physiology of Behavior,* 5/e. Boston, Allyn & Bacon, 1994.

Casals T, Bassas L, Egozcue S, et al: "Heterogeneity for mutations in the CFTR gene and clinical correlations in patients with congenital absence of the vas deferens," *Human Reproduction* 15(7): 1476–1483, 2000.

Chandrasoma P, Taylor CR: *Concise Pathology,* 3/e. Stamford, CT, Appleton & Lange, 1998.

Coe FL, Favus MJ (eds): *Disorders of Bone and Mineral Metabolism.* New York, Raven, 1992.

Cotran RS, Kumar V, Collins, T: *Robbins Pathologic Basis of Disease,* 6/e. Philadelphia, W.B. Saunders, 1999.

Craig CR, Stitzel RE (eds): *Modern Pharmacology with Clinical Applications,* 6th ed. Philadelphia, PA, Lippincott Williams & Wilkins, 2004.

Damjanov I, Linder J (eds): *Anderson's Pathology,* 10/e. St. Louis, Mosby, 1996.

Feldman M, Friedman LS: *Sleisenger and Fordtran's Gastrointestinal and Liver Disease,* 7/e. Philadelphia, Saunders, 2002.

Gilroy, J: *Basic Neurology,* 3/e. New York, McGraw-Hill, 2000.

Goetz CG (ed): *Textbook of Clinical Neurology,* 2/e. Philadelphia, Saunders, 2003.

Goldman L, Bennett JC: *Cecil's Textbook of Medicine,* 21/e. Philadelphia, Saunders, 2000.

Greenberg DA, Aminoff MJ, Simon RP: *Clinical Neurology,* 5/e, New York, McGraw-Hill, 2002.

Greenspan FS, Gardner DG: *Basic and Clinical Endocrinology,* 6/e. New York, Lange Medical Books/McGraw-Hill, 2001.

Guyton AC, Hall JE: *Textbook of Medical Physiology,* 10/e. Philadelphia, W.B. Saunders, 2000.

Hardman JG, Limbird LE: *Goodman & Gilman's the Pharmacological Basis of Therapeutics,* 10th ed. New York, McGraw-Hill, 2001.

Henry JB, et al (eds): *Clinical Diagnosis and Management by Laboratory Methods,* 20/e. Philadelphia, Saunders, 2001.

Hoffman R, Benz EJ, Shattil SJ: *Hematology: Basic Principles and Practice,* 3/e. New York, Churchill Livingstone, 2000.

Hughes M, Kroehler CJ, Vander Zanden JW: *Sociology: The Core,* 5/e. New York, McGraw-Hill, 1999.

Junqueira LC, Carneiro J: *Basic Histology: Text and Atlas,* 10/e. New York, Lange Medical Books/McGraw-Hill, 2004.

Kandel ER, Schwartz JH, Jessel TM: *Principles of Neural Science,* 4/e. New York, McGraw-Hill, 2000.

Katzung BG: *Basic and Clinical Pharmacology,* 9th ed. New York, McGraw-Hill, 2004.

Kierszenbaum AL: *Histology and Cell Biology,* St. Louis, Mosby, 2002.

Kumar V, Cotran RS, Robbins SL: *Basic Pathology,* 7/e. Philadelphia, W.B. Saunders, 2003.

Levinson W, Jawetz E: *Medical Microbiology and Immunology: Examination and Board Review,* 7/e. New York, McGraw-Hill, 2002.

Mandell GL, et al (eds): *Principles and Practice of Infectious Diseases,* 5/e. New York, Churchill Livingstone, 1998.

McKenzie JC, Klein RM: *Basic Concepts in Cell Biology and Histology.* New York, McGraw-Hill, 2000.

McPhee SJ, Lingappa VR, Ganong WF (eds): *Pathophysiology of Disease: An Introduction to Clinical Medicine,* 4/e. New York, McGraw-Hill, 2003.

Moore KL and Persaud TVN: *Before We Are Born: Essentials of Embryology and Birth Defects*, 6/e. Philadelphia: W.B. Saunders, 2003.

Moore KL, Dalley AF: *Clinically Oriented Anatomy*, 4/e. Baltimore, Williams & Wilkins, 1999.

Moore KL, Persaud TVN: *The Developing Human: Clinically Oriented Embryology*, 7/e. Philadelphia, W.B. Saunders, 2003.

Murray PR, et al (ed): *Manual of Clinical Microbiology*, 8/e, Washington, DC, ASM Press, 2003.

Murray PR, et al: *Medical Microbiology*, 4/e, St. Louis, Mosby, 2002.

Murray RK, Granner DK, Mayes PA, Rodwell VW: *Harper's Illustrated Biochemistry*, 26/e. New York, McGraw-Hill, 2003.

Nolte J: *The Human Brain: An Introduction to Its Functional Anatomy*, 4/e. St. Louis, MO, Mosby, 1999.

Parslow TG, et al: *Medical Immunology*, 10/e, New York, McGraw-Hill, 2001.

Ravel R: *Clinical Laboratory Medicine*, 6/e. St. Louis, Mosby-Year Book, 1995.

Rowland, LP (ed): *Merritt's Textbook of Neurology*, 10/e. Philadelphia, Lippincott, Williams & Wilkins, 2000.

Rubin E, Farber JL: *Pathology*, 3/e. Philadelphia, Lippincott, 1999.

Ryan KJ, et al (ed): *Sherris Medical Microbiology*, 4/e, New York, McGraw-Hill, 2001.

Sack GH Jr: *Medical Genetics*, New York, McGraw-Hill, 1999.

Sadler TW: *Langman's Medical Embryology*, 9/e. Philadelphia, Lippincott Williams & Wilkins, 2004.

Scriver CR, Beaudet AL, Sly WS, Valle D: *The Metabolic and Molecular Bases of Inherited Disease*, 8/e. New York, McGraw-Hill, 2001.

Siegel GJ, Agranoff BW, Albers RW, Fisher SK, Uhler MD: *Basic Neurochemistry*, 6/e. Philadelphia, Lippincott, Williams & Wilkins, 1999.

Sierles FS (ed): *Behavioral Science for Medical Students*, Baltimore, Williams & Wilkins, 1993.

Taylor SE: *Health Psychology*, New York, McGraw-Hill, 1995.

Townsend CM, et al: *Sabiston's Textbook of Surgery*, 16/e. Philadelphia, WB Saunders, 2001.

Waxman SG: *Correlative Neuroanatomy*, 24/e. New York, McGraw-Hill, 2000.

Wedding D: *Behavior and Medicine*, 2/e. St. Louis, Mosby-Year Book, 1995.

Wilson JD, Larsen PR, Shlomo M: *Williams Textbook of Endocrinology*, 10/e. Philadelphia, WB Saunders, 2002.

Young B, Heath JW: *Wheater's Functional Histology,* 4/e. New York, Churchill Livingstone, 2000.

Young PA, Young PH: *Basic Clinical Neuroanatomy,* 1/e. Philadelphia, Lippincott, 1997.